"The *Therapist's Notebook for Systemic Teletherapy* is the premier guide for systemic therapists engaging in telebehavioral health. With chapters written by the top scholars in the field of technology and treatment, this comprehensive resource shows therapists how to work highly effectively with various populations, presenting problems, and through theoretical orientations. Further, the inclusion of clinical examples makes this book a go-to for any level of treatment professional. This text is a must-have for today's therapists."

Katherine Hertlein, PhD, *professor of couple and family therapy, Kirk Kerkorian School of Medicine, University of Nevada, Las Vegas, author of* The Internet Family and The Couple and Family Technology Framework, *and editor of* The Couple and Family Therapist's Notebook *and* The Therapist's Notebook for Family Healthcare

"An invaluable resource for mental health professionals! The authors seamlessly integrate creativity into teletherapy, offering a treasure trove of innovative interventions for diverse clients. This guide delivers practical insights, ethical considerations, and creative strategies that transcend the virtual divide. A must-read for therapists navigating the digital landscape, it not only enriches therapeutic practice but also redefines the possibilities of connection and healing. A true gem for those seeking to enhance their teletherapy toolkit."

Sophia Ansari, LPCC, RPT, *owner of Let's Play Therapy Institute*

"Rebecca Cobb has done a magnificent job of bringing together a notable group of experienced authors to write about one of the most important topics of our time, teletherapy. This text is a resource to all therapists, especially those who practice systemically. Teletherapy is relatively new, and it is further complicated when therapists are required to assess and intervene systemically online. This text is both practical and informative and is a rich resource for therapists who practice teletherapy."

Adrian Blow, PhD, *professor of couple and family therapy, Michigan State University, and author of* Deliberate Practice in Systemic Family Therapy *and* Bringing Common Factors to Life in Couple and Family Therapy

"A virtual treasure trove of clinical innovation, practice focused intervention, and ethical guidance for bringing your systemic practice into the online world of your clients with focus and impact. Rich with practical wisdom, this compendium captures the 'how to's', 'what if's', and 'now what's' found in the everyday practice of systemic based telehealth. Clear, accessible, and informative, this notebook provides a handy guide for flourishing in the online clinical space."

James Furrow, PhD, *author of* Emotionally Focused Family Therapy *and* Becoming an Emotionally Focused Therapist, *Seattle University*

THE THERAPIST'S NOTEBOOK FOR SYSTEMIC TELETHERAPY

Many therapeutic activities that engage clients in in-person therapy rooms are not obviously available via telehealth. Yet there are creative, practical, and easy ways to intervene in teletherapy that go beyond talk therapy.

The Therapist's Notebook for Systemic Teletherapy: Creative Interventions for Effective Online Therapy provides systemic teletherapy activities and interventions for a variety of topics and presenting problems. Forty chapters are arranged into seven parts: setup and preparation, self of the therapist, children and adolescents, adults, intimate relationships, families, and training and supervision. Leading experts provide step-by-step guidelines on setup, instructions, processing, and suggestions for follow-up for interventions that are grounded within foundational therapy theories/models and evidence-based practice. This book explores both new intervention strategies and ways to adapt in-person therapy interventions for telehealth.

This book provides creative inspiration and practical advice for novice and experienced family therapists, clinical social workers, counselors, play therapists, psychologists, psychiatrists, and others in related fields.

Rebecca A. Cobb, PhD, LMFT, is a clinical professor for Seattle University's Master of Arts in Couples and Family Therapy program. She also has her own Seattle-based private practice, where she provides supervision as an American Association for Marriage and Family Therapy (AAMFT) approved supervisor and supervision mentoring to AAMFT approved supervisor candidates. She has authored numerous journal articles and book chapters, is a former president of the Washington Association for Marriage and Family Therapy (WAMFT), and has won awards from AAMFT, WAMFT, and the National Council on Family Relations. When she isn't working, she enjoys hot yoga, hosting dinner parties, hiking with Laney the Aussiedoodle, and spending time with her partner and the small humans that keep attempting to make her a morning person.

THE THERAPIST'S NOTEBOOK FOR SYSTEMIC TELETHERAPY

Creative Interventions for Effective Online Therapy

Edited by Rebecca A. Cobb

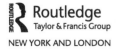

Routledge
Taylor & Francis Group

NEW YORK AND LONDON

Designed cover image: © Christine Walsh Borst

First published 2025
by Routledge
605 Third Avenue, New York, NY 10158

and by Routledge
4 Park Square, Milton Park, Abingdon, Oxon, OX14 4RN

Routledge is an imprint of the Taylor & Francis Group, an informa business

Library of Congress Cataloging-in-Publication Data
Names: Cobb, Rebecca A., editor.
Title: The therapist's notebook for systemic teletherapy : creative interventions for effective online therapy / edited by Rebecca A. Cobb.
Description: New York, NY : Routledge, 2024. | Includes bibliographical references and index. |
Identifiers: LCCN 2024001299 (print) | LCCN 2024001300 (ebook) | ISBN 9781032267937 (pbk) | ISBN 9781032267944 (hbk) | ISBN 9781003289920 (ebk)
Subjects: LCSH: Internet in psychotherapy.
Classification: LCC RC489.I54 T44 2024 (print) | LCC RC489.I54 (ebook) |
DDC 616.89/140285—dc23/eng/20240313
LC record available at https://lccn.loc.gov/2024001299
LC ebook record available at https://lccn.loc.gov/2024001300

ISBN: 978-1-032-26794-4 (hbk)
ISBN: 978-1-032-26793-7 (pbk)
ISBN: 978-1-003-28992-0 (ebk)

DOI: 10.4324/9781003289920

Typeset in Stone Serif
by Apex CoVantage, LLC

Access the Support Material: www.routledge.com/9781032267937

For Addison, who inspires me daily with his creativity and confidence in it.

CONTENTS

Contributors   xiv

Foreword   xx

Preface   xxii

Acknowledgments   xxv

PART 1: SETUP AND PREPARATION   **1**

■ **CHAPTER 1**   Can We Meet Remotely? Legal and Ethical
                   Considerations for Systemic Teletherapy   3

                   Eric L. Ström

■ **CHAPTER 2**   Managing Multiple Therapeutic Environments   11

                   *Paul R. Springer, Nathan C. Taylor, and
                   Richard J. Bischoff*

■ **CHAPTER 3**   Confidentiality in Systemic Teletherapy   18

                   Eric L. Ström and Rebecca A. Cobb

■ **CHAPTER 4**   Building Therapeutic Relationships Via Teletherapy 21

                   *Lisa Rene Reynolds, Paul R. Springer, Nathan C. Taylor,
                   Richard J. Bischoff, and Rebecca A. Cobb*

■ **CHAPTER 5**   Overcoming Lack of Visual and Auditory Cues
                   in Online Sessions   25

                   Paul R. Springer, Nathan C. Taylor, and Richard J. Bischoff

■ **CHAPTER 6**   Using Background Images to Signal Messages
                   Via Teletherapy   29

                   Amanda Veldorale-Griffin

PART 2:   SELF OF THE THERAPIST   **33**

■ **CHAPTER 7**   Managing Distractions and Remaining Present:
                   Suggestions for Online Therapists   35

                   Jessie Everts

■ **CHAPTER 8**   The "Commute Home": End-of-Day Letting-Go
                   Rituals for Online Therapists   38

                   Deborah Koons-Beauchamp

■ **CHAPTER 9**   Teletherapist Self-Care Assessment   41

                   Rebecca A. Cobb and Monique Willis

■ **CHAPTER 10**   Burnout for Online Therapists   44

                   Veronica P. Viesca and Parker Leukart

■ **CHAPTER 11**   Self-Care Tips and Tricks for Online Therapists   47

                   Monique Willis and Rebecca A. Cobb

■ **CHAPTER 12**   Bumpin' Into Teletherapy: Planning for
                   Parental Leave   52

                   *Veronica P. Viesca, Parker Leukart, Amanda Rausch,
                   and Whitney Molitor*

PART 3:   CHILDREN AND ADOLESCENTS   **59**

■ **CHAPTER 13**   Digital Sand Therapy: Cognitions and
                   the Underworld   61

                   Jessica Stone

■ **CHAPTER 14**   Virtual Puppet Play Therapy   70

                   Karen Fried

■ **CHAPTER 15**   Chess and Telemental Health: A Structural
                   Therapy Approach   79

                   Amy Marschall

■ **CHAPTER 16**   The Solution-Focused Scavenger Hunt   86

                   Jacob Priest

■ **CHAPTER 17**   Teletherapy Poetry   91

*Tiffany Alexis Leal, Molly P. Downes, and
Rebecca A. Cobb*

PART 4:   ADULTS   **99**

■ **CHAPTER 18**   Transformational Teletherapy Chairs   101

George A. Garcia III

■ **CHAPTER 19**   Changing Narratives With Virtual Vision Boards   107

Deneisha S. Scott-Poe and Khushbu S. Patel

■ **CHAPTER 20**   Guided Grounding in Teletherapy Intervention   115

Kayla Sellers

■ **CHAPTER 21**   Solution-Focused Teletherapy for Suicide
Intervention   121

*Benjamin T. Finlayson, Jaclyn Cravens Pickens,
and Ethan Jones*

■ **CHAPTER 22**   A Peek Inside: Virtual Home Visits for
Hoarding Disorder   130

Jennifer M. Sampson and Leslie Shapiro

■ **CHAPTER 23**   Virtual Cognitive Stimulation Therapy:
A Group Intervention for Older Adults With
Memory Loss   137

*Matthew Amick, Max Zubatsky, and
Marla Berg-Weger*

PART 5:   INTIMATE RELATIONSHIPS   **147**

■ **CHAPTER 24**   Structural Interventions for Intimate
Relationship Therapy: Capitalizing on the
Limitations of Telehealth   149

Veronica P. Viesca and Parker Leukart

■ **CHAPTER 25**   Doorbells, Babies, and Dogs, Oh My: Distractions as Metaphors in Teletherapy With Intimate Relationships   155

Racine R. Henry

■ **CHAPTER 26**   Intimate Relationship Deescalation for Teletherapy: The Structured Pause   160

Charity Francis Laughlin

■ **CHAPTER 27**   Mapping the Cycle: A Virtual Emotion-Focused Intervention for Clients Practicing Consensual Nonmonogamy   165

Kk O. Lightsmith

■ **CHAPTER 28**   Mindfulness-Based Sex Therapy: Setting the Stage for Sensate Focus via Telehealth   174

Tina M. Timm

■ **CHAPTER 29**   Assessing Appropriateness of Teletherapy for Intimate Partner Violence   180

Jaclyn Cravens Pickens and Aaron Norton

PART 6:   FAMILIES   187

■ **CHAPTER 30**   Digital Play Genograms   189

Rebecca A. Cobb

■ **CHAPTER 31**   Telehealth Family Sculpt: So Many People, So Little Space   195

Nathan C. Taylor, Paul R. Springer, and Richard J. Bischoff

■ **CHAPTER 32**   Stacking the Deck: A Strategic Approach to the Ungame   202

Rebecca A. Cobb

■ **CHAPTER 33**   Virtual Altar-Making for Grief and Loss   208

Christie Eppler, J. Maria Bermúdez, and Rebecca A. Cobb

■ **CHAPTER 34**   Migration Journeys: Increasing Bonds With
Shared Stories and Geographical Maps   213

Jacqueline Florian and Rebecca A. Cobb

■ **CHAPTER 35**   Medical Family Teletherapy: Expanding Care
to Promote Health Equity   219

*Angela L. Lamson, Jennifer L. Hodgson,
Betül Küçükardalı Cansever, and Irma Abrego Lappin*

PART 7:   TRAINING AND SUPERVISION   **227**

■ **CHAPTER 36**   Supporting Therapists Through Deliberate
Practice in Systemic Teletherapy   229

*Debra L. Miller, Gianna M. Casaburo,
and Melissa M. Yzaguirre*

■ **CHAPTER 37**   Round-Robin Case Conceptualization for
Theoretically Grounded Virtual Supervision   235

Kelly Duggan Shearer

■ **CHAPTER 38**   Virtual Reflecting Teams: A Milan Approach
to Teletherapy Intervention   244

*Rebecca A. Cobb, Stephanie Brownell,
Samantha J. Camera, and Camille Chapin*

■ **CHAPTER 39**   Plurilinguistic Virtual Reflecting Teams With
Latino/a Families   251

Carlos A. Ramos, Julian F. Crespo, and Ezequiel Peña

■ **CHAPTER 40**   "Real" Practice With Clients: Using Simulation
in Virtual Group Supervision   257

Dana J. Stone and Deborah J. Buttitta

Index   266

CONTRIBUTORS

Cover Contributor

Christine Borst, PhD, LMFT, is an artist, therapist, and creative entrepreneur. She left her role as an assistant professor in family therapy to pursue a creative career, which includes but is not limited to writing and illustrating children's books and tearing up old magazines to make pretty pictures. Her published books include *What Is Coronavirus?*, *For the Love of Organs: A Quasi-Educational Collection of Poems*, *Us: An Introduction to Pronouns*, and *Drawing the Sun*, a book about the journey to the authentic self. Additionally, she runs a private coaching practice, where she supports clients in connecting with their wild selves. When she isn't having fun at work, she is hanging out in Colorado with her husband (the other Dr. Borst), her three wonderful children, and their two dogs, kitten, and hedgehog. You can find her on Instagram at @thechristineborst or at www.christineborst.com.

Chapter Contributors

Matthew Amick, PhD, LMFT, was conferred a PhD in medical family therapy from Saint Louis University School of Medicine. His research and clinical interests include caregiver wellness and cognitive health of older adults. He practices in an Atlanta-based private practice.

Marla Berg-Weger, PhD, LCSW, is professor emerita for the Saint Louis University School of Social Work and is executive director of the Gateway Geriatric Education Center. Her scholarship focuses on family caregiving, nonpharmacologic interventions for persons with dementia, loneliness/social isolation, and older drivers. She has authored four books and 100+ publications.

J. Maria Bermúdez, PhD, LMFT, is an associate professor of couple and family therapy at the University of Georgia. She is the co-author of the book *Socioculturally Attuned Family Therapy: Guidelines for Equitable Theory and Practice* (2018, 2023), an AAMFT clinical fellow and approved supervisor, and a feminist-informed scholar and therapist who uses narrative and creative approaches in her clinical practice.

Richard J. Bischoff, PhD, is a professor and associate vice chancellor of the Institute of Agriculture and Natural Resources at the University of Nebraska-Lincoln (UNL). He and colleagues at UNL created a training program in collaborative rural mental health care that maximizes the use of telemental health to address mental health access disparities.

Stephanie Brownell, MA, LMFTA, has a private psychotherapy practice supporting individuals, couples, and families with acute and complex trauma and relational issues. She is based in the Pacific Northwest.

Deborah J. Buttitta, PsyD, LMFT, is an assistant professor and AAMFT-approved supervisor in the Marriage and Family Therapy Program at California State University, Northridge. Her collective work centers on addressing diversity issues in clinical practice and creating educational opportunities that foster personal and professional growth. She utilizes postmodern and strength-based approaches in her private practice in Los Angeles, California.

Samantha J. Camera, MA, LMFTA, is a psychotherapist at Bloom and Blossom group practice. She also runs a private practice, helping individuals, families, and couples in Bellingham, Washington.

Betül Küçükardalı Cansever, MA, MFT, is a PhD candidate in the Medical Family Therapy Program at East Carolina University (ECU). She is a medical family therapist fellow at ECU Health Medical Center's inpatient rehabilitation unit, where she provides individual, family, and couple therapies, serves on an interdisciplinary treatment team, and supervises master's-level MFT interns.

Gianna M. Casaburo, PhD Candidate, LMFT, is the director of Student Counseling Services at Purdue University Fort Wayne and an adjunct professor in the Counselor Education Program.

Camille Chapin, MA, LMFTA, is a therapist working with individuals and couples navigating life transitions, peri- and postpartum mood disorders, and relationship to self and others. Camille runs a private practice and also works with clients part-time in a group practice setting.

Julian F. Crespo, PhD, LMFT, is an assistant professor for Our Lady of the Lake University's master's program in marriage and family therapy. He is also the director of the marriage and family therapy clinic at La Feria Campus. He provides supervision as an AAMFT-approved supervisor and supervision mentoring to AAMFT-approved supervisor candidates.

Molly P. Downes, MA, LMFT, works in private practice in the greater Seattle area. She previously worked in a Seattle-based community mental health clinic, providing systemic individual, couples, and family therapy in King County.

Christie Eppler, PhD, LMFT, is the program director and professor of Seattle University's Master of Arts in Couples and Family Therapy program. She is an AAMFT-approved supervisor who has a private practice in Seattle, Washington. The focus of her clinical practice and research is systemic resilience and narrative therapy.

Jessie Everts, PhD, LMFT, PMH-C, is owner and founder of Empower Mental Health. She is the author of two books, *Brave New Mom: A Survival Guide for Mindfully Navigating Postpartum Motherhood* and *Connecting With Loneliness: A Guided Journal*.

Benjamin T. Finlayson, PhD, MFTC, is an assistant professor of marriage and family therapy at Regis University. His research centers around solution-focused brief therapy, sexual and gender identity, medical family therapy, and suicide prevention/intervention. He owns and operates his own practice, Benjamin Taylor Therapy, PLLC, specializing in family therapy for LGBTQIA+ families.

Jacqueline Florian, MA, LMFT, provides therapy to the BIPOC community in both English and Spanish in Los Angeles, California. In addition, she is a clinical training coordinator for Alliant International University in the Couples and Family Therapy program.

Karen Fried, PsyD, LMFT, is a licensed marriage and family therapist and an educational therapist and consultant in Los Angeles, California. Karen uses the Oaklander Model of child therapy in her private practice and is the president of the Violet Solomon Oaklander Foundation. She trains child and adolescent therapists and educators in the United States and internationally.

George A. Garcia III, PhD, LMFT, is a clinical professor and clinical training director for Hope International University's Master of Arts in Marriage and Family Therapy program, Master of Science in Counseling, and Doctor of Marriage and Family Therapy programs. He is licensed in California and Ohio and works in private practice, specializing in working with children and young adults from an experiential model.

Racine R. Henry, PhD, LMFT, is an AAMFT clinical fellow, approved supervisor, and faculty member of the Family Institute at Northwestern University. Dr. Henry is the founder of Sankofa Marriage & Family Therapy, PLLC and the creator of the A Palate For Love™ series.

Jennifer L. Hodgson, PhD, LMFT, served as an AAMFT-approved supervisor, professor, co-creator, and former director of the Medical Family Therapy doctoral program at East Carolina University. She is a principal consultant with Health Management Associates and an elected member of her county's board of education.

Ethan Jones, PhD, LMFT, is a faculty lecturer at Utah Valley University, where he teaches and mentors students. In addition to his role at the university, he is the clinical director for Zest for Life Counseling, where he finds great fulfillment in supporting new clinicians in reaching their potential.

Deborah Koons-Beauchamp, PhD, MBA, LMFT, is a clinical assistant professor at Northern Illinois University, where she teaches in the Human Development and Family Sciences program. She blends both in-person and telehealth in her clinical practice and has a unique history of working both in-office and virtually as an executive director for nonprofit and corporate organizations.

Angela L. Lamson, PhD, LMFT, is an AAMFT-approved supervisor, professor, co-creator, and former director of the Medical Family Therapy doctoral program at East Carolina University (ECU). She has served as the director of the Marriage and Family Therapy program, director of ECU's Family Therapy Clinic, and director of the Medical Family Therapy Research Academy.

Irma Abrego Lappin, MSW, is a bilingual, licensed clinical social worker-associate and licensed addiction specialist. She operates a thriving private practice based in Greenville, North Carolina, offering therapeutic services to individuals, couples, and families.

Charity Francis Laughlin, MA, LMFT, CST, specializes in sexuality and distressed intimate relationships, providing clinical services as part of a Seattle-based private group practice. She is an AAMFT-approved supervisor candidate, and her clinical work is influenced by system thinking, differentiation theory, attachment theory, and interpersonal neurobiology.

Tiffany Alexis Leal, MA, LMFTA, is a graduate of Seattle University's Master of Arts in Couples and Family Therapy program. She owns and operates a Seattle-based private practice, Bloom Therapy PNW, and is pursuing a certificate in play therapy.

Parker Leukart, MA, AMFT, is a graduate student working toward her doctorate in psychology at the Graduate School of Education and Psychology at Pepperdine University. Her research interests center around the connection between psychosocial factors and health across the life span. Parker has trained in numerous settings, working with children, adults, and families.

Kk O. Lightsmith, MA, MEd, LMFT, owns their own private practice in Seattle, Washington. Through group, individual, and relationship therapy, they are passionate about providing effective and attuned services to LGBTQAI+ community members, polyamorous relationships, kinky clients, and clients from the Global Majority. They also provide supervision as an AAMFT-approved supervisor candidate.

Amy Marschall, PsyD, is a licensed psychologist, speaker, and author specializing in telemental health, trauma, and neurodiversity-affirming care. She has a private practice, RMH Therapy, and provides resources for therapists or anyone who wants to learn more at her website, Resiliency Mental Health.

Debra L. Miller, PhD, LMSW, is the director of Family Services for Community Mental Health for Central Michigan and faculty with the Family Therapy Training Institute of Miami. Dr. Miller is committed to improving outcomes for youth and families through evidence-based-practice training, implementation, research, and clinical practice.

Whitney Molitor, MA, LMFT, is a clinician at a group psychotherapy private practice called Good Therapy San Diego. Areas of expertise include the treatment of eating disorders, trauma, and issues pertaining to women's health and well-being.

Aaron Norton, PhD, LMFT, is an associate professor at Texas Woman's University. His research focuses on the role of technology in couples and families and the practice of relational teletherapy.

Khushbu S. Patel, MS, is a doctoral candidate at Virginia Tech, specializing in marriage and family therapy. She is an instructor in Valdosta State University's master's in MFT program and works as a therapist at Turning Point Hospital in Moultrie, Georgia. She approaches her research on caregiving and intergenerational relationships from a systemic perspective.

Ezequiel Peña, PhD, is an associate professor at Our Lady of the Lake University in the Marriage and Family Therapy and Counseling Psychology graduate programs. His clinical and scholarly interests are in strengths-based Spanish-English bilingual therapy, training, and supervision. His scholarship focuses on the intersections of Latinx identity, class, gender, sexual orientation, spirituality, and individual voice.

Jaclyn Cravens Pickens, PhD, LMFT, is an associate professor at Texas Tech University. Her research focuses on the intersection of technology and romantic relationships (internet infidelity) as well as within the mental health profession (relational teletherapy education and training).

Jacob Priest, PhD, LMFT, is an associate professor and director of the Couple and Family Therapy program at the University of Iowa. He is also a clinical associate professor in the LGBTQ and Weight Management Clinics in the Department of Internal Medicine at the University of Iowa Carver College of Medicine.

Carlos A. Ramos, PhD, LMFT, is an assistant professor in the psychology department at Our Lady of the Lake University in San Antonio. He is also the certificate director of Psychological Services for Spanish Speaking Populations. His theoretical orientation is grounded in Ericksonian and systemic concepts. His interests include clinical hypnosis, bilingual supervision and therapy, and qualitative research.

Amanda Rausch, MA, LMFT, is the owner and founder of NoStressNoStigma Telehealth Practice. She also provides supervision as an AAMFT-approved supervisor and supervision mentoring to AAMFT-approved supervisor candidates.

Lisa Rene Reynolds, PhD, LMFT, is a faculty member of The Family Institute at Northwestern University's master of science in couples and family therapy program, is an AAMFT-approved supervisor, and has private practices in New York and Connecticut. She is also the author of *Parenting Through Divorce: Helping Your Kids Thrive During and After the Split.*

Jennifer M. Sampson, PhD, LMFT, CST, is the program chair for Antioch University's Master of Arts in Couples and Family Therapy program in Seattle, Washington. Her research has included work on hoarding disorder and families and the use of mixed-reality simulation software in marriage and family therapy training programs.

Deneisha S. Scott-Poe, PhD, LMFTA, is an assistant professor and clinic director at Converse University. She uses an intergenerational systemic approach in her clinical work. Dr. Scott-Poe holds a certificate in gerontology, and her research focuses on aging Black families, Alzheimer's disease caregiving, and how clinicians can better work with older Black adults and their families.

Kayla Sellers, MA, tLMFT, is a couple and family therapy doctoral student at the University of Iowa. She also works for an Iowa City-based private practice, where she provides couple and family therapy services and supervision as an AAMFT-supervisor candidate.

Leslie Shapiro, MA, LMFT, is a therapist and skills group leader at Thira, a renowned mental health treatment center specializing in dialectical behavioral therapy. She provides continuing-education courses on hoarding disorder through Northwest Relationships. Leslie also co-authored a chapter on hoarding in *The SAGE Encyclopedia of Marriage, Family, and Couples Counseling.*

Kelly Duggan Shearer, LMFT, LPCC, is an assistant professor of marriage and family therapy at Azusa Pacific University. She has been in private practice since 2008 and is an AAMFT-approved supervisor. Her areas of expertise include Aponte's Person of the Therapist Training model, DIRFloortime®, and implementing relationally attuned teaching practices.

Paul R. Springer, PhD, LMFT, is a professor in the Marriage and Family Therapy Program at Virginia Tech. As an AAMFT-approved supervisor, he has worked with students in how to deliver telemental health services to rural underserved communities since 2008.

Dana J. Stone, PhD, LMFT, is an associate professor and fieldwork coordinator for the Marriage and Family Therapy program at California State University Northridge. She is an AAMFT-approved supervisor and supervisor mentor and has a telehealth private practice. Her work contributions to the field focus on students and early-career MFTs with marginalized identities bringing their whole selves into their clinical work.

Jessica Stone, PhD, RPT-S, is a licensed psychologist with experience in private practice, academia, and tech innovation. She has pioneered the use of digital tools in therapy, is an affiliate of the East Carolina University College of Education Neurocognition Science Laboratory, and holds various key board positions.

Eric L. Ström, JD, PhD, LMHC, is a licensed attorney and a licensed mental health counselor in Seattle, Washington. Eric has taught as an adjunct instructor at a range of clinical graduate programs. His clinical experience has been focused on working with combat veterans, and he currently provides clinical counseling, clinical supervision, and legal/ethical consultation through his private practice.

Nathan C. Taylor, PhD, is an assistant professor for University of Northern Iowa's Department of Families, Aging, and Counseling. He has researched, supervised, and trained clinicians to use telemental health for systemic clients for almost a decade, seeking to improve access and acceptability of mental health care in underserved areas.

Tina M. Timm, PhD, LMSW, LMFT, is an associate professor in the School of Social Work at Michigan State University. She has been a sex therapist for more than 30 years. Her research and clinical work focus on the integration of sexuality into clinical practice, affair recovery, and LGBTQ+ well-being.

Amanda Veldorale-Griffin, PhD, LMFT-S, is a professor of marriage and family sciences at National University. She also has a private practice in which she specializes in working with transgender individuals and their families.

Veronica P. Viesca, PhD, LMFT, is an assistant professor of psychology in the Graduate School of Education and Psychology at Pepperdine University, where she teaches theories of couple and family therapy. She is a licensed MFT in California, Texas, and Washington. She is recognized as an AAMFT-approved supervisor and regularly mentors AAMFT-approved supervisor candidates.

Monique Willis, PhD, LMFT, is an assistant professor at Loma Linda University's School of Behavioral Health. She specializes in culturally sensitive therapy training and self-care competencies. She offers telehealth services to underserved populations and caregivers affected by chronic health conditions.

Melissa M. Yzaguirre, PhD, LMFT, is an assistant professor for the Department of Counseling and Marital and Family Therapy at the University of San Diego. Dr. Yzaguirre's research and clinical interests are to improve mental health outcomes and strengthen family relationships in systematically marginalized communities, primarily Latino communities, through increased culturally relevant practices available to mental health providers.

Max Zubatsky, PhD, LMFT, is an associate professor for Saint Louis University's Department of Family and Community Medicine and the associate director for the Gateway Geriatric Education Center. Dr. Zubatsky is also an AAMFT-approved supervisor. His research and clinical interests include caregiving, geriatrics, integrated behavioral health, residency education, and provider wellness.

FOREWORD

Prior to COVID, telehealth had been viewed with skepticism and disdain and was largely sidelined as an inferior way to deliver psychotherapy. Then a transformation occurred, with many of us therapists tucked into our newly converted home offices, navigating this new medium, embracing the fact that we could now do therapy *and* laundry all at once (even while navigating our own anxiety about the pestilence lurking in the background). The use of technology to deliver telehealth has had far-reaching impact – it is not going away, and we need to know how to deliver from this e-platform effectively and ethically. It is with great pleasure that I introduce you to a book that will do exactly that, *The Therapist's Notebook for Systemic Teletherapy: Creative Interventions for Effective Online Therapy*, edited by my talented former student, Dr. Rebecca Cobb.

I created the *Therapist's Notebook* series 25 years ago with the goal of educating therapists on practical techniques that would bring theory into living practice. I am happy the baton has been passed and Dr. Cobb was inspired to take up this mantle. She has done this by compiling an inspiring and unique volume that addresses this movement of therapy onto e-platforms. While in-person therapy is certainly not dead, online therapy has been found to be effective, enjoyable, convenient, and a unique way to reach our clientele. In fact, telehealth has allowed us to reach more clientele who might not otherwise be able to access therapy. Most of us have experienced a burgeoning client population as the stress of a pandemic *and* online availability of mental health assistance coincided. This book addresses both the challenges and potential triumphs in telehealth that can occur when therapists have adequately addressed those challenges by being informed and putting action plans in place to protect clients, ourselves, and our practices.

The unique ethical challenges of online therapy are detailed in these pages; knowing these will save you much grief down the road. There is practical advice provided on how to navigate both legal and ethical challenges of teletherapy from a systemic lens. Building the therapeutic relationship online and helping clients build healthy relationships from an online platform are all addressed. The authors address how to overcome limitations of cues in online therapy (see Chapter 5 by Springer, Taylor, & Bischoff) but also how to use technology productively in ways in-person therapy cannot do (see Chapter 6 by Veldorale-Griffin). A systemic view of the e-environment is provided in and of itself; this includes an analysis of the virtual environment, the therapist's physical environment, and the physical environment of the client(s).

Readers will also appreciate the attention to self-of-the-therapist issues that arise in the context of telehealth. The authors give practical suggestions and advice to help therapists navigate the drains that are ever present for therapists but also the unique challenges brought by delivering therapy remotely. While we often give lip service to self-care, the authors take this topic very seriously, as most of us have experienced more emotional stress in this transition. The authors provide soothing salve for these wounds with sound suggestions.

This unique book also addresses what I consider the most challenging aspect of telehealth – how to deliver telehealth to children. As a supervisor, I have seen some people do this brilliantly, while others flounder, unable to make play therapy accessible in this format. There are five chapters in this book that give very clear instructions and ideas that allow therapists to make this difficult transition. They bring *fun* into the online platform and allow children, who have often been ignored in telehealth, to flourish. If you want children to *want* to come to your sessions, study these chapters that teach you this important teleskill.

The Therapist's Notebook for Systemic Teletherapy also provides solid information on how to transform the emotional process of therapy in an electronic format when working with adults. I believe *this* is what we feared we would lose doing telehealth, and in this section, the authors teach us how to stay connected with clients and how to help them connect and navigate their own affect in ways that are deeply therapeutic. The authors teach you how to ground clients, process emotions, make connections, and establish goals by using an e-format *as an advantage and not a detriment to therapy*.

Lastly, this book addresses our fears as therapists: How do we keep clients alive? How do we keep them safe in an online format? How can I possibly work on relationships online? These issues are all addressed in this book: suicidal intervention, intimate partner violence, deescalation of conflict, and addressing sexual relationships, with the various authors *teaching* the reader solid conceptualization and intervention in these areas. It is rare that a book provides relief, but this book does just that as we navigate this new era of therapy. It also inspires us to be solid online therapists to our "virtual" clients in the reality of their lives.

Lorna Hecker, PhD, LMFT
Professor Emerita, Marriage and Family Therapy, Purdue University Northwest

PREFACE

Like most other university instructors, I was tasked with quickly transferring my courses to online format at the start of the pandemic. Most of my courses relied heavily on experiential activities to model creative ways in which to engage client systems in the therapy room. I struggled to think of how I was going to lead engaging online courses that relied so heavily on systemic experiential therapeutic activities.

I was a new mom at the time, just returning from maternity leave. Sleepless nights provided time to come up with some ideas. I consulted with a fabulous attorney/licensed mental health counselor colleague who helped me navigate the rapidly changing laws that related to this quick transition (see Chapters 1 and 3). I transferred the play genogram activity that I normally conducted to a clip art play genogram (see Chapter 30), figured out how to play the Ungame even more creatively via online platforms (see Chapter 32), and began conducting virtual reflecting teams in online supervision (see Chapter 38).

But I also wondered how therapists across the world were navigating this transition. What creative ideas were others coming up with? I did some research and discovered online platforms created for use in virtual therapy, such as Dr. Jessica Stone's Virtual Sandtray®© App (see Chapter 13) and Dr. Karen Fried's Online Puppets platform (see Chapter 14). Professionals across the globe were quickly figuring out how to transfer in-person practices to online formats at the start of the pandemic (e.g., Crockett et al., 2020; Sammons et al., 2020). Some therapists had already been doing online work for years and were in a position to share coveted knowledge on navigating online therapy environments with others who were just encountering these platforms for the first time (see Chapters 2 and 5 by Springer, Taylor, & Bischoff). Many also specifically attended to the application of systems theory in figuring out how to actively engage individuals, intimate relationships, families, and supervision groups via online platforms (e.g., Allan et al., 2021; Levy et al., 2021; Taylor et al., 2021). In doing this research and in navigating my own challenges with the transition to online therapy, I was inspired to create a practical resource that would compile creative ideas that could be used in working with children, adolescents, adults, intimate relationships, and families specifically via teletherapy.

As a family therapy student, I found *The Therapist's Notebook* series to be an invaluable resource in coming up with creative systemic therapy interventions for working with a variety of clientele. These books remain at arm's reach in my office and have continued to provide inspiration throughout my career. When this book was just an idea in my head, I reached out to my mentor, Dr. Lorna Hecker, who created this series 25 years ago. With her encouragement, this book was on its way to becoming an extension of her work and that series.

There are 40 chapters in this book, written by over 50 talented clinicians/authors, each of whom has contributed their own unique and creative teletherapy ideas to this text. They have personally inspired me with what they have shared. I anticipate they will do the same for you. Their work in this book is divided into seven sections: *Setup and Preparation, Self of the Therapist, Children and Adolescents, Adults, Intimate Relationships, Families*, and *Training and Supervision*.

Section 1: Setup and Preparation addresses practical considerations that systemic teletherapists can take to create a successful online therapy practice. Chapters in this section are written by expert clinicians who have been practicing and teaching how to do online therapy since well before the pandemic shifted most therapists to online practice. Chapter 1 addresses legal and ethical considerations of systemic teletherapy, focusing on how to determine whether it is appropriate to practice online therapy. Chapter 2 brings to light the complexities of online practice as it relates to managing multiple therapeutic environments and step-by-step procedures for navigating these environments for successful systemic practice. Chapter 3 provides practical advice on setting up confidential spaces from which to conduct and attend teletherapy. Chapters 4 and 5 focus on practical steps that therapists can take to build therapeutic relationships via teletherapy and specifically how to overcome common visual and auditory cue deficits in online sessions. Finally, Chapter 6 gives advice on how to set up physical and online therapy spaces to create a welcoming online environment and to communicate other important messages to clients.

Section 2: Self of the Therapist addresses unique personal considerations for therapists who practice online. Topics in this section include ways in which to manage distractions and remain present during teletherapy sessions (Chapter 7), create end-of-day letting-go rituals to use in place of a typical commute home (Chapter 8), assess and attend to unique considerations of self-care that relate to teletherapy practice (Chapters 8–11), and plan for parental leave in the absence of visual cues, such as a "baby bump," that might otherwise naturally tip clients off to an impending break from therapy (Chapter 12).

Sections 3–6 focus on specific teletherapy interventions/approaches for working with particular populations (i.e., children and adolescents, adults, intimate relationships, families). The organization of these chapters is inspired by that of the original *Therapist's Notebook* series. Most chapters provide an objective, a rationale for use that is grounded in research/evidence-based practice, steps necessary for setup, instructions for conducting the intervention, guidance on how to process the intervention with client systems, an example vignette (in which client names and identifying features from any actual cases have been altered), suggestions for follow-up, and possible contraindications. Each chapter also lists materials required for both therapists and clients. This text assumes that both clients and therapists have access to a computer or another device that has a working camera and audio, has a screen large enough to adequately see the video of another person/people, and can be used to connect to working Wi-Fi and/or the Internet. It also assumes that therapists have access to and use a teletherapy platform that is consistent with required HIPAA laws and regulations. Though most chapters are grounded in a particular systemic therapy theory or model, they can be adapted and used from your own approach.

Section 3: Children and Adolescents provides step-by-step instructions on how to conduct creative teletherapy interventions using digital sand therapy (Chapter 13), virtual puppet play (Chapter 14), online chess using a structural therapy approach (Chapter 15), a solution-focused scavenger hunt capitalizing on children and adolescents being in their own physical environment(s) (Chapter 16), and poetry via teletherapy using a narrative approach (Chapter 17).

Section 4: Adults presents instructions on how to conduct a virtual adaptation of the Gestalt empty-chair technique (Chapter 18), create virtual vision boards using a narrative therapy approach (Chapter 19), use guided grounding in teletherapy (Chapter 20), conduct solution-focused teletherapy for suicidal intervention (Chapter 21), conduct virtual home visits for hoarding disorder (Chapter 22), and conduct virtual cognitive stimulation therapy for groups of older adults with memory loss (Chapter 23).

Section 5: Intimate Relationships addresses creative structural and strategic interventions for working with intimate relationships in ways that capitalize on the limitations of telehealth (Chapters 24–26). Chapter 27 provides instructions on using an emotion-focused intervention for mapping cycles with clients practicing consensual nonmonogamy. Chapter 28 applies internal family systems theory and mindfulness-based sex therapy to set the stage for sensate focus work via telehealth. Chapter 29 provides practical steps to assess the appropriateness of teletherapy with clients experiencing intimate partner violence.

Section 6: Families presents instructions on conducting digital play genograms (Chapter 30), guiding clients to do family sculpts (Chapter 31), strategically playing the Ungame (Chapter 32), creating altars for grief and loss (Chapter 33), using virtual maps to share stories of migration journeys (Chapter 34), and practicing medical family therapy (Chapter 35), all via teletherapy platforms.

Section 7: Training and Supervision includes chapters aimed at therapy supervisors and educators, though information contained within this section is informative for any practicing clinician, especially those who may be interested in implementing virtual reflecting teams with groups of other clinicians. Chapters provide advice on supporting therapists through deliberate practice in systemic teletherapy (Chapter 36), round-robin case conceptualization for theoretically grounded virtual supervision (Chapter 37), conducting virtual reflecting teams using the Milan approach (Chapter 38), adapting virtual reflecting teams for use with Latino/a families (Chapter 39), and using simulation in virtual group supervision (Chapter 40).

With creative thinking, teletherapy allows for the application of unique and engaging systemic interventions. If you have struggled in conducting creative teletherapy interventions, my hope is that this book provides you with a starting point that inspires more of your own creative ideas for online intervention. If you already have an established regimen of creative teletherapy interventions, I hope that the chapters within this text provide continued inspiration and ideas for your practice.

References

Allan, R., Wiebe, S. A., Johnson, S. M., Piaseckyj, O., & Campbell, T. L. (2021). Practicing emotionally focused therapy online: Calling all relationships. *Journal of Marital and Family Therapy, 47*(2), 424–439. https://doi.org/10.1111/jmft.12507

Crockett, J. L., Becraft, J. L., Phillips, S. T., Wakeman, M., & Cataldo, M. F. (2020). Rapid conversion from clinical to telehealth behavioral services during the COVID-19 pandemic. *Behavior Analysis in Practice, 13*(4), 725–735. https://doi.org/10.1007/s40617-020-00499-8

Levy, S., Mason, S., Russon, J., & Diamond, G. (2021). Attachment-based family therapy in the age of telehealth and COVID-19. *Journal of Marital and Family Therapy, 47*(2), 440–454.

Sammons, M. T., VandenBos, G. R., & Martin, J. N. (2020). Psychological practice and the COVID-19 crisis: A rapid response survey. *Journal of Health Service Psychology, 46*, 51–57. https://doi.org/10.1111/jmft.12509

Taylor, N. C., Springer, P. R., Bischoff, R. J., & Smith, J. P. (2021). Experiential family therapy interventions delivered via telemental health: A qualitative implementation study. *Journal of Marital and Family Therapy, 47*(2), 455–472. https://doi.org/10.1111/jmft.12520

ACKNOWLEDGMENTS

I offer my deepest appreciation to the incredible clinicians and authors whose collective work made this book a reality. Thank you for your creativity, time, effort, and encouragement throughout the process.

A special thanks to Dr. Lorna Hecker, editor of *The* [original] *Therapist's Notebook*, who encouraged me and provided guidance in submitting the proposal for this book.

Thank you to Heather Evans at Routledge for her enthusiastic support in following through with that submission. And to Julia Giordano, who stepped in for Heather, answered dozens of last-minute questions, and helped in the finishing stages of the editing process.

Thank you to Seattle University's College of Arts and Sciences for supporting this project through the Dean's Research Fellowship and Student Assistantship Award. And to Tiffany Alexis Leal, who was steadfast in her work well beyond her time as a graduate student research assistant. Thank you not only for your keen attention to detail and continued help but for your "can do it" attitude and generous uplifting spirit.

Jacob and Christine, my academic life partners, it's been extra special having you be a part of this project. Fifteen years after the publication of CAGRIC (Cobb et al., 2009), it warms my heart knowing that we can still find ways to collaborate, albeit sans *Guitar Hero* and the Cocomotion.

To friends who checked in on the status of this book time and time again, thank you for supporting me.

And finally, to Adam, Addison, and Charlie, thank you for supporting Mama in the completion of her book. Just now, you barged into the room and saw me working. I promise I'm almost done and will come out to play soon.

Reference

Cobb, R. A., Walsh, C. E., & Priest, J. B. (2009). The cognitive-active gender role identification continuum. *Journal of Feminist Family Therapy*, *21*(2), 77–97. https://doi.org/10.1080/08952830902911339

Part 1
Setup and Preparation

CHAPTER 1

CAN WE MEET REMOTELY? LEGAL AND ETHICAL CONSIDERATIONS FOR SYSTEMIC TELETHERAPY

Eric L. Ström

Teletherapy is defined as any use of technology as a medium for delivering clinical services to a client who is in a physical location separate from the clinician. Under this definition, teletherapy can refer to services delivered via synchronous audio/video telehealth platforms, phone, email, text, or even clinical services delivered through virtual environments. Thus, the defining features of teletherapy are the use of technology and physical separation of the clients' and clinician's locations.

When determining how best to apply legal and ethical standards in the context of technology, it's often best to start by analogizing the situation to the "physical" world. Generally, ethical and legal standards of clinical work in the physical world apply to clinical work in the virtual world. However, teletherapy presents several unique issues to consider regarding ethical and legal aspects of practice. Among the most important of these is determining when it is appropriate to conduct teletherapy with a client or client system.

When considering whether it is appropriate to conduct teletherapy, clinicians should ask themselves the following questions:

1. Is it legal for me to conduct teletherapy given my physical location and the physical location of my clients?

2. Have I received the proper training to conduct teletherapy?

3. Is teletherapy sufficiently effective for this client in this situation?

4. Are there other contextual factors that might make in-person therapy a better option for my clients?

5. Do clients have accessibility to alternative services if in-person therapy is a better option for them or if I'm not legally allowed to provide teletherapy to them given jurisdictional limitations?

To help answer these questions, the following outlines the necessary considerations when assessing working within jurisdictional limitations, teletherapy training, the effectiveness of teletherapy services, contraindications of teletherapy given particular presenting problems, and accessibility of alternative services.

Jurisdictional Limitations

When providing teletherapy, health care is legally considered to occur in both the clients' and the clinician's physical locations simultaneously. Therefore, the laws and regulations of the jurisdiction the

DOI: 10.4324/9781003289920-2

clinician is physically located in and the jurisdiction(s) the clients are physically located in during teletherapy both apply (American Association for Marriage and Family Therapy, 2015; American Counseling Association, 2014; American Mental Health Counselors Association, 2020). Accordingly, to determine what legal standards apply, clinicians must consider (1) the clinician's physical location, (2) the physical location of clients, and (3) the clinician's location of licensure.

The Clinician's Physical Location

Generally, clinicians must be licensed in and follow all applicable laws and regulations regarding teletherapy practice in the location in which they are physically located while teletherapy services are taking place. This means that if a clinician is physically located outside of the jurisdiction of their license, they might be restricted from providing teletherapy from that location. This is true even if the clients are in the location of the clinician's licensure and even if the clinician is just temporarily in that location (e.g., Alaska Admin. Code, 2022).

The Client's Physical Location

Likewise, clinicians must follow all applicable laws and regulations regarding teletherapy practice in the locations in which their clients are physically located while teletherapy services are taking place. This usually includes a requirement for the clinician to be licensed by the state(s) their clients are located in. Many states have clear statutory requirements for licensure when providing teletherapy to clients located in those states. Other states express this requirement as policy rather than statutory law (e.g., New York State Office of the Professions, 2021). In many cases, this means that if a client is outside of the location in which the therapist is licensed, they must have permission from that other state before they can provide teletherapy services to anyone located there. This is true even if the client is just temporarily in that location.

These jurisdictional issues are compounded when a clinician engages in systemic teletherapy. When a family or relationship is the identified client and members are in different locations, the clinician needs to comply with applicable laws and regulations for all jurisdictions (i.e., state and/or country) members of the family or relationship are located in. For example, an identified client consisting of a family with the biological mother, stepmother, and daughter all present in different states would require the therapist to comply with licensure rules in all three states at once. Dependent on the rules of each state, this may require the therapist to be licensed in all three states to provide therapy to this family. If the clinician were physically present in another state, this could mean that the clinician might need to be licensed in up to four different jurisdictions all at once.

Some states, however, have provisions that allow for temporary practice. This means that under certain circumstances, those states will allow a clinician to provide teletherapy, under a license from the clinician's state, to a client located within that other state. These temporary practice rules range anywhere from 15 to 90 days (Exceptions to Licensure: Jurisdiction, 2015; Regulation of Professions and Occupations – Exemptions, 2013). Similarly, some states allow temporary practice only for specific purposes, such as the recent relocation of a client (Exemptions from Licensure, 2021) or in case of an emergency (Exemptions, 2018). Defining what situations may constitute a valid "emergency" is up to the discretion of applicable regulatory board(s).

Therefore, if either the daughter, biological mom, or stepmother in the aforementioned example was only temporarily located in one of the states in which there are temporary practice rules, the therapist may only be required to be licensed in two of the three states in which the family members are located, though they would still need to comply with licensure rules for all three states while practicing with this family. However, let's say that the daughter, rather than the family, has been identified as the sole client and that the therapist and daughter simply involve the biological mother and stepmother to participate in a session for support. In that case, the healthcare is being delivered only in the locations of the therapist and the daughter. In this situation, the jurisdictions each of the mothers are located in would generally not have a legal basis to regulate the therapy.

Just as when delivering clinical services in person, the client must be explicitly identified prior to providing systemic therapy, and all participants must have a shared understanding of that identification. Identification of the client defines who has entered into a clinical relationship with the clinician and, therefore, the location(s) in which therapy is taking place. Issues of legal jurisdiction and licensure requirements then flow directly from the physical location of the identified client(s).

The Clinician's Location of Licensure

Within the United States, healthcare largely continues to be regulated on a state-by-state basis. When providing teletherapy across state lines, the rules and regulations (including licensure requirements) require a state-by-state analysis due to the variation between states. For example, some states have temporary practice provisions, some allow for temporary licensure, and some simply require full licensure. With a temporary practice provision, a state may allow an out-of-state clinician to provide services to a client located in that state for a limited amount of time or for a limited number of sessions. Temporary licensure, on the other hand, would be when a state would grant a license to an out-of-state therapist for a limited time, context, or purpose (e.g., natural disaster or crisis-response work).

There are a few federal legal provisions allowing clinicians to provide teletherapy across state lines while being exempted from state regulation in very limited contexts. One such example applies to clinicians providing healthcare services as employees of the United States Department of Veterans Affairs (Health Care Providers Practicing via Telehealth, 2018). Most (if not all) states have implemented exceptions to state licensure requirements for employees of the federal government when providing healthcare services as part of their federal employment.

However, there are no general national policies or rules that allow the delivery of teletherapy across state lines. Some multistate agreements, or "compacts," have been created to facilitate state-to-state credential portability for clinicians with equivalent licenses in different states. These compacts apply only to clinicians who hold specific types of licenses in states that have joined the compacts. The types of licenses covered and the number of member states increase year by year.

Many teletherapy clinicians choose to become licensed in more than one jurisdiction to allow them the flexibility of travel. For example, a clinician who spends summers in Washington and winters in Florida may choose to seek licensure in both states to continue their clinical work throughout the year. This also allows them access to a wider array of clientele (i.e., clients who are physically located in both Washington and Florida). Other clinicians may maintain licensure in several jurisdictions simultaneously simply to allow access to a larger pool of clients with whom they can work. This can be particularly important for clients who are in long-distance relationships or travel often between different jurisdictions. For example, a couple who lives primarily in Kansas but travels often to Illinois to help care for their grandchildren may avoid large gaps in treatment by having a therapist who is licensed in both Kansas and Illinois.

In the case of international teletherapy, laws and regulations of the jurisdiction the clinician is physically located in and the jurisdictions clients are physically located in during teletherapy both also apply just as they do with teletherapy that crosses state lines. While many other nations regulate the practice of psychology, very few countries specifically regulate the practice of counseling or marriage and family therapy. However, it is possible that another country might limit or restrict the services a clinician licensed elsewhere can provide either when they themselves are physically located in that country or when a client is physically present in that country.

The bottom line is that if the clinician and client(s) are physically located in different jurisdictions (countries or U.S. states) during a teletherapy session, the clinician has an obligation to ensure the clinical work is in compliance with all local laws, rules, and policies of all jurisdictions involved. The best way to maintain practice within appropriate legal and ethical boundaries is to:

1. Include a statement in the informed consent indicating what jurisdiction(s) the clinician is licensed in.

2. Identify who is the client (versus support people who may be present during sessions).

3. Identify the location(s) of the identified client(s) during each teletherapy session.

4. In advance of conducting therapy, verify authorization to provide clinical services in each client location.

5. When in doubt about another state's licensure requirements or temporary practice provisions, contact that state's licensing board for more specific guidance about licensure and any applicable exceptions.

Given these jurisdictional complexities when providing services via teletherapy, it is vital for clinicians to have a plan in place to support effective continuity of care and/or transfer care in response to jurisdictional restrictions. An example of this could be if the client or the clinician needs to temporarily travel outside of the state of the clinician's licensure. In this case, it would be important for the clinician to have a plan in place to request temporary practice permission from that other state, to temporarily pause the clinical services, or to terminate care or refer the client to a different provider.

Teletherapy Supervision

All of these same jurisdictional considerations apply within supervisory relationships as well. This means that if a therapist is under supervision, the therapist and supervisor need to ensure that supervision is in compliance with the laws and regulations of the client's location, the supervisee's location, and the supervisor's location. For example, consider a clinical supervisor who is licensed in Kansas and is supervising a candidate for LMFT licensure who temporarily relocates to Texas to be with family over the holidays. The supervisor would need to verify that Texas permits the supervisee to provide supervised teletherapy from Texas and that Kansas permits the licensure candidate's supervised experience to occur outside of Kansas. They would also need to verify that the state in which the client is located allows the service to be provided by the supervisee.

Teletherapy Training

Just as the specific requirements for licensure vary from jurisdiction to jurisdiction, so do the requirements for specific training and continuing education in teletherapy. Some states have requirements regarding specific teletherapy training that must be completed before a clinician may deliver teletherapy services. Some states have a teletherapy continuing-education requirement. Some states have both requirements.

Even in jurisdictions in which specific training in teletherapy is not required, the ethical standard of care still requires that clinicians develop competency for safe and effective delivery when providing clinical services via teletherapy (American Association for Marriage and Family Therapy, 2015; American Counseling Association, 2014; American Mental Health Counselors Association, 2020).

Clinicians should therefore:

1. Be aware of and follow any relevant jurisdictional regulations regarding training and continuing education in teletherapy.

2. Seek training opportunities to develop and enhance practice specifically as it relates to teletherapy.

Effectiveness of Teletherapy

In addition to these applicable laws and regulations, services should be provided via teletherapy only when such services are effective and appropriate for individual clients (American Association for Marriage and Family Therapy, 2015; American Counseling Association, 2014; American Mental Health Counselors Association, 2020). Research indicates that teletherapy is just as effective as in-person services for many clinical conditions including adjustment disorder, anger management, anxiety, depression, eating disorders, posttraumatic stress, and substance use (Braeuer et al., 2022; Lazur et al., 2020; Slone et al., 2012; Turgoose et al., 2018; Varker et al., 2019). In fact, teletherapy may be even more effective than in-person therapy for some clinical presentations such as depression (Luo et al., 2020). Teletherapy may be particularly effective in the formation of the therapeutic alliance between client and clinician, especially when working with children and adolescents (Braeuer et al., 2022; Slone et al., 2012; Stiles-Shields et al., 2014). While these studies demonstrate the potential effectiveness of teletherapy as a modality, it is still imperative that clinicians assess the applicability and effectiveness of this modality on a client-by-client basis.

Contraindications of Teletherapy

Despite the effectiveness of teletherapy, there may be instances in which teletherapy is contraindicated or in-person services may be more effective than teletherapy for particular clients. Teletherapy may not be appropriate for clients with severe mental illness or when there is a safety risk for the client or others. For example, unless the clients are currently involved in other in-person treatments, therapists should carefully consider referring clients to in-person service providers if any of the following are of concern within the client system:

- There is a serious mental health diagnosis.

- There are indicators of severe dysregulation or profound dissociation.

- There is a history of self-harm.

- The client demonstrates indicators of uncontrolled substance abuse or dependence (Wrape & McGinn, 2019).

- There are indicators that domestic violence may be taking place (Myers et al., 2017).

- There are indicators that the confidentiality of teletherapy is compromised and the client's safety may be at risk as a result (see Chapter 29 for more information on cyberstalking and assessing the appropriateness of teletherapy for intimate partner violence).

Accessibility of Alternative Services

As more and more clinicians transfer their practice to telehealth, fewer in-person services may be available. Finding specialists for particular presenting problems may be extra challenging, especially for those in rural communities. If affordable in-person services necessary to meet the client's needs are not currently available due to limitations of client mobility, geographic availability of services, or cost of travel, it may be in the client's best interest to participate in teletherapy services, at least until other services become available. This may help to avoid situations in which clients have no services at all.

Questions to Consider

As it relates to determining whether teletherapy is appropriate, therapists should ultimately consider:

- Who is the identified client?

- Where are all members of the client system physically located?

- Am I legally allowed to practice with all members of the client system given each of their physical locations?

- Are there provisions allowing temporary practice in any of the locations in which members of the client system are located?

- Is teletherapy appropriate for the client given their presenting problem and other unique factors? Why or why not?

- If in-person services would be better suited for the client, is there an accessible option for this available to them?

- What are the positive and negative implications if services are temporarily paused or terminated?

- If services must legally be paused or terminated, how might you address the client's need for continuity of care?

Resources for Identifying State Regulatory Boards

Person-Centered Tech

https://personcenteredtech.com/teletherapy-practice-rules-by-state/

Telehealth Certification Institute

https://telementalhealthtraining.com/states-rules-and-regulations

As with all state-by-state guides, be sure to verify that these resources are current and accurate. This area of state regulation is evolving and developing quickly. A state-by-state guide to teletherapy regulations is a good starting point for your research but is potentially out of date as soon as it is written down.

Ethics Codes Provisions

Ensuring That Teletherapy Is Used Only When Effective for the Client

American Association for Marriage and Family Therapy, 2015, 6.1

American Counseling Association, 2014, H.4.c

American Mental Health Counselors Association, 2020, I.B.6.c

Teletherapy Crossing Jurisdictions

American Association for Marriage and Family Therapy, 2015, 6.1, 6.5

American Counseling Association, 2014, H.1.b

American Mental Health Counselors Association, 2020, I.B.6.e

Teletherapy Training

American Association for Marriage and Family Therapy, 2015, 6.1

American Counseling Association, 2014, H.1.a

American Mental Health Counselors Association, 2020, I.B.6.d

References

American Association for Marriage and Family Therapy. (2015). *2015 AAMFT code of ethics*. www.www.aamft.org/Legal_Ethics/Code_of_Ethics.aspx

American Counseling Association. (2014). *2014 ACA code of ethics*. www.counseling.org/docs/default-source/default-document-library/2014-code-of-ethics-finaladdress.pdf

American Mental Health Counselors Association. (2020). *2020 AMHCA code of ethics*. www.amhca.org/HigherLogic/System/DownloadDocumentFile.ashx?DocumentFileKey=24a27502-196e-b763-ff57-490a12f7edb1

Braeuer, K., Noble, N., & Yi, S. (2022). The efficacy of an online anger management program for justice-involved youth. *The Journal of Addictions & Offender Counseling, 43*(1), 26–37. https://doi.org/10.1002/jaoc.12101

Distance Professional Services, Alaska Admin. Code, 12 § 62.400. (2022).

Exceptions to Licensure: Jurisdiction, Ariz. Rev. Stat., 32–3271. (2015).

Exemptions from Licensure, Utah Code 58-60-107. (2021).

Exemptions, Code of the Dist. of Columbia, §3-1205.02. (2018).

Health Care Providers Practicing via Telehealth, 38 C.F.R. § 17.417 (2018).

Lazur, B., Sobolik, L., & King, V. (2020). *Telebehavioral health: An effective alternative to in-person care*. Milbank Memorial Fund.

Luo, C., Sanger, N., Singhal, N., Pattrick, K., Shams, I., Shahid, H., Hoang, P., Schmidt, J., Lee, J., Haber, S., Puckering, M., Buchanan, N., Lee, P., Ng, K., Sun, S., Kheyson, S., Chung, D. C., Sanger, S., Thabane, L., & Samaan, Z. (2020). A comparison of electronically-delivered and face to face cognitive behavioural therapies in depressive disorders: A systematic review and meta-analysis. *EClinicalMedicine, 24*, Article 100442. https://doi.org/10.1016/j.eclinm.2020.100442

Myers, K., Nelson, E. L., Rabinowitz, T., Hilty, D., Baker, D., Barnwell, S. S., Boyce, G., Bufka, L. F., Cain, S., Chui, L., Comer, J. S., Cradock, C., Goldstein, F., Johnston, B., Krupinski, E., Lo, K., Luxton, D. D., McSwain, S. D.,

McWilliams, J., . . . Bernard, J. (2017). American telemedicine association practice guidelines for telemental health with children and adolescents. *Telemedicine Journal and E-Health: The Official Journal of the American Telemedicine Association, 23*(10), 779–804. https://doi.org/10.1089/tmj.2017.0177

New York State Office of the Professions. (2021). *Guideline 9: Engaging in telepractice.* www.op.nysed.gov/prof/mhp/mhppg9.htm

Regulation of Professions and Occupations – Exemptions, Fl. Stat. 32 § 491.014. (2013).

Slone, N. C., Reese, R. J., & McClellan, M. J. (2012). Telepsychology outcome research with children and adolescents: A review of the literature. *Psychological Services, 9*(3), 272–292. https://doi.org/10.1037/a0027607

Stiles-Shields, C., Kwasny, M. J., Cai, X., & Mohr, D. C. (2014). Therapeutic alliance in face-to-face and telephone-administered cognitive behavioral therapy. *Journal of Consulting and Clinical Psychology, 82*(2), 349–354. https://doi.org/10.1037/a0035554

Turgoose, D., Ashwick, R., & Murphy, D. (2018). Systematic review of lessons learned from delivering tele-therapy to veterans with post-traumatic stress disorder. *Journal of Telemedicine and Telecare, 24*(9), 575–585. https://doi.org/10.1177/1357633X17730443

Varker, T., Brand, R. M., Ward, J., Terhaag, S., & Phelps, A. (2019). Efficacy of synchronous telepsychology interventions for people with anxiety, depression, posttraumatic stress disorder, and adjustment disorder: A rapid evidence assessment. *Psychological Services, 16*(4), 621–635. https://doi.org/10.1037/ser0000239

Wrape, E. R., & McGinn, M. M. (2019). Clinical and ethical considerations for delivering couple and family therapy via telehealth. *Journal of Marital and Family Therapy, 45*(2), 296–308. https://doi.org/10.1111/jmft.12319

CHAPTER 2

MANAGING MULTIPLE THERAPEUTIC ENVIRONMENTS

Paul R. Springer, Nathan C. Taylor, and Richard J. Bischoff

In systemic teletherapy, clinicians need to manage multiple therapeutic environments. Unlike in-person therapy, in which therapists only need to worry about the physical environment in which therapy is occurring, telemental health becomes more complex as therapists need to manage three (or more) unique environments to be effective. These environments include (1) the virtual environment, (2) the therapist's physical environment, and (3) the physical environment(s) of clients. In addition, therapists need to consider implications of each of these environments for client safety.

The Virtual Environment

To provide quality therapy via videoconferencing, adapt the virtual environment to facilitate treatment outcomes. This can be accomplished by (1) choosing the best platform for treatment, (2) assessing and monitoring clients' experiences with the chosen platform, and (3) planning for technological difficulties.

Choose the Platform

There are a multiplicity of online platforms for conducting teletherapy. Different platforms provide different levels of communication options (i.e., chat options, video sharing, sharing documents, delivery of assessments), are more or less user friendly, and support different levels of security and anonymity. When selecting an online therapy platform, consider the following.

Of utmost importance, the selected platform must ensure confidentiality and be HIPAA consistent (see Chapter 3). For therapists who accept insurance, this platform should also ideally offer documentation options that lead to improved billing to insurance companies. For example, some platforms such as Simple Practice and Theranotes provide: (1) a centralized client portal, where clients can complete all paperwork and initial assessments prior to session, (2) a scheduling function that sends free email and/or text reminders, (3) a function that simplifies client payment, and (4) the ability to file primary and secondary insurance claims in seconds.

Select a platform that can easily be used through a variety of technology mediums (e.g., computer, smartphone, tablet) to increase access of services. Many clients have limited experience using technology. Others may not have access to reliable internet service or own a computer, smartphone, or other electronic device. Clients who may need to connect to therapy from varying locations (e.g., work, multiple residences, while traveling) must be able to access therapy utilizing different devices at different times. It is important that clients can use whatever electronic devices are available.

DOI: 10.4324/9781003289920-3

Specifically for systemic teletherapists, this platform must also allow people to connect from different locations simultaneously. This lets family members participate in therapy regardless of where they live. Even when all members are present within the same household, this provides greater flexibility in online sessions for members to join from separate devices or spaces within the household. For example, when doing therapy with large families, multiple devices may be used to allow therapists a better field of view of all family members at once. Alternatively, therapists may ask volatile partners to join session from separate devices in separate rooms (see Chapter 24).

Other important things to consider when choosing a platform include the ability to:

- Share screens

- Share files that can be downloaded by the end user

- Collaborate in using a whiteboard function for doing activities such as a family genogram (see Chapter 30)

- Put clients joining from different devices into "breakout rooms" to allow therapists to meet with one or more clients separately for a brief period

- Enable closed captioning or live transcript options for clients who are hearing impaired

- Record sessions for interventions in which therapists may want to replay session clips to clients or for the purpose of clinical supervision

Additional considerations should be based on client needs and preferences (Hertlein et al., 2021).

Assess and Educate About the Client Experience

To ensure that client needs are met and to prevent disruptions to the therapeutic process, assess client comfort with both the therapy platform and devices used to access the platform (Hertlein et al., 2021). Then, based on client responses, provide education about any aspects of online therapy that may be needed. For example, consider asking the following questions prior to the first session:

- How comfortable are you using technology?

- What is your comfort level using a tablet or phone to join into therapy?

- Have you ever attended virtual or online therapy?

   - If yes, what platforms have you used?

   - If no, what concerns you the most about online therapy?

- Do you know how to mute audio and turn off your video?

These questions allow therapists to understand the extent to which they need to educate clients about the platform and the device used to access it. For example, it can be helpful to teach clients how to:

- Download the therapy platform on their device(s)

- Turn the camera on and off

- Adjust the volume

- Use the mute function

- Use the chat function

- Share their screen

In addition to providing education about the general experience of the therapeutic platform, explain how the platform they are using will ensure their privacy, can facilitate the efficacy of treatment, and can enhance their overall virtual experience (Hertlein et al., 2021). When therapists take the time to have these conversations, clients tend to gain a greater sense of confidence in the modality, clients are more engaged in treatment, and many technological problems can be averted.

Throughout treatment, continue monitoring clients' comfort and personal fit with the treatment modality. Periodically and frequently asking for feedback about a client's experience helps clients feel understood. It also provides valuable information about how comfortable clients feel using this modality, which impacts their overall investment and engagement in online therapy (Burgoyne & Cohn, 2020). Examples of questions you can ask include:

- What has been working well doing therapy online?

- What are some things you enjoy about online therapy?

- Are there concerns you have about doing online therapy?

- What are some things that make online therapy challenging for you?

- What are some things I could do to improve your online experience?

- How comfortable are you disclosing sensitive information about yourself doing online therapy?

- I am noticing that you seem distracted or are not looking at the screen. Is there something on your mind?

Plan for Technological Difficulties

Technology can be unreliable and stop working at inopportune times. Common challenges therapists need to plan for when engaging clients in systemic teletherapy include:

- Audio stops working

- Video stops working

- Internet connections fail

- There is a dramatic lag in conversation

If therapists do not plan for these difficulties with clients in advance, these disruptions can negatively impact the flow of therapy and have the potential to be traumatic for clients disclosing vulnerable information. To avoid inadvertent consequences of technological difficulties, the following suggestions may be addressed at the onset of therapy:

- Teach clients how to troubleshoot when their camera or microphone is not working.

- Develop a protocol where clients will restart their computer and log back on when facing technological challenges.

- If another device with video and audio capabilities is available (e.g., computer, tablet, smartphone), create a plan to rejoin sessions utilizing that device to quickly continue therapy when other devices fail.

- Create a plan to call clients on a mobile device or landline when technology with video capabilities is not working and/or the internet connection cannot be fixed.

Ultimately, failure to plan with clients risks allowing technological problems to overshadow the positive experiences and growth that clients may experience in teletherapy. Set realistic expectations, and normalize occasional disruptions to help clients be more resilient when technological problems inevitably occur.

The Therapist's Physical Environment

Research shows that the physical environment in which face-to-face psychotherapy is provided (e.g., décor, cleanliness) impacts treatment (Jackson, 2018). It would therefore stand to reason that parts of the therapist's physical environment that are visible and audible to clients have similar therapeutic impacts. Some have argued that the therapist's physical environment should closely resemble that of in-person therapy (Hertlein et al., 2021; Springer et al., 2020; Taylor et al., 2021). Consider the following as it relates to the physical environment in which you conduct teletherapy:

- Of utmost importance, do everything in your power to ensure confidentiality in your physical space, especially if you are working from home (see Chapter 3).

- Organize your space in such a way that it creates a private, warm, and calming environment (see Chapter 6).

- Use noise-canceling headphones to limit noises in your physical location (e.g., ambulance, construction, barking dogs) from being disruptive.

As therapists maximize ways to improve their physical environment and to disrupt interruptions in this space, they are better able to focus on ways to help clients adapt and improve their online experience.

Client Physical Environments

Just as the therapist's physical environment has the potential to impact treatment, the client's physical environment has the potential to impact treatment. Ambient noise, where clients are physically positioned in the room, and other distractions in the physical location where clients are situated impact treatment progress and outcomes. Likewise, the probability of interruptions or the ability to have confidential conversations all affect treatment. For example, a child, roommate, or intimate partner entering the room during therapy can be incredibly disruptive to the therapeutic process, especially when talking about sensitive issues or participating in an activity that requires the client's undivided attention (e.g., EMDR, guided meditation, trauma work). This can be especially problematic when discussing sensitive topics and therapists don't know that someone else is nearby and listening because they're positioned outside of view of the camera. Even just the possibility of interruption (e.g., knowing that someone else is present within the household) may inhibit clients from discussing sensitive topics.

Unfortunately, physical locations of clients are often not set up in ways that are conducive to therapy and may inherently have potential for disruption to the therapeutic process. To make matters even more complicated, when working with partners or families who have members join sessions from different physical locations, opportunities for environmental disruptions are exponential. However, there are things that therapists can do to help clients set things up in the best possible way.

To mitigate any negative effects of the client's environment, discuss the best time and space from which to attend therapy. If multiple physical locations are available from which to attend sessions, discuss with clients the best place for them to use for teletherapy. For example, though it may be more convenient for some clients to attend sessions from their work office, this may not be the best option if clients don't have a private office or are concerned about others overhearing their conversations. Alternatively, an individual who has come out to their co-workers as being gay may prefer to join therapy from a work office rather than attending sessions from home if they haven't shared this with all members of the household who may be present during their scheduled sessions. Also discuss with clients the best day and time for them to schedule sessions. For example, clients who have small children in the household may be more likely to have a distraction-free environment on weekdays during times that their children are at school or daycare. To further support clients in maintaining a distraction-free environment, offer the following suggestions:

- Lock doors to rooms where clients will be while therapy is taking place.

- Put "do not disturb" signs on doors.

- Place noise machines just inside the doors of rooms where therapy will take place.

- Use noise-cancelling headphones if attending session individually.

- Ensure that children in the home have what they need prior to sessions so they are less likely to interrupt.

Once this has been discussed, share with clients how to best organize their equipment and space (Hertlein et al., 2021; Springer et al., 2020). Consider offering the following suggestions:

- Set up the room to have optimal lighting. For example, avoid sitting directly in front of windows and lamps to prevent shadows from impairing the view of facial expressions on the screen.

- Position chairs to allow a clear view of each person's face and body.

- In instances where everyone attending session cannot be clearly seen on one screen, have some family members join session from a second device (e.g., laptop, tablet, phone) in the same room if a second device is available. If either or both devices are portable, advise clients to place devices in strategic locations so you can see all clients in relation to one another.

- If using multiple devices in the same room, mute all but one device. This is critical because if multiple devices are on at the same time, it will distort the audio.

As you work with clients on enhancing their physical environment, do not assume that clients have access to private spaces to do therapy. Many clients do not have access to private spaces for this purpose. This is especially true when working with clients from marginalized communities. Be flexible with whatever is safe and comfortable for clients. For example, clients may not feel safe or have a separate space in their home to do therapy, so they may choose to join therapy sessions from a parked car.

Safety Considerations in Therapeutic Environments

Most importantly, safety should be considered as it relates to both the virtual environment and the client's physical environment.

Consider the following as it relates to the virtual environment:

- Assess the potential of cyberstalking, especially when working with clients who have a history of being in violent relationships (see Chapter 29).

- Discuss with clients the importance of continued audio and visual contact throughout teletherapy sessions as a means of ensuring client safety. Though some clients may prefer to turn their camera off or to walk out of the camera's view during difficult conversations, encourage clients to allow visual contact for the purpose of continued assessment of dissociation or other key safety signals.

- Have a backup plan for when technology stops working or for when clients disconnect from teletherapy without notice, especially when working with those who struggle with dissociation, domestic abuse, suicidal ideation, or other concerns regarding the safety of self or others.

Consider the following as it relates to the physical environment(s) of clients:

- Assess the physical location of clients at the start of each session so you know where to send law enforcement or other appropriate sources for a wellness check.

- Regularly assess for the presence of other people in the client's physical location during teletherapy sessions, especially if there are safety concerns such as intimate partner violence or child abuse. If there are others present who may overhear therapeutic conversations, avoid discussing anything that could put clients at risk of harm. When safe to do so, discuss other options for communicating if confidentiality is a concern (e.g., using the chat function).

- In advance of emergencies, identify and discuss appropriate resources for clients (e.g., domestic violence shelters) that are within physical proximity to clients. In comparison with in-person therapy sessions, this may take extra planning on the part of the therapist since therapists may need to familiarize themselves with resources in the areas surrounding each client's physical location.

- Set clear boundaries regarding the physical location of clients during teletherapy sessions as it relates to the safety of clients or others. For example, clients should not join teletherapy sessions while they are operating heavy machinery (e.g., driving a car). This puts both clients and others at risk, especially as clients discuss emotional or traumatic topics and may be less capable of focusing on the physical task at hand and on the therapeutic process simultaneously.

Finally, recognize that there may come a time when telemental health is no longer effective for particular clients. Assess for effectiveness of teletherapy services and make referrals to appropriate in-person service providers within the client's local community when necessary.

References

Burgoyne, N., & Cohn, A. S. (2020). Lessons from the transition to relational teletherapy during COVID-19. *Family Process*, *59*(3), 974–988. https://doi.org/10.1111/famp.12589

Hertlein, K. M., Drude, K. P., Hilty, D. M., & Maheu, M. M. (2021). Toward proficiency in telebehavioral health: Applying interprofessional competencies in couple and family therapy. *Journal of Martial and Family Therapy*, *47*(2), 359–374. https://doi.org/10.1111/jmft.12496

Jackson, D. (2018). Aesthetics and the psychotherapist's office. *Journal of Clinical Psychology*, *74*(2), 233–238. https://doi.org/10.1002/jclp.22576

Springer, P. R., Bischoff, R. J., Taylor, N. C., Kohel, K., & Farero, A. (2020). Collaborative care at a distance: Student therapists' experiences of learning and delivering relationally focused telemental health. *Journal of Marital and Family Therapy*, *46*(2), 201–217. https://doi.org/10.1111/jmft.12431

Taylor, N. C., Springer, P. R., Bischoff, N. C., & Smith, J. (2021). Experiential family therapy interventions delivered via telemental health: A qualitative implementation study. *Journal of Marital and Family Therapy*, *47*(2), 455–472. https://doi.org/10.1111/jmft.12520

CHAPTER 3

CONFIDENTIALITY IN SYSTEMIC TELETHERAPY

Eric L. Ström and Rebecca A. Cobb

Just as with in-person services, confidentiality is a critical aspect of providing safe and effective teletherapy services. While all rules of confidentiality that apply to conventional practice settings apply to teletherapy service (American Association for Marriage and Family Therapy, 2015; American Counseling Association, 2014; American Mental Health Counselors Association, 2020), there are some important additional considerations regarding confidentiality in teletherapy practice. These special considerations include the teletherapy platform, use of any external websites or applications during therapy, privacy on devices used by clients to access teletherapy services, the therapist's physical environment, and the client's physical environment. It's also important to consider any specific state laws, regulations, or requirements with regard to confidentiality in teletherapy.

HIPAA-Consistent Platform

All services must be provided via a platform that is consistent with HIPAA standards. Some videoconferencing services have HIPAA-consistent and non–HIPAA-consistent versions of the platform. Ensure that the version of the platform that you are using is consistent with HIPAA standards. This means that at a minimum, the platform must issue a HIPAA business associate agreement to the therapist.

Use of External Websites and Applications

Some creative therapeutic interventions may require access to websites and applications that may not be HIPAA consistent (e.g., see Chapter 14 on virtual puppet play therapy and Chapter 15 on chess and teletherapy). When this occurs, explain to clients the difference between the HIPAA-consistent therapy platform and use of any other websites or applications that may be accessed during therapy. If non–HIPAA-consistent chat functions are available through the website or application being used, instruct clients to dialogue with their therapist in a way that is HIPAA compliant. You may use only HIPAA-consistent technologies for client communications and must use them in a HIPAA-compliant way. Explicitly share information with clients regarding confidentiality and any identified risks to confidentiality so that clients can make informed decisions regarding their interactions within these interventions.

DOI: 10.4324/9781003289920-4

Privacy on Client Devices

Additionally, therapists should have sufficient technical understanding to help clients assess whether their device and online environment are sufficiently secure and private. For example, if you know that a client is joining teletherapy from work, you could discuss how data relating to teletherapy that is stored on the client's work computer might be vulnerable to being accessed by the client's employer. When intimate partner violence or other forms of abuse appear likely, discuss any potential access that others may have to their device to assess for the potential of cyberstalking without further endangering the client (see Chapter 29 on assessing the appropriateness of teletherapy for intimate partner violence).

Therapist's Physical Environment

For the most part, confidentiality in the therapist's physical environment should be similar to that of in-person services. However, clinicians working from home offices should consider taking additional measures to support confidentiality if other people are physically present in their home environment. Consider the following:

- Lock office door(s) while in session.

- Effectively soundproof the space being used to deliver teletherapy.

- Use a headset so only your side of the conversation may be heard in your physical location.

- Use noise machines or take other additional steps as necessary to prevent your side of the conversation from being heard.

You may also consider scanning the room with your camera to provide clients with a visual of your physical location to ease any concerns that clients may have over confidentiality via teletherapy.

If special circumstances necessitate supervisors or other healthcare providers being present in your physical location (e.g., see Chapter 35 on medical family teletherapy), explicitly disclose this information to clients prior to beginning teletherapy, especially if the other third party is not visible on screen. This allows clients to have full informed consent to the treatment circumstances.

Client Physical Environments

A key fundamental consideration that may be unique to the teletherapy setting is that therapists are only able to manage half of the physical space in which therapy occurs. The client's physical environment is generally outside of the therapist's control. This means that the therapist needs to explicitly assist clients in assessing who might be able to see or overhear clients from their location during the session.

To assist clients in setting up their physical environment in a way that supports their confidentiality, you may offer the following suggestions:

- Identify a space to engage in teletherapy sessions where privacy may be maximized.

- Close and, as appropriate, lock door(s) to the room(s) where you will be during session.

- Use a headset so only your side of the conversation may be heard in your physical location. This may only work if clients attend the session individually (e.g., would not work with a family therapy session with multiple members present in the same room).

- Use noise machines to prevent others from overhearing your side of the conversation. If a noise machine isn't available, an application can be downloaded on your phone or tablet that can be used to make white or brown noise. This device can then be placed on the inside of your door at the start of the session.

To assess for confidentiality in the client's physical location, therapists should begin sessions by asking:

- Where are you joining therapy from today?
- Is there anyone else there with you?
- Do you think anyone else might be able to overhear our conversation?

At times, you might consider having members of the client system join a session from separate physical locations. This may be particularly important to assure each member of the client system that their discussions will remain private. When confidentiality cannot be maintained by one or more member of the client system, discuss with all members of the client system their comfort in moving forward with the therapy session and which topics they are comfortable discussing given the identified limitations to confidentiality. Provide each member of the client system with the option of postponing the session until additional confidentiality precautions can be implemented.

Not all clients have the resources or privilege to make use of a private space to access teletherapy. When the presence of others cannot be avoided, help clients assess whether teletherapy is appropriate and if it will be clinically effective given the circumstances. Empower clients to take the lead in determining which topics they are or are not comfortable addressing while others may be present or able to overhear the session. When others are able to overhear a session, use caution in initiating discussion of topics addressed in previous sessions that may be more sensitive. Also consider alternative or adjunct forms of communication that may add an additional level of confidentiality. For example, the client may choose to type more sensitive information into the teletherapy platform chat function rather than discuss that information out loud.

Ethics Codes Provisions

American Association for Marriage and Family Therapy, 2015, 6.3

American Counseling Association, 2014, H.2.b, H.2.d

American Mental Health Counselors Association, 2020, I.A.2.n

References

American Association for Marriage and Family Therapy. (2015). *2015 AAMFT code of ethics*. www.www.aamft.org/Legal_Ethics/Code_of_Ethics.aspx

American Counseling Association. (2014). *2014 ACA code of ethics*. www.counseling.org/docs/default-source/default-document-library/2014-code-of-ethics-finaladdress.pdf

American Mental Health Counselors Association. (2020). *2020 AMHCA code of ethics*. www.amhca.org/HigherLogic/System/DownloadDocumentFile.ashx?DocumentFileKey=24a27502-196e-b763-ff57-490a12f7edb1

CHAPTER 4

BUILDING THERAPEUTIC RELATIONSHIPS VIA TELETHERAPY

Lisa Rene Reynolds, Paul R. Springer, Nathan C. Taylor, Richard J. Bischoff, and Rebecca A. Cobb

Positive therapeutic relationships are paramount for successful outcomes in therapy (DeAngelis, 2019). Research on the effectiveness of telemental health shows that this modality can lead to a therapeutic alliance that's comparable with that of in-person treatment (Richardson et al., 2009). However, components of building therapeutic alliance that may come easily for in-person therapy may be more challenging in a remote format. Developing a strong therapeutic relationship takes more time and intentionality on the part of the therapist when using technology to deliver treatment (Springer et al., 2020). It is incumbent on therapists to employ a myriad of intentional efforts to effectively manage and maintain online therapeutic relationships. The following offers suggestions for building therapeutic relationships via teletherapy by maintaining "eye contact," making the covert overt, slowing down, and using physical environments to enhance connection.

Maintaining "Eye Contact"

Eye contact and leaning one's body forward are linked to clients' perceptions of therapist empathy and therapeutic alliance (Dowel & Berman, 2012). Likewise, intentional "high eye contact" (i.e., intending to make eye contact most of the time) is associated with higher ratings of perceived empathy in teletherapy sessions (Grondin et al., 2022). Although direct eye-to-eye contact is impossible in virtual settings, both clients and therapists can experience what feels like eye contact if things are set up correctly.

To attend to client nonverbal behaviors, it is critical to keep focused on the client's video. This allows for continued client observation, which offers opportunities for making connection by commenting on key facial expressions, body movements, or other things that might be observed via video. This also allows therapists to experience their own felt connection with clients more fully.

Unfortunately, the therapist's camera isn't necessarily located in the same place as the client's image on the screen. Unless the two are aligned, it may appear on the client's end that the therapist is looking away from them, which may ultimately lead to a feeling of disconnection with the therapist. To avoid this from happening, the therapist can center the client's video under the camera. This allows for continued visual contact on the client's image while keeping eyes centered near the camera, therefore allowing for the client's felt experience of eye contact while maintaining client observation.

DOI: 10.4324/9781003289920-5

Likewise, avoid attempts to multitask during session unless the task is directly involved in the immediate implementation of a therapeutic intervention. Even if the therapist maintains mental focus on both clients and the task at hand, multitasking inevitably results in lost focus as well as eye movements that signal to clients that they are not fully being attended to.

Making the Covert Overt

Make the covert more overt by discussing the difficulty in connecting in sessions. For example, in response to a client who is crying in a remote session, the therapist might say, "Times like these are when teletherapy isn't ideal. If you were in my office, I would be able to hand you a box of tissues or offer you a safe and supportive space away from your home to process this. I'm sorry I can't do those things, but is there something you need right now that we could figure out how to get for you?" You can also use the following techniques to make the covert more overt:

- *Nod to signal appreciation, agreement, or otherwise provide affirmation to clients.* Note that in some cultures (e.g., Bulgaria, Cyprus, Greece, Iran, Turkey), a nod of the head up and down may indicate "no," or the meaning between nodding and shaking one's head may be switched. Be attuned to clients' cultural backgrounds, and have open discussions about the meaning of nonverbal communication such as head nodding.

- *Pay attention to parts of the body that could send nonverbal and affirming messages to clients that can be seen on camera.* For example, you might clasp your hands together under your chin in a hopeful gesture when a client expresses optimism about an effort, a change, or a potentially favorable outcome. Likewise, you could briefly cover your face with your hands when responding to clients' disclosure of something meant to shock or "wow" them.

- *Mirror body language and expression.* Although teletherapy affords less exposure of body parts, the concept of mimesis in systemic therapy suggests the importance of imitating the style and mannerisms of clients in ways such as verbal pacing, joking, or matching expressions of family members.

- *Consider your distance from the camera.* Sitting farther back from the camera allows therapists to lean in and move closer to make connective gestures with clients. For example, a therapist bending the trunk of their body forward is linked to higher client perceptions of a strong alliance (Dowel & Berman, 2012).

- *Practice verbal transparency, monitor tone of voice, and exaggerate facial expressions and body movements.* See Chapter 5 for more details on how to overcome lack of visual and auditory cues using these methods.

Slowing Down

Teletherapists need to intentionally take time to build the client–therapist relationship and slow down the therapeutic process (Springer et al., 2020). This helps clients feel that their therapist is genuinely interested in them and cares about their success in treatment. The following suggestions can help with this:

- *Spend more time in the initial stages of therapy.* Get to know clients and their experience of presenting problems.

- *Reserve a minute or two at the beginning of each session for casual chitchat.* The rituals of entering and exiting a physical office do not occur in online sessions (Burgoyne, 2020). This typically leads to a quick start and blunt ending to online sessions, which can result in a less relaxed meeting time. By making a regular practice of casually talking with clients at the start of each session, an organic personal connection is fostered, much like what would normally occur as therapists and clients meet in an in-person waiting room.

- *Take time to talk about the client's experience of the virtual environment.* Having a conversation about how clients are feeling about the treatment modality normalizes anxiety and helps clients trust the therapist as well as the online therapeutic process.

- *Avoid rushing into problem solving.* Since therapists may lack nonverbal cues in teletherapy sessions that might support a solid understanding of what clients are sharing, take special care to ensure that you fully understand client problems and their goal(s) prior to intervention and problem solving.

Using Physical Environments to Enhance Connection

The following suggestions may help in using the clients' physical environment to enhance connectivity and alliance in the therapeutic relationship:

- *Invite clients to make themselves comfortable.* Teletherapy clients often attend sessions from their own chosen environment, so therapists may not think to consider inviting clients to make themselves comfortable. However, clients themselves may not consider this, especially if therapy is uncomfortable for them. You may encourage clients to create a space from which it feels good for them to attend teletherapy sessions, find a comfy space on the couch instead of sitting upright in an office chair, or go grab a cup of water or hot tea.

- *Invite clients to share things of significance from their physical environment.* Allow clients to give you a tour of their home or to show you things that are important to them within their physical environment (e.g., animals, toys). Alternatively, if clients join therapy from a space other than their home, you may invite clients to share their screen to show photos documenting topics of discussion like their favorite pet or a recent family outing.

- *Share things from your own physical environment with clients.* Likewise, therapists might share with clients appropriate things within their own physical environment (e.g., animals, books, toys). This may help clients to picture the therapist more fully within their current setting and to connect with them in ways that are more typical for in-person therapy sessions.

- *Comment on the client's change of setting if they appear to be attending therapy from a new location.* This serves as a casual opening to the session that best mimics in-person sessions. There may also be helpful information gleaned from the backstory of this change. For example, you might casually say, "Oh, is this your kitchen?" to a client who usually attends therapy from their home office. They may share that their partner is out of town for the week and begin discussing increased anxiety that occurs when their partner is away.

- *Comment on other things that you might see in the client's physical environment.* You may compliment clients on a new haircut or a new pair of glasses. You might also reference something that you see in the client's background, such as a painting on the wall, and ask them to share what it is, how they got it, or the significance that it has to them.

This chapter aims to offer ideas for remote therapists' consideration, with the enthusiastic suggestion that they adjust to the needs of each unique client, situation, and personality.

References

Burgoyne, N. (2020). Lessons from the transition to relational teletherapy during COVID-19. *Family Process, 59*(3), 974–988.

DeAngelis, T. (2019). Better relationships with patients leads to better outcomes. *American Psychological Association, 50*(10), 38–43.

Dowel, N. M., & Berman, J. S. (2012). Therapist nonverbal behavior and perceptions of empathy, alliance, and treatment credibility. *Journal of Psychotherapy Integration, 23*(2), 158–165.

Grondin, F., Lomanowska, A. M., Poire, V., & Jackson, P. L. (2022). Clients in simulated teletherapy via videoconference compensate for altered eye contact when evaluating therapist empathy. *Journal of Clinical Medicine, 11*(12), 3461. https://doi.org/10.3390/jcm11123461

Richardson, L. K., Frueh, B. C., Grubaugh, A., L., Egede, L. E., & Elhai, J. D. (2009). Current directions in video conferencing tele-mental health research. *Clinical Psychology, 16*(3), 323–338. https://doi.org/10.1111/j.1468-2850.2009.01170.x

Springer, P. R., Bischoff, R. J., Taylor, N. C., Kohel, K., & Farero, A. (2020). Collaborative care at a distance: Student therapists' experiences of learning and delivering relationally focused telemental health. *Journal of Marital and Family Therapy, 46*(2), 201–217. https://doi.org/10.1111/jmft.12431

CHAPTER 5

OVERCOMING LACK OF VISUAL AND AUDITORY CUES IN ONLINE SESSIONS

Paul R. Springer, Nathan C. Taylor, and Richard J. Bischoff

One of the most significant challenges therapists encounter when providing service via videoconferencing is adjusting to the limited scope of visual and auditory cues. With videoconferencing platforms, it is not uncommon for therapists to miss the nuances of nonverbal communication such as vocal intonations, facial expressions, and other body-language cues that are more easily seen in in-person sessions. These signals can be critical in providing a clear picture of the client's state of being. Missing these visual and auditory cues may result in greater potential for miscommunication that could negatively impact the therapeutic relationship and therapeutic outcomes. Similarly, clients may also miss the therapist's visual and auditory cues that are crucial to therapeutic communication. To overcome these challenges: (1) help clients set up an ideal environment from which to attend therapy, (2) frequently use client names, (3) practice verbal transparency, (4) monitor tone of voice, and (5) exaggerate facial expressions and body movements.

Client Environment

The physical locations from which clients attend teletherapy are often set up in ways that prevent therapists from seeing and hearing things that are important in the therapeutic process. To set up the best possible environments, share with clients how to organize their equipment and space (Hertlein et al., 2021; Springer et al., 2020) by offering the following suggestions:

- Position cameras and seating so each person's face and body can be seen on screen.

- If everyone cannot be clearly seen on one screen at once, and if another device is available, have some people join session from a second device in the same room.

- If clients use multiple devices in the same room, request that they mute all but one device to avoid audio distortions and provide guidance on how to position devices so you can see everyone in relation to one another.

- Create optimal lighting conditions by opening blinds or curtains, turning on lights, and not sitting directly in front of light sources.

For more information on setting up ideal teletherapy environments, see Chapter 2.

DOI: 10.4324/9781003289920-6

Frequently Using Clients' Names

Frequently using clients' names can help to make up for reduced visual and auditory cues and is particularly impactful in teletherapy. Use of client names clearly indicates who the therapist is speaking to, captures the attention of clients, emphasizes important points, and slows down the therapeutic process (Taylor et al., 2021).

When simultaneously working with multiple members of the same system in in-person therapy, the therapist can look at one person in the room and speak to them directly, with everyone generally knowing who they're speaking to. With online therapy, it's less clear who the therapist is looking at on their computer screen. When speaking to one person in particular via teletherapy, say the person's name to clearly indicate who you are talking to.

Likewise, you may effectively use names in session to help capture attention and reengage clients as needed. Research has shown that certain parts of the brain light up when people hear their own name (Carmody & Lewis, 2006). Because people respond so strongly to hearing their name, they tend to listen more closely to your thoughts and ideas when you use it. Hearing one's own name also causes their brain to react as if they're engaging in behaviors and thought patterns that are part of their core identity (Carmody & Lewis, 2006). This may be particularly important in online therapy because visual and auditory cues from the therapist are more limited, and clients may be more likely to be distracted by things in their environment or tempted to multitask on the computer. For example, when a client is struggling to engage in a change behavior, the therapist may interrupt this negative cycle by using the client's name, leaning closer to the camera, and then encouraging the client to visualize themself engaging in this change behavior.

Beyond this, the use of client names highlights things that you may want to emphasize, such as key moments of empathetic reflection, validation, or things that are important for clients to understand. You may use a client's name, followed by a brief pause, to further emphasize important points. This technique also offers a way to slow down the therapeutic process, especially when clients are emotional or agitated in session.

Verbal Transparency

One primary adaptation that therapists can make in addressing lack of visual and auditory cues is verbal transparency (Taylor et al., 2021). Verbal transparency is the skill of intentionally identifying and describing what would normally be communicated nonverbally. This can be applied to both client- and therapist-initiated communication.

To encourage client verbal transparency, ask them to describe why they looked away, sighed, or performed any other form of nonverbal communication that you may have noticed. You might also ask clients to describe nonverbal auditory cues, such as changes in tone of voice or the volume with which they speak to you, partners, or family members. The goal is to have clients verbally describe why they are acting certain ways. With further prompting, you may ask clients specifically to address any feelings that are associated with their nonverbal communication. This makes covert actions clearer and allows clients to more easily tie these actions back to their emotional experience. For example, asking a client to describe why they looked away helps you make the connection that this was due to feeling uncomfortable rather than being distracted by something outside of your frame of view.

Verbal transparency can also include what you can't see. For example, you can ask clients to describe what they are seeing or hearing as well as their overall experience of their physical environment.

Likewise, therapists should be more verbally transparent in their own feelings and actions. For example, a therapist might highlight the challenge they are experiencing with connecting with their client because the client is constantly moving outside of their field of vision. The goal is to create a dialogue around the overt or covert behaviors so one can get to the underlying meaning associated with the behaviors.

Client engagement increases when therapists talk about nonverbal behaviors, both their own and that of their clients. Client engagement in online interventions is also positively associated with the degree to which therapists intentionally explain why they want clients to do certain things and their intended outcome(s). Explain your intentions for the use of verbal transparency in online sessions. Doing this also models behavior that many clients will then emulate, further improving the therapeutic conversation.

Monitoring Tone of Voice

When using telemental health, therapists also need to be aware of how they balance their tone of voice to improve communication of emotion (e.g., portray empathy when clients are upset). The challenge with effectively using one's tone of voice via teletherapy is that technology (i.e., microphones) may have difficulty picking up sounds and nuances of speech. To overcome this barrier, speak louder or at a slower, more even pace. Alternatively, manipulate tone of voice for a more dramatic effect when attempting to show empathy or make what you're saying better understood. For example, a therapist may speak more softly when they highlight attachment-based injuries and more loudly when they need to intervene in a family's argument.

Exaggerating Facial Expressions and Body Movements

Therapists who do telemental health well also tend to exaggerate their facial expressions and body movements to increase the likelihood that nonverbal behaviors will be noticed by clients (Taylor et al., 2021). For example, you may exaggerate hand expressions to emphasize a point, such as pointing at the screen. You may also move more closely to the camera to exaggerate a stern look when setting boundaries around appropriate behavior in session. These techniques are important because the limited size of the video screen, quality of the image, and distance to the camera can make it otherwise difficult for clients to see what therapists are doing. Exaggerating facial expressions and body movements can also benefit effective communication and the therapeutic alliance. At times, it may also serve as a therapeutic intervention. For example, when partners or families are arguing, you may lean in closer to the camera, black out the screen, or play music at the start of an argument to intervene and shut down unwanted behaviors or destructive cycles of interaction. Hand or facial expressions can also be exaggerated to communicate the importance of a statement or to challenge a client's verbal behavior. The goal of these techniques is to increase your presence and influence in therapy when you are not physically in the room so you can intervene in productive ways.

Make modifications to each of the aforementioned techniques for overcoming lack of visual and auditory cues based on the needs of each client and any relational or cultural factors that may need to be considered. For example, you could limit the number of people who participate in a therapy session if it becomes visually too difficult to see and follow too many people in session at the same time. To address language barriers, have software that provides closed captioning to help family members follow the conversations better.

References

Carmody, D. P., & Lewis, M. (2006). Brain activation when hearing one's own and others' names. *Brain Research*, *1116*(1), 153–158.

Hertlein, K. M., Drude, K. P., Hilty, D. M., & Maheu, M. M. (2021). Toward proficiency in telebehavioral health: Applying interprofessional competencies in couple and family therapy. *Journal of Martial and Family Therapy*, *47*(2), 359–374. https://doi.org/10.1111/jmft.12496

Springer, P. R., Bischoff, R. J., Taylor, N. C., Kohel, K., & Farero, A. (2020). Collaborative care at a distance: Student therapists' experiences of learning and delivering relationally focused telemental health. *Journal of Marital and Family Therapy*, *46*(2), 201–217. https://doi.org/10.1111/jmft.12431

Taylor, N. C., Springer, P. R., Bischoff, N. C., & Smith, J. (2021). Experiential family therapy interventions delivered via telemental health: A qualitative implementation study. *Journal of Marital and Family Therapy*, *47*(2), 455–472. https://doi.org/10.1111/jmft.12520

CHAPTER 6

USING BACKGROUND IMAGES TO SIGNAL MESSAGES VIA TELETHERAPY

Amanda Veldorale-Griffin

Visual cues provided by a therapist's physical or virtual background in teletherapy offer a unique opportunity to enhance client comfort and facilitate strong therapeutic relationships. This can be especially impactful for clients from minoritized populations who have more barriers to care and may enter therapy unsure if their therapist will understand and accept them.

A strong therapeutic alliance is the foundation upon which the therapeutic process is built. The therapist's ability to develop that relationship is a major component in creating successful therapeutic outcomes (Del Re et al., 2012). There are many ways that therapists foster a sense of comfort in session, including the language they use and the ways in which they structure the therapy space. In physical spaces, this includes the way the therapy room is set up, books, toys, and any art that might be on display. In digital spaces, this can include the platform used, digital content offered to clients, and background images displayed by the therapist (Yamamoto et al., 2021). Visual cues presented in teletherapy practice can nonverbally communicate messages regarding the therapist's interests and ultimately foster a sense of comfort to clients if done strategically. The following steps can be taken to achieve this goal:

1. Determine what message(s) you want to cultivate within your teletherapy space.

2. Decide whether you will present a digital background or the actual physical space behind you.

3. Display in that space images that communicate your intended message(s).

4. Process with clients their experience of your teletherapy space.

Determining the Message(s)

Consider what message(s) you want to share with clients through images seen in your teletherapy practice. Therapists in specialized practices may want to show images that are particularly relevant to their clientele. For example, therapists who work primarily with particular populations may want to display images that communicate acceptance and inclusion of those communities. Likewise, therapists who specialize in working with children may want to communicate that their therapy practice is a place for young people and offers a sense of playfulness.

DOI: 10.4324/9781003289920-7

In addition, some therapists may intentionally use objects and other images to communicate things that are more personal about them. Sharing things that tell clients a bit about the therapist, such as a picture of a favorite animal or cartoon character, can also be a way to help build rapport and set clients at ease.

Determining the Space

Once you have decided what message(s) you want to communicate using images in your space, decide whether you will use a digital background or display the actual physical space that is behind you during sessions. Consider the following when making this decision:

- Do you have physical objects available to you that could communicate your intended message(s)?

- Do you have the physical space available to display those objects behind you during sessions (e.g., a large bookcase for objects or wall space for artwork)?

Another factor to consider, especially for therapists who work with a wide range of clientele, is that digital images can easily be changed between sessions for each client. For example, a therapist working with children could display a virtual background pertaining to a child's favorite television show in one session and quickly change their virtual background to an image pertaining to another child's favorite video game in the next.

Displaying Images

Images can be powerful in conveying messages quickly and without having to rely on verbal sharing. Images can be shared as part of both physical and digital spaces.

If you choose to show the physical space you are in, test your video to determine what will be seen on the client's screen. Then, set up items behind you in the camera's field of view that provide desired cues. For example, therapists may curate a bookshelf behind them with texts representing diverse topics addressed in their practice such as antiracism, anxiety, LGBTQ+ issues, neurodiversity, or books by authors from minoritized populations. When setting up an LGBTQ+ affirmative space, therapists might include a Pride flag on the wall, artwork that displays gender diversity, and relevant books on shelves behind them.

Digital Images

If using a digital background, get acquainted with the virtual background options available through your HIPAA-consistent video platform. There are also many background images that can be found online and used as digital backgrounds. For example, Pride backgrounds are available through the Human Rights Council (Human Rights Council, n.d.), and antiracism backgrounds are available through the University of California's End Racism Initiative (End Racism Initiative, 2020).

Many platforms, however, allow therapists to select or create their own image to use as a background. Creating a personalized background allows for greater intentionality in selecting images that communicate intended messages. Consider including symbols that may be relevant to your populations, such as Black Lives Matter posters, gay Pride flags, autism awareness symbols, or quotes related to diversity, equity, and inclusion.

Many teletherapy platforms also allow therapists and clients to input their names to display on screen. Displaying your pronouns along with your name can signal to clients that they can feel comfortable sharing their pronouns with you.

Furthermore, therapists can encourage clients to create their own virtual background or physical background to display behind them, which can show symbols that are important to them. These could be relevant to their identities or presenting issues or other things that they value in their lives.

Processing

Once visual cues have been integrated into teletherapy sessions, offer clients the opportunity to discuss the space created and to provide feedback. Examples of processing questions include the following:

- How is this virtual platform working for you?

- What helps you feel comfortable in this space?

- Are there things you would like me to add or take away?

- What other visual reminders would be helpful for you during sessions?

- Are there other images you'd like to see in future sessions?

- How do you think [other member(s) of the client's system] might respond to the visuals we've created?

Responses provided to these questions can then be used to inform adjustments to background images as needed. These questions may be revisited as images, clients, and therapists evolve and change over time.

Contraindications

Some clients may be in a situation in which their safety could be compromised if the therapist is seen as promoting a particular value. For instance, in states where gender-affirmative care for minors is not accepted or with families who are particularly rejecting, the presence of a Pride flag or other materials showing support for LGBTQ+ communities could increase risk if clients attend therapy from a location where others might enter their physical space during session and potentially see the therapist and their background on screen. In such cases, it is recommended that you engage in more subtle signals, such as introducing themselves using their pronouns or simply including books on gender identity and sexual orientation in the background, without the inclusion of more overt symbols like the Pride flag.

References

Del Re, A. C., Fluckiger, C., Horvath, A. O., Symonds, D., & Wampold, B. E. (2012). Therapist effects in the therapeutic alliance-outcome relationship: A restricted-maximum likelihood meta-analysis. *Clinical Psychology Review, 32*(7), 642–649. https://doi.org/10.1016/j.cpr.2012.07.002

End Racism Initiative. (2020, November 19). *New Zoom virtual backgrounds.* https://sites.uci.edu/endracism/2020/11/19/new-zoom-virtual-backgrounds/#

Human Rights Council. (n.d.). *Zoom with pride using our digital backgrounds.* www.hrc.org/resources/zoom-with-pride-using-our-digital-backgrounds

Yamamoto, F. R., Voida, A., & Voida, S. (2021). From therapy to teletherapy: Relocating mental health services online. *Proceedings of the ACM on Human-Computer Interaction, 5*(CSW2), Article 364.

Part 2
Self of the Therapist

CHAPTER 7

MANAGING DISTRACTIONS AND REMAINING PRESENT

SUGGESTIONS FOR ONLINE THERAPISTS

Jessie Everts

Magda is a telehealth therapist working from home. As she sits down at her desk with a cup of tea, she realizes that her neighbors are doing construction work. Not only is the noise audible, but it's causing Magda's dog to bark incessantly. Magda gets a text from her child's daycare provider, saying that daycare will be closing early due to a staffing shortage. Before Magda can make plans for an early pickup, she gets a notification that her clients are in the virtual waiting room. Magda rushes to log onto her computer and knocks over her tea, spilling everywhere.

The benefits of teletherapy are many. However, maintaining focus can be challenging for therapists and clients. While some distractions are unavoidable, therapist engagement and attunement are critical in creating secure therapeutic relationships (DeAngelis, 2019; Hilty et al., 2020). The following suggestions will help you set up an environment for teletherapy that minimizes distractions and maximizes your ability to focus. Suggestions focus on minimizing external noise, setting up a distraction-free environment, allowing time to process after each session, taking care of your own personal needs, and addressing unavoidable distractions as needed.

Minimizing External Noise

To avoid auditory distractions, think about how you can minimize concerns related to external noise in your physical environment.

- If working from home, discuss with everyone in the household ways to reduce noise during working hours.

- Leave a sign on your door indicating when you are in session as a reminder to keep noise at a minimum.

- Close and lock your office door(s).

- Place a white noise machine just inside your office door(s).

- Wear noise-canceling headphones.

- If there is unavoidable noise or sensory input, prepare yourself to ignore it as much as possible. Acknowledge it to yourself and clients (if necessary) and bring attention to your clients.

DOI: 10.4324/9781003289920-9

Setting Up a Distraction-Free Environment

Prepare yourself before sessions. Set yourself up to be distraction free and avoid multitasking during sessions.

- Put your phone on silent or "do not disturb." If you are tempted to look at your phone during sessions, place it out of reach.

- Close computer windows and applications that aren't necessary for the activities that you plan to perform during the current session.

- Turn off automatic notifications that might pop up on your computer (e.g., incoming email).

- Have a writing utensil and notepad nearby to document during sessions any follow-ups you might need to do.

- Set aside a few minutes before each session to center yourself. You might set an intention for your work, set aside concerns about other clients, or review files in preparation for your next session.

Allowing Time to Process After Each Session

Allow processing time after sessions. Take a few moments to bring personal closure to each session before starting the next.

- You may not have time to complete your case note, but write down critical information that you might be worried about remembering so you don't need to hold mental space for it during your next session.

- Take a few deep breaths or stretch to release physical tension created from challenging or emotional sessions.

- Take a moment to honor the work that you and your client(s) just did.

Taking Care of Personal Needs

Consider how you take care of your needs so that you are in your best frame of mind.

- Optimize your sleep.

- Make time for breaks throughout the workday.

- Consider the timing of eating, physical movement, using the restroom, or taking medications. It's difficult to focus with a growling stomach or a full bladder! Build time into your schedule to attend to physical needs.

- Participate in continual self-care and other self-of-the-therapist work (see Chapters 9 and 11). Self-awareness and attunement allow you to bring your best self to the therapeutic relationship (Aponte, 2022).

Addressing Unavoidable Distractions

Some distractions are unavoidable. Even with the best plans, you can't guarantee that you will be completely distraction free.

- When your attention has wandered from where you want it, gently bring it back to the task at hand (Hasenkamp et al., 2011). You might notice that your mind has drifted from what your client is saying to a sound in the background or a spider on the wall. When you recognize that you have become distracted, bring your mind gently back to your client(s) and focus on what is being said. If you miss something, ask them to repeat it. Doing this without self-judgment models mindful attention for your client as well.

- If you get an urgent message or something alarming happens in your environment or your client's environment, acknowledge the distraction, take care of it if needed, and then move on. Talking this through with clients builds trust and recognizes natural human responses.

- If distractions become too difficult to overcome, consider responsibly bringing the session to a close by saying, "I'm sorry; I don't think we can continue today. Can we reschedule so we can both focus on this important work together?"

Facing a multitude of distractions, Magda might first need a moment to collect herself and decide how to proceed. She takes a deep breath and lets her clients know she will be a moment late. She cleans the spilled tea and sends a message to see if someone can pick her child up from daycare early. She moves her dog to a room away from her office to minimize distraction from its barking. Then, she logs in with her clients. She apologizes for the delay, acknowledges that there is some construction noise, and says, "Let's do our best to ignore it and keep our attention on what we need to talk about today. If the noise is too distracting, please let me know, and we can reschedule for another time."

References

Aponte, H. J. (2022). The soul of therapy: The therapist's use of self in the therapeutic relationship. *Contemporary Family Therapy, 44*(2), 136–143. https://doi.org/10.1007/s10591-021-09614-5

DeAngelis, T. (2019). Better relationships with patients lead to better outcomes. *Monitor on Psychology, 50*(10), 38–43.

Hasenkamp, W., Wilson-Mendenhall, C. D., Duncan, E., & Barsalou, L. W. (2011). Mind wandering and attention during focused meditation: A fine-grained temporal analysis of fluctuating cognitive states. *NeuroImage, 59*(1), 750–760. https://doi.org/10.1016/j.neuroimage.2011.07.008

Hilty, D. M., Randhawa, K., Maheu, M. M., McKean, A. J. S., Pantera, R., Mishkind, M. C., & Rizzo, A. (2020). A review of telepresence, virtual reality, and augmented reality applied to clinical care. *Journal of Technology in Behavioral Sciences, 5*(2), 178–205. https://doi.org/10.1007/s41347-020-00126-x

CHAPTER 8

THE "COMMUTE HOME"

END-OF-DAY LETTING-GO RITUALS FOR ONLINE THERAPISTS

Deborah Koons-Beauchamp

Some people identify their end-of-day commute home from work as an opportunity to process emotions and to avoid "taking work home" with them (Jain & Lyons, 2008). For therapists providing teletherapy services from a home office, the traditional commute home is not an option. And yet the physical, mental, and emotional stressors unique to performing teletherapy make self-care even more important.

End-of-day rituals performed in lieu of a commute home can provide an important transition from work to personal life. It's easy to skip this transition period when the realities of life are standing outside your home-office door, demanding full attention. But before walking out of the home office, therapists might consider practicing a ritual that allows them to be more fully present the remainder of the day.

Rituals can be any intentional practice performed systematically and decisively in a repeatable pattern, helping the action become second nature (Tharp & Reiter, 2003). The secret to a useful ritual is that it means something. An end-of-the-day ritual signifies a transition from one mindset to another. End-of-the-day rituals might also signify a process of letting go of the day's challenges and any accompanying worries or other challenging emotions. They can be practiced in lieu of a traditional commute home from the office. Therapists working from out-of-home offices might also practice an end-of-day ritual before leaving the office if their commute home doesn't provide the time, space, or conditions needed to transition from work to personal life. Intentional end-of-day rituals can be a form of self-care that helps to increase resiliency and prevent burnout, ultimately allowing therapists to offer their therapeutic best (Eppler, 2021).

The following offers instructions on how to create a personalized end-of-day ritual. Example rituals that have been implemented by teletherapists are also provided.

Creating an End-of-Day Ritual

Creating an end-of-day ritual can be performed in two steps:

1. Select a ritual that has meaning, is personally motivating, is simple to perform, and can easily be repeated at the end of each workday. This ritual may involve just one activity or action, or it may consist of more than one activity or action.

2. Mindfully and intentionally perform the ritual.

DOI: 10.4324/9781003289920-10

End-of-Day Rituals for Teletherapists

Anecdotal data collected from teletherapists offers example end-of-day rituals that can be categorized into four themes: reflection and gratitude, moving the body, personal maintenance, and closure.

Reflection and Gratitude

Reflection and gratitude rituals are meant to create space to reflect on the day and provide opportunities for self-compassion, self-improvement, and professional growth. Example rituals include the following:

- At the close of each session, share with clients how you honor them and their journey.
- Purposefully reflect on the day, journal, or write at least one item of gratitude.
- Lie down for a few minutes or snuggle on a chair with a blanket, quietly practicing gratitude.
- Perform a guided meditation or breathing exercise.
- Repeat a mantra or affirmation.
- Light a candle to memorialize the work performed and entrance into the next phase of the day.

Moving the Body

Moving-the-body rituals involve the practice of meaningful movement with an intention to release energy and connect the body and mind. Example rituals include the following:

- Perform a few yoga poses or stretches.
- Sit on the porch, lanai, or somewhere outside.
- Take a walk or run, even if it's just around the block.
- Go to the gym.
- Turn on music and dance.
- Change clothes.
- Watch, read, or listen to something that will make you laugh.

Personal Maintenance

Personal-maintenance rituals involve purposefully performing productive tasks that do not have work-related consequences. Personal-maintenance rituals allow time to release the day while creating a positive transition into personal life. Example rituals include the following:

- Organize your work desk.
- Wash your coffee cup or water bottle.
- Create a priority list for the next day.
- Update a grocery list.

- Feed the fish, cat, dog, or any other animal that might need feeding.

- Play a game on your phone, do a crossword puzzle, or play sudoku.

- Call or visit a friend or family member.

Closure

Closure rituals mindfully bring closure to a day of teletherapy and purposefully transition to personal life. An example of a closing ritual may include a series of small rituals performed in sequential order:

- Sign out of programs with confidential client information.

- Turn off the computer.

- Put away your headphones.

- Purposefully place notepads and other loose paper in storage areas.

- Lock file cabinets.

- Set an intention for the remainder of the day.

- Turn off lights in methodical order.

- Walk out of the room, shut the door, and lock it.

The benefit of even small rituals like the ones described here is in creating intentional transition from one environment to the next. It is important to identify a ritual that meets your own unique needs and preferences. When a ritual no longer works for you, simply adjust as needed.

References

Eppler, C. (2021). Systemic teletherapists' meaningful experiences during the first months of the coronavirus pandemic. *Journal of Marital and Family Therapy*, *47*(2), 244–258. https://doi.org/10.1111/jmft.12515

Jain, J., & Lyons, G. (2008). The gift of travel time. *Journal of Transport Geography*, *16*(2), 81–89. https://doi.org/10.1016/j.jtrangeo.2007.05.001

Tharp, T., & Reiter, M. (2003). *The creative habit: Learn it and use it for life*. Simon & Schuster.

CHAPTER 9

TELETHERAPIST SELF-CARE ASSESSMENT

Rebecca A. Cobb and Monique Willis

Due to the intense emotional demands often faced by therapists, self-care is critical. Foundationally, self-care involves establishing consistent routines that aim to reduce the adverse effects of clinical work while supporting optimal functioning crucial for the success of therapy (Barnett & Homany, 2022). Therapists who maintain regular self-care experience improved well-being and quality of life and can better handle personal and professional stressors. Consequences of not practicing self-care may include burnout, secondary traumatic stress, vicarious trauma, and compassion fatigue. Moreover, poor self-care may ultimately lead to diminished quality of care for clients (Delgadillo et al., 2018; Yang & Hayes, 2020).

In addition to job stressors typically faced by therapists, online therapists face a unique set of challenges. For example, teletherapists may be more likely to remain stationary in front of a computer screen for extended periods of time, which can have negative physical consequences. In addition, they may be more likely to encounter frustrating technical difficulties that can increase stress (Lin et al., 2022), especially if technology is not an area of expertise. Therapists who work primarily from home may face challenges in finding a dedicated space for therapy, potentially blurring the boundaries between home life and work (Steidtmann et al., 2021). Teletherapists who work remotely may also experience limited face-to-face personal exchanges throughout the workday (Steidtmann et al., 2021), hindering discussions with colleagues who deeply understand the profession and who might otherwise be available to provide consultation between therapy sessions at an in-person workplace setting. The lack of in-person contact may ultimately lead to feelings of isolation. Due to these circumstances, teletherapists may need to develop unique self-care strategies.

The following assessment is designed to help teletherapists evaluate their current self-care practices. It is not a comprehensive assessment but focuses on how often you engage in activities related to six dimensions of self-care (i.e., physical, intellectual, emotional, spiritual, relational, professional) specifically associated with practicing online therapy. This assessment may be used as an initial check-in and revisited over time.

Instructions

Circle the number that best represents the frequency with which you do each of the following self-care-related acts. Then, total your score for each dimension of self-care. It is not necessary to tally a total score for all dimensions of self-care. Rather, use the scores provided in each domain to identify dimensions of self-care in which you excel and areas with room for improvement.

DOI: 10.4324/9781003289920-11

0 – I never do this
1 – I rarely do this
2 – I occasionally do this
3 – I frequently do this

Physical				
• I work from an ergonomic workstation, move my body between teletherapy sessions, and/or use a standing desk.	0	1	2	3
• I limit excessive screen time outside of work hours and before going to sleep.	0	1	2	3
• I take a sick day if I'm unwell.	0	1	2	3
Physical Score: _____				
Intellectual				
• I maintain realistic expectations for myself regarding my technological abilities.	0	1	2	3
• I consult with experts as needed when setting up new platforms and devices.	0	1	2	3
• I seek continuing education and/or supervision opportunities related to teletherapy practice.	0	1	2	3
Intellectual Score: _____				
Emotional				
• I do telehealth from a comfortable and enjoyable workspace.	0	1	2	3
• I'm gentle with myself when telehealth tasks involving technology don't go as expected.	0	1	2	3
• I regularly check in with my feelings and recognize the emotional challenges that arise when providing telehealth services.	0	1	2	3
Emotional Score: _____				
Spiritual				
• I start my day with mindfulness and/or engage in mindful moments between teletherapy sessions.	0	1	2	3
• I ground myself in nature, even when I'm working inside on a computer.	0	1	2	3
• I ethically incorporate parts of my faith and/or spirituality into my daily work practice.	0	1	2	3
Spiritual Score: _____				
Relational				
• I regularly connect with friends, family, and colleagues in person.	0	1	2	3
• I attend in-person conferences and networking meetings when available.	0	1	2	3
• I utilize technology to maintain connections with supportive colleagues who may be physically distant.	0	1	2	3
Relational Score: _____				
Professional				
• I have a separate workspace at home and avoid using my rest space for work.	0	1	2	3
• I use separate spaces for different activities or during specific times throughout my day.	0	1	2	3
• I have distinct boundaries between my teletherapy practice and personal time.	0	1	2	3
Professional Score: _____				

Instructions for Follow-Up

After evaluating your current self-care practices, consider the areas you want to improve. Then, come up with a strategic plan. Consider adding a monthly or quarterly check-in to your calendar to complete the self-assessment and strategize ways to improve current practices. For tips and tricks explicitly aimed at online therapists' self-care, see Chapter 11.

References

Barnett, J. E., & Homany, G. (2022). The new self-care: It's not all about you. *Practice Innovations*, *7*(4), 313–326. https://doi.org/10.1037/pri0000190

Delgadillo, J., Saxon, D., & Barkham, M. (2018). Associations between therapists' occupational burnout and their patients' depression and anxiety treatment outcomes. *Depression and Anxiety*, *35*(9), 844–850. https://doi.org/10.1002/da.22766

Lin, L., Stamm, K. E., Ferenz, K., Wright, C. V., Bethune, S., & Conroy, J. (2022). Relationship between challenges with the use of telehealth and psychologists' response during the coronavirus pandemic. *Professional Psychology: Research and Practice*, *53*(6), 596–605. https://doi.org/10.1037/pro0000481

Steidtmann, D., McBride, S., & Mishkind, M. C. (2021). Experiences of mental health clinicians and staff in rapidly converting to full-time telemental health and work from home during the COVID-19 pandemic. *Telemedicine and e-Health*, *27*(7), 785–791. https://doi.org/10.1089/tmj.2020.0305

Yang, Y., & Hayes, J. A. (2020). Causes and consequences of burnout among mental health professionals: A practice-oriented review of recent empirical literature. *Psychotherapy*, *57*(3), 426–436. https://doi.org/10.1037/pst0000317

CHAPTER 10

BURNOUT FOR ONLINE THERAPISTS

Veronica P. Viesca and Parker Leukart

Teletherapy offers therapists the opportunity to work remotely and provide services to clients who might not otherwise have therapy access. This may yield a higher caseload, longer hours, increased emotional demand, or blurred boundaries between work and home. Without careful attention to the management of work stress, teletherapists are at risk of burnout, characterized by emotional exhaustion, depersonalization, and a decreased sense of accomplishment (Nagoski & Nagoski, 2020).

Burnout may lead to mental health concerns (e.g., anxiety, depression), physical concerns (e.g., fatigue), interpersonal consequences (e.g., irritability, isolation), and professional consequences (Awa et al., 2010). Professional consequences may manifest in what dialectical behavioral therapy (DBT) refers to as "therapy interfering behaviors," or anything that hinders one's ability to engage in clinical work. For example, teletherapists may join sessions late, multitask on the computer during sessions, end sessions early, or conduct sessions while sick with a distracting cough or while unable to think clearly enough to practice effectively.

According to the DBT framework, addressing therapy interfering behaviors is critical (Chapman & Rosenthal, 2016) and comes only second to addressing life-threatening behaviors (Rizvi et al., 2013). For their clients' well-being, therapists have an ethical responsibility to assess burnout's influence on their work and address concerns as they arise (Simionato et al., 2019). The following self-assessment questions may be used to evaluate your own levels of burnout as a teletherapist. Suggestions to address these concerns are also offered.

Self-Assessment

Use the following questions to assess burnout's impact on your well-being and ability to provide care via teletherapy services. This is not an exhaustive list of questions to consider. Rather, questions have been adapted from Kulik's (2010) *Volunteer Burnout Questionnaire* and Montero-Marín and García-Campayo's (2010) *Burnout Clinical Subtype Questionnaire* to focus specifically on signs of burnout for therapists providing services via online platforms. You may reflect on these items individually, in peer consultation, or in supervision.

Emotional Exhaustion

- Do basic work tasks feel overwhelming (e.g., difficulty responding to emails in a timely manner)?

- Am I angered or irritated by things that never before bothered me (e.g., a weak internet connection)?

DOI: 10.4324/9781003289920-12

- Do I feel trapped in my job as a teletherapist?

- Do I lack insight into personal scheduling boundaries (e.g., work outside of "work hours" or forget to schedule breaks during the workday)?

- Is my energy low during teletherapy sessions?

- Is my energy low outside of teletherapy sessions?

Depersonalization

- Do I struggle to identify and address personal needs amidst teletherapy work obligations (e.g., not notice when I'm hungry or need to use the restroom)?

- Do I lack inspiration from my work as a teletherapist?

- Is it difficult for me to take in appreciation shown by others for the work that I do as a teletherapist?

Sense of Accomplishment

- Do I feel unaccomplished in my work as a teletherapist?

- Do I overattribute telehealth blunders (e.g., technical glitches) as "proof" of professional failure?

- Do I believe my telehealth interventions are generally unsuccessful?

- Does my teletherapy work feel meaningless or like my career as a teletherapist is going nowhere?

- Do I lack pride in my work as a teletherapist?

- Do I lack passion for my work as a teletherapist?

Therapy Interfering Behavior

- Does lack of adequate transition times lead to inadequate preparation for online sessions (e.g., waking up right before an appointment)?

- Do I procrastinate in planning for online sessions or writing notes?

- Do I log in late to online sessions?

- Do I end online sessions early?

- Do I lack focus on client needs or multitask (e.g., check email) during online sessions?

- Do I fail to adequately apply important attending skills during online sessions (see Chapter 4)?

- Am I unable to effectively manage emotional expression and monitor tone of voice during online sessions (see Chapter 5)?

- Do I experience a decreased sense of professionalism (e.g., conduct teletherapy from a vehicle, frequently reschedule sessions at the last minute)?

- Do I believe that most of my teletherapy sessions are bad or that most of my clients are not improving?

Suggestions for Follow-Up

If you responded yes to two or more questions in one category, consider the extent to which burnout is impacting your ability to provide teletherapy services. Should you find yourself emotionally exhausted, lacking empathy, care, or compassion for self or others, are experiencing a decreased sense of accomplishment in your work as a teletherapist, or you notice therapy interfering behaviors making their way into your practice, take steps towards accessing support. A benefit of telehealth is accessibility to personal therapy, virtual supervision, and peer consultation groups, all of which can reduce burnout (Carney & Jefferson, 2014). However, consider what modality of support (e.g., in person or online) is most helpful for you. When burnout arises for telehealth providers, seeking support online may feel like "more work." In this case, in-person therapy, supervision, or peer consultation may be of greater benefit in mitigating burnout. For an assessment of self-care practices and tips and tricks for self-care specific to online therapists, see Chapters 9 and 11.

References

Awa, W. L., Plaumann, M., & Walter, U. (2010). Burnout prevention: A review of intervention programs. *Patient Education and Counseling, 78*(2), 184–190. https://doi.org/10.1016/j.pec.2009.04.008

Carney, J., & Jefferson, J. (2014). Consultation for mental health counselors: Opportunities and guidelines for private practice. *Journal of Mental Health Counseling, 36*(4), 302–314. https://doi.org/10.17744/mehc.36.4.821133r0414u37v7

Chapman, A. L., & Rosenthal, M. Z. (2016). *Managing therapy-interfering behavior: Strategies from dialectical behavior therapy*. American Psychological Association. https://doi.org/10.1037/14752-000

Kulik, L. (2010). *Volunteer Burnout Questionnaire* [Database record]. APA PsycTests. https://dx.doi.org/10.1037/t31927-000

Montero-Marín, J., & García-Campayo, J. (2010). A newer and broader definition of burnout: Validation of the "burnout clinical subtype questionnaire (BCSQ-36)." *BMC Public Health, 10,* Article 302. https://doi.org/10.1186/1471-2458-10-302

Nagoski, E., & Nagoski, A. (2020). *Burnout: The secret to unlocking the stress cycle*. Ballantine Books.

Rizvi, S. L., Steffel, L. M., & Carson-Wong, A. (2013). An overview of dialectical behavior therapy for professional psychologists. *Professional Psychology: Research and Practice, 44*(2), 73–80. https://doi.org/10.1037/a0029808

Simionato, G., Simpson, S., & Reid, C. (2019). Burnout as an ethical issue in psychotherapy. *Psychotherapy, 56*(4), 470–482. https://doi.org/10.1037/pst0000261

CHAPTER 11

SELF-CARE TIPS AND TRICKS FOR ONLINE THERAPISTS

Monique Willis and Rebecca A. Cobb

The following offers tips and tricks focused on self-care practices specific to online therapists. The suggested strategies are organized by various dimensions of self-care (i.e., physical, intellectual, emotional, spiritual, relational, professional) to help you prioritize your self-care as a teletherapist. These suggestions may be used as a starting point in your self-care journey, as a reentry point, or perhaps simply as an opportunity to check in with yourself on practices that already work for you. You may choose to implement suggestions that feel fitting for you and disregard those that may not be applicable. Because self-care looks unique to each person, space is provided to include your ideas and potential next steps in your self-care journey.

Physical

The physical dimension of self-care involves fitness, diet, sleep habits, medical health, and well-being. The following suggestions may support physical wellness as you engage in teletherapy practice:

- Set up an ergonomic workstation. For example, ensure that your computer screen is at eye level, your head and neck remain straight, and your shoulders are relaxed throughout your workday.

- Move your body between sessions. Take a quick walk, stretch, or do chair yoga to stay active and energized.

- Consider using a standing desk or alternating sessions between sitting and standing.

- End your workday at a reasonable time to engage in healthy sleep practices. Maintaining suitable work hours is particularly important due to the association between screen time before bed and poor sleep.

- Limit excessive screen time outside of work hours.

- Take a sick day if you're unwell, even if working remotely prevents you from getting anyone else sick.

- _____

- _____

DOI: 10.4324/9781003289920-13

Intellectual

The intellectual dimension of self-care involves education and learning. The following offers ideas for staying intellectually engaged in topics relevant to teletherapy practice:

- If technology is not one of your areas of expertise, maintain realistic expectations regarding what you can and cannot do yourself.

- Consult with experts as needed when setting up new platforms or devices.

- Seek continuing education or supervision opportunities that will advance your engagement with clients, specifically in teletherapy practice.

- _____

- _____

Emotional

Emotional self-care involves tending to personal feelings and emotions and cultivating compassion for oneself and others. The following suggestions offer opportunities for enhancing emotional wellness as you engage in teletherapy practice:

- Create a comfortable and enjoyable workspace. Prioritize the quality of your environment and add things that bring you joy, like a painting or plant.

- Select cheerful desktop backgrounds and screensavers to brighten your day.

- Be gentle with yourself when things like client progress or technology may not go as expected.

- Check in with your feelings regularly and recognize any emotional challenges that might come up when providing telehealth services. Consider the possible causes of these challenges and address them as needed.

- Create a "feelgood" file on your desktop for easy access during challenging times. Fill it with things that uplift your mood.

- Schedule sessions with your therapist as needed. A benefit of engaging in teletherapy for yourself is that it doesn't require additional travel time and typically only requires you to block off the time it takes to see one client.

- _____

- _____

Spiritual

Spiritual self-care involves beliefs and values about life and the nourishment of the soul. Spiritual practices may or may not include religious activities and rituals. The following offers ideas for ethically incorporating spirituality throughout your teletherapy workday:

- Start your day with mindfulness and/or engage in mindful moments between sessions (Norcross & Phillips, 2020). Mindfulness may include the use of:

  - Meditation apps

  - Breathing exercises

  - Two minutes of mindfulness (Geller, 2017)

- Ground yourself in nature (Norcross & Phillips, 2020), even when working inside and on a computer.

  - Take a moment to gaze out of an office window.

  - Walk outside between sessions.

  - Bring plants or cut flowers into your office. Aromatic plants such as rosemary and lavender may have particularly calming effects. A benefit of teletherapy practice is that you don't need to worry about client allergies or sensitivities to scents that you find particularly appealing.

  - Place images of nature on your desktop or in your office.

- If you're religious, consider incorporating grounding parts of your faith into your daily work practice. A benefit of teletherapy is that you can keep your spiritual and/or religious items nearby without revealing them to clients if you prefer privacy. For example, depending on your faith tradition, you might:

  - Place a statue of the Buddha within your view as a reminder of peace, wisdom, enlightenment, compassion, and care for the clients you serve.

  - Keep a rosary within reach to hold onto during challenging sessions or between clients.

  - Light a candle at your desk for grieving clients.

  - Between sessions, pray for the clients you see and for yourself as a healing guide.

- _____

- _____

Relational

The relational dimension of self-care involves the nurturance of relationships and connections with friends, family, and colleagues. The following offers ideas for staying connected with others in person and virtually:

- Consider ways to connect with people beyond online interactions and include in-person engagement. Meet with friends, family, or colleagues for coffee, tea, lunch, or a yoga break.

- Attend in-person conferences and networking meetings when offered to connect with colleagues in the same physical environment.

- Utilize technology to maintain connections with supportive colleagues who may be physically distant by setting up regular meetings and reunions. Creating and maintaining a self-care network by connecting with supportive colleagues and sharing helpful recommendations for clients and colleagues (Barnett & Homany, 2022) promotes relational resilience (Walsh, 2010).

- _____
- _____

Professional

Those with an active career may also need to attend to their professional self-care. This dimension of self-care involves tending to work environments and setting realistic boundaries and expectations for self and others. The following suggestions offer opportunities for enhancing professional wellness as a teletherapist:

- When working from home, create a separate workspace. If possible, avoid using your bedroom or other rest spaces for work. If your bedroom is the only private space from which you can work, create a separate area in your bedroom dedicated to your work. At the end of your workday, put your computer and other work things away or cover them so that they are out of sight until you are ready to begin working again the next day.

- Utilize separate spaces for various activities or during specific times of the day when possible. For example, take lunch and other breaks away from your desk.

- Establish distinct boundaries between teletherapy practice and personal time. For example, you might avoid checking email 30 minutes after your last session of the day and not check it again until 30 minutes before your first session the next day.

- _____
- _____

Regardless of the dimension of self-care, self-compassion plays a significant role by acting as a buffer against stress (Geary et al., 2023). It involves showing kindness to oneself in tough times, recognizing that these experiences are part of the human condition, and being mindful of difficult emotions without becoming overly invested (Neff, 2003). As you contemplate how to care for yourself, consider the advice that you might give to the people you serve. Pause for a moment, think about the valuable gift you offer your clients, and ask yourself, "What would I encourage clients to do to care for themselves when working online?" Then, lean on your gifts and knowledge to develop a sustainable plan for your care and wellness.

Since achieving wellness goes beyond oneself, establish a community of supportive telemental health professionals to aid you in maintaining your wellness. Having peer support relationships can prevent burnout throughout your professional career, as it can provide honest, supportive, and nurturing feedback (Barnett & Homany, 2022).

References

Barnett, J. E., & Homany, G. (2022). The new self-care: It's not all about you. *Practice Innovations*, *7*(4), 313–326. https://doi.org/10.1037/pri0000190

Geary, M. R., Shortway, K. M., Marks, D. R., & Block-Lerner, J. (2023). Psychology doctoral students' self-care during the COVID-19 pandemic: Relationships among satisfaction with life, stress levels, and self-compassion. *Training and Education in Professional Psychology*, *17*(4), 323–330. https://doi.org/10.1037/tep0000444

Geller, S. M. (2017). *A practical guide to cultivating therapeutic presence.* American Psychological Association. https://doi.org/10.1037/0000025-000

Neff, K. D. (2003). Self-compassion: An alternative conceptualization of a healthy attitude towards oneself. *Self and Identity*, *2*(2), 85–101. https://doi.org/10.1080/15298860309032

Norcross, J. C., & Phillips, C. M. (2020). Psychologist self-care during the pandemic: Now more than ever. *Journal of Health Service Psychology*, *46*(2), 59–63. https://doi.org/10.1007/s42843-020-00010-5

Walsh, F. (2010). A family resilience framework for clinical practice: Integrating developmental theory and systemic perspectives. In W. Borden (Ed.), *Reshaping theory in contemporary social work: Toward a critical pluralism in clinical practice* (pp. 146–176). Columbia University Press.

CHAPTER 12

BUMPIN' INTO TELETHERAPY

PLANNING FOR PARENTAL LEAVE

Veronica P. Viesca, Parker Leukart, Amanda Rausch, and Whitney Molitor

Readying teletherapy practice for parental leave and navigating self-disclosure to clients requires careful planning and consideration. In a virtual setting, it can be difficult for clients to detect physical signs of pregnancy (e.g., the "baby bump"), making a therapist-initiated transition process even more critical. When preparing for parental leave, therapists should take the following steps: (1) determine when and how to disclose the upcoming leave to clients, (2) create plans for client care, (3) consider additional business management needs that may need to be addressed during leave, (4) troubleshoot alternative plans in the event that the baby arrives early or leave needs to be extended beyond the originally planned time, (5) take leave, and (6) return to work. The following provides step-by-step guidance on these actions.

Disclosure

Generally, it is best for clinicians to share their news of impending parental leave at least one to three months before their planned absence. This allows time to discuss any client concerns and to create a plan for the leave of absence. Many childbearing clinicians report disclosing to clients during the second trimester or once they start "showing" and clients might naturally start wondering or asking about a potential pregnancy. Telehealth, however, affords some flexibility with this since the physical signs of pregnancy may not be visible if the therapist is only seen on screen from the shoulders up. Additionally, some nonchildbearing clinicians may choose not to disclose the news of expecting a child for professional or personal reasons and instead simply share they will be taking a planned leave of absence. Consulting with clinical supervisors, mentors, or peers can be helpful to discern whether to disclose and how much to disclose based on individual providers' and clients' needs.

In addition, it is crucial to consider each client's particular needs when determining timing of disclosure. Some clients may need more time to transition. Others may be okay with less notice. For example, clients with abandonment wounds typically need more time to process in subsequent sessions.

You may disclose your plans for parental leave during session, or choose to share the news via email a few days before session to allow clients time to process prior to meeting. Again, consider the needs of each client when deciding the best approach.

DOI: 10.4324/9781003289920-14

Sample Disclosure

The following example may be shared verbally in session or via email. Make edits to personalize the disclosure as you see fit.

"I have personal news to share. I am [expecting a baby/adopting a child next year]. I plan to be available as usual until [month] unless the baby comes early. Then, I'll take parental leave until [date]. While I'm away, you have a few options: (1) You can take a break from therapy, utilizing this time to practice the skills you have learned, (2) you can transfer to a new therapist to gain a fresh perspective, or (3) if you sign a release of information, I can connect you with one of my colleagues for the interim. I can fill them in on what we've been working on so you can pick up where we leave off, and then we can transition back to working together when I return. If you decide to transfer to a new therapist, I can provide a list of referrals. There is no need to decide now. Think it over and let me know what you prefer by [date] so we can formalize a plan. Let me know if you have any questions or concerns or if you'd like to discuss your options in further detail. Until then, business as usual!"

Because visual cues of pregnancy and natural reminders of impending leave may not be available via telehealth, consider providing verbal or written reminders of the upcoming leave if the initial disclosure occurred well in advance.

Processing

Many clients will express opposing reactions to the news, sharing happiness for the clinician and/or sadness or anxiety about the transition. Normalizing this and presenting options for a collaborative plan can be reassuring.

The following questions can be used in session to help clients process the news:

- How do you feel about the news of my pregnancy?

- What thoughts or emotions does my pregnancy bring up for you?

- Do you have any questions and/or concerns about how my news may impact our therapeutic relationship?

- As we collaboratively come up with your care plan prior to my leave, is there anything important you'd like me to know and/or take into consideration?

- Are there ways in which you would like our sessions to be adjusted during this time?

- What support or resources can I provide to help you feel comfortable and supported during this period?

- If a client has struggled or is struggling with their own fertility:

  - I know that you have struggled with your own fertility. What, if any, feelings are present regarding your own journey?

  - Is there anything in particular that I can do to be sensitive and supportive to your experience?

  - Are there any boundaries you'd like me to be sensitive to before and/or after my leave?

Developing Plans for Client Care

It is essential to consider client needs when developing each plan for client care (Gerber, 2005). A successful transition should be therapist led, and termination should typically be client initiated. Consider exploring the following questions with clients when discussing the plan for leave.

If clients consider transferring to a new therapist:

- Is the transfer temporary or final? What are the dates of treatment with the new therapist?

- Will clients connect directly with the new therapist, or will they sign a release of information and have you initiate contact?

- Would a release of information and consultation with the new therapist support a better transition?

- Would it be beneficial for you and the new therapist to meet together with the client(s) for a transfer session?

If clients consider pausing therapy:

- Do(es) the client(s) want to schedule a return appointment in advance of leave or develop a plan for scheduling this appointment after leave?

If clients consider terminating care:

- What led them to reach out initially? Has this presenting problem been resolved?

- What goals were met during treatment?

- What can they continue doing to ensure long-term success?

- What are the signs that might signal the need for a "tune-up session"?

- Would it be helpful to schedule a check-in session upon your return?

- If you were not going on leave, would treatment still be ending?

For clients who decide to pause therapy or entirely terminate care, consider doing each of the following in closing sessions:

- Provide a list of emergency contacts.

- Provide contact information for a covering clinician.

- Develop a list of other resources (e.g., groups, books, podcasts, friends) that clients can turn to for support in the absence of therapy.

- Develop a personalized plan with each client to navigate stressors or challenging events that do not warrant the use of emergency contacts.

Business Management

There are many ancillary considerations in telehealth that may need to be addressed prior to parental leave. Depending on the treatment setting, plan for appropriate business management while on leave.

Make plans for paying bills and renewing necessary renewals, set an automatic reply on email, and leave an appropriate voicemail message indicating temporary absence from practice and outlining other important details.

Renewals and Bill Payments

Though clinicians may pause therapy sessions while on parental leave, some tasks cannot be paused. Consider how any necessary bills and renewals will be managed while on leave. Consider the following:

- License renewal(s)

- Malpractice insurance renewal(s)

- Professional membership renewal(s)

- Other business bills including rent, internet, teletherapy platform subscriptions, advertising platforms, etc.

If possible, put bills on automatic payment/renewal prior to going on leave. If this isn't possible, determine a plan for paying/renewing during leave. Many people don't look at their calendars regularly during leave, so you might need to consider alternative options. Build in safeguard reminders upon return to make sure that these were completed during what is often a sleep-deprived state.

Email Away Message

Prepare an email away message in advance of going on leave. If leave needs to begin sooner than anticipated, having a message already prepared will allow for a faster and easier task of simply turning the automatic message on during a special time when you may want to be as present as possible. The following example may be edited to personalize your own away message as you see fit:

> "I am currently away on leave with an anticipated return date of [date]. Clients, please contact [name of covering clinician and/or administrative staff] in the interim. Supervisees, please contact [name of covering supervisor]. If this is an urgent need or emergency, or you need immediate assistance, please call 911.
>
> [resource line, suicide hotline]"

Voicemail Message

Also prepare an outgoing voicemail message in advance of going on leave. The following example may be edited to personalize your own voicemail message as you see fit:

> "Thank you for calling [practice/therapist name]. If this is a medical or psychiatric emergency, please hang up and dial 911. I am currently away on leave with an anticipated return date of [date]. Clients, please contact [name of covering clinician and/or administrative staff] in the interim. Supervisees, please contact [name of covering supervisor]. This voicemail is [not being monitored during my leave/being monitored by (name of covering clinician and/or administrative staff)]. The call will be returned [within two business days/after my return on (date)]."

Troubleshooting

Unfortunately, plans don't always go accordingly. Consider plans to adjust your expected leave or return dates as needed based on unforeseen circumstances. Create flowcharts for the following three conditions:

- The "according to plan" plan
- The "early arrival" plan
- The "need to extend leave" plan

For each plan, include dates of expected leave and the names and contact information for individuals who will be providing coverage along with a description of their role (i.e., billing, scheduling, business operations, clinical supervision). Provide these flow charts to whoever is responsible for implementing the adjustments, keeping confidentiality in mind.

Taking Leave

Addressing necessary considerations before taking leave is critical for success. Actually taking leave is also important! One benefit of telehealth is the ease of accessibility. This means that while on leave, it may be easy to slide back into working because laptops, emails, and text messages are an arm's reach away. However, it's important to maintain clear boundaries during this time (Gerber, 2005). The following offers considerations for determining boundaries and structure that best suit your own personal needs:

- In addition to having an out-of-office response, consider staying completely out of your email account. To achieve this, it might be helpful to log out of all work email accounts and only use a personal email account while on leave.
- Consider turning off or muting any work-related notifications or alerts that may be sent to your personal phone(s). If you are using an app-based phone service, consider removing or hiding the app or its alerts while you are on leave.
- For any personnel who may be covering or filling in for you, consider asking them not to contact you about work-related matters during your leave. It may help to provide contacts for other people who may be able to answer any work-related questions while you are away.
- Provide a point person who acts as your proxy and only contacts you in the event of a serious matter. Upon return to work, this person could also debrief you on relevant information.

Returning to Work

In addition to considering the factors that must be addressed before and during leave, it is equally important to consider one's return-to-work plan. The following questions should be considered to help with reentry into clinical work:

- How will you plan to be debriefed on what happened during your time away?
- Will you begin by seeing a full caseload again or ease back into work by titrating this process (Novotney, 2014)? One option for an eased transition is to start seeing existing clients and to slowly reintroduce new clients with time.

- Will clients virtually "meet" baby or receive an announcement?

- How might telehealth sessions be scheduled to accommodate any necessary breaks for lactation and/or feeding?

Parental leave in the context of teletherapy practice demands careful planning and client-centered considerations. While the timing of disclosure and the nature of client's care planning varies based on situation and need, both should occur with thorough planning and care for clients. During leave, maintaining clear boundaries is vital, a boundary some find difficult to maintain in the context of teletherapy. Finally, the return to work should be planned with consideration of client needs, the therapist's capacity, and the nature of the treatment in mind.

References

Gerber, J. (2005, July 21). *The pregnant therapist: Caring for yourself while working with Clients*. APA Services. www.apa services.org/practice/ce/self-care/pregnancy

Novotney, A. (2014). Having a baby? *Monitor on Psychology, 45*(3), 58–61.

Part 3
Children and Adolescents

CHAPTER 13

DIGITAL SAND THERAPY

COGNITIONS AND THE UNDERWORLD

Jessica Stone

Materials for Therapists and Clients: Hardware and software to access a digital sand therapy program. An additional device (e.g., computer, tablet, phone) for teletherapy platform access is optional.

Objective

Sandtray therapy is an effective therapy assessment and intervention used with children, adolescents, adults, intimate relationships, families, and groups to express inner worlds without the use of words. Digital sand therapy programs combine the flexibility and customizability of technology with the power of sand therapies. As a contemporary take on a traditional therapeutic tool, digital sand therapy offers a space where clients can construct, deconstruct, and reconstruct narratives, feelings, and experiences. This virtual realm becomes an external representation of their internal world, enabling clients to give form to abstract thoughts, emotions, and memories, thereby facilitating greater understanding, communication, and self-awareness. This chapter offers instruction on how to conduct two different sand therapy interventions utilizing virtual platforms that are compatible with online therapy.

Rationale for Use

Sandtray therapy involves the processing of intra- and interpersonal matters using a sand tray and miniature objects (Homeyer & Sweeney, 2011). Categories of miniature objects typically provided with sand trays include living creatures, fantasy and folklore, scenery, transport, equipment, and miscellaneous objects (Homeyer & Lyles, 2022; Lowenfeld, 1993). The use of these objects allows clients to represent their experiences while a therapist observes. The use of sand therapies promotes safety and control by allowing clients to address emotionally charged issues through the medium without the need to verbally explain their experience.

Sandtray therapy can be successfully used with children, adolescents, and adults. It is adaptable for therapy with individuals, intimate relationships, families, and groups and has been used as a successful intervention for child abuse and neglect (Cunningham et al., 2000; Ismail et al., 2019; Maharjan, 2019),

DOI: 10.4324/9781003289920-16

intergenerational trauma (Ayres, 2016), military combat trauma (Popejoy et al., 2020), neurological changes (Akimoto et al., 2018; Foo et al., 2020), and autism disorder (Lu et al., 2010; Parker & O'Brien, 2011).

The adaptability, flexibility, and customizability of digital sand therapies allows this powerful intervention to be used in online therapy when the traditional version is not a viable option. Digital sand therapy should retain the core tenets of traditional sand therapies.

The digital platform affords an expansive array of choices concerning object types, backgrounds, and settings, facilitating a nearly limitless selection of symbolic mediums. This vastness augments the expressive avenues available to clients, enabling them to delve into and navigate intricate emotional terrains, which might be restricted in a traditional setup limited by tangible objects and a static sand tray environment. The rich variety of available elements and features can render the therapeutic experience more captivating and potentially foster a deeper probing of psychological facets.

In addition, some clients may not like the tactile sensation of physical sand, feeling dirty, or the mess often created through use of physical sand trays. People who have experienced complex trauma may not be able to utilize physical sand trays due to overwhelm of the sensory experience, which can be triggering. Others may be unable to reach the sand tray because of mobility issues such as degenerative disorders or due to being in a wheelchair, which may prevent them from moving close enough to the tray. Digital sand therapy is an excellent alternative to the use of physical sand trays, even in in-person therapy settings.

The capacity to store, modify, and revisit sessions conducted in digital sand work extends its therapeutic potential by furnishing a dynamic chronicle of a client's journey over sessions. This mode of digital documentation proves invaluable to both therapists and clients as it aids in tracking growth and regressions and discerning patterns or shifts in the therapeutic process.

Setup

1. ***Select the platform that you will use to conduct the sand tray activity.*** This intervention is powerful and allows access to important emotions, perspectives, and experiences. Therapists must ensure that the digital version of sand work encompasses key tenets, capabilities, and protections. Features may include moving, resizing, and knocking over items. An ideal platform includes key tenets of sand therapy fundamentals and is electronically secure. Consider components such as end-to-end encryption, whether or not data is stored on a server, password/login protections, and whether or not clients can access the program outside of session. Some platforms may require a one-time purchase and may need to be downloaded prior to use.

   The Virtual Sandtray®© App includes the unique ability to create a world on top of the sand and underneath the sand (Stone, 2020). The worlds can be seen simultaneously with the tilt feature or only one at a time as desired. One world can be hidden until the user chooses to reveal its contents.

   The first of the two interventions described in this chapter (i.e., positive/negative cognitions) may be used with any digital sand tray that the therapist deems appropriate. The second (i.e., Underworld Technique) is specific to the Virtual Sandtray®©, in that it requires the ability for clients to create a multidimensional, multilayered digital depiction of their world.

2. ***Practice.*** Prior to using a digital sand tray in teletherapy, practice using the platform. Practice creating trays and discovering features to gain the knowledge and experience necessary to guide clients during use.

3. ***Discuss the use of digital sand trays with legal guardians.*** When working with children and adolescents, discuss the use of digital sand trays with legal guardians prior to implementing them in session.

4. ***Determine whether clients will use one or two devices during the intervention.*** Digital sand trays may be used with one device. However, when using via telemental health, the windows on the device's screen may be layered, only allowing the viewer to see one program at a time. With the use of one device, users may be able to hear the other person while using the sand tray but cannot see them until the window for the telehealth platform is brought to the forefront. If one device can be used for the digital sand tray and another for the telemental health platform, clients and therapists can see one another while using the sand tray application. This is ideal for allowing therapists to attend to nonverbal cues. If using two devices, explain which device should be used for accessing the digital sand tray prior to providing more detailed instructions.

5. ***Provide guidance for setting up the platform on the client's device.*** Explain how to access the digital sand tray application. Some platforms simply require clients to access a website to use the application. Others may require an application to be downloaded onto their device.

Overall, the ways clinicians conduct traditional sand therapy is translated directly to the digital version. The use of prompts, directives, themes, questions, and more can be used with the traditional and digital versions of sand work. The following are two examples of specific interventions for use with digital sand trays.

Positive/Negative Cognitions

Positive and negative cognitions from eye movement desensitization and reprocessing (EMDR) and neurolinguistic programming (NPL) can be effectively integrated into sand therapy interventions (Andreas, 2021; Marques, 2023; Rosen, 2023).

In EMDR, negative cognitions are core beliefs about oneself that are often linked to traumatic experiences. These beliefs are identified and targeted during therapy. In digital sand therapy, clients are invited to create a symbolic representation of their emotions or experiences using sand and virtual objects. Negative cognitions can be represented in this digital sand world through the choice of objects, colors, or the arrangement of the sand. For example, a client might place a figurine representing themselves in a trapped or helpless position to symbolize a negative cognition.

NLP emphasizes the importance of positive self-talk and beliefs. Positive cognitions cultivated through NLP techniques, such as affirmations and reframing, can be introduced into the digital sand therapy process. Clients can incorporate positive cognitions by creating scenes in the digital sand that reflect their desired beliefs or self-concept. For instance, they may build a scene in which they are depicted as confident and in control.

As the negative and positive cognitions shift over the course of treatment, clients can enlarge or shrink the chosen object according to the desired representation of power, meaning, impact, etc. If the digital sand tray platform offers the feature, objects can also be knocked over, buried, levitated, recycled, or blown up as desired by the client. When these features are available, camera filters can be applied to depict a black-and-white scene that becomes colorful or, conversely, a colorful scene that becomes devoid of color. Effects such as rain, snow, earthquakes, and more can further allow for the representation of positive and negative cognitions, their impact, and their prevalence.

The following offers step-by-step instructions on integrating elements from EMDR and NLP into digital sand therapy to help clients explore, process, and transform their cognitions in creative and meaningful ways.

1. ***Access a digital sand tool.*** Therapists and clients should simultaneously access a digital sand tool.

2. ***Share screen.*** Prior to beginning the intervention, share your screen with clients. Some platforms, such as the Virtual Sandtray®©, allow therapists and clients to see the same sand tray simultaneously through an encrypted connection without needing to share screens. This is done by providing login credentials to clients when this feature is available.

3. ***Provide general instructions on features of the digital sand tray.*** Some clients may intuitively explore the application and may not need specific instructions. Others may need more guidance. Provide instructions and demonstrate features of the sand tray as needed.

4. ***Instruct clients to share their screen.*** Stop sharing your own screen and ask clients to share their screen to allow you to see the sand tray on their device. This step may be skipped if using a sand tray platform that does not necessitate screen sharing.

5. ***Identify positive and negative cognitions.*** Clients and therapists should work together to identify positive and negative cognitions related to a client's situation, emotion, or experience. The following questions may be used to process these cognitions:

   • What thoughts or beliefs come to mind when you think about the specific situation or emotion we are working on?

   • Can you describe any negative thoughts or self-talk that you notice in relation to this issue?

   • Are there any positive thoughts or beliefs that you currently hold about yourself or the situation?

6. ***Select and place digital representations of cognitions.*** Instruct clients to choose digital representations of the positive and negative cognitions and place them in the tray. Inform clients that they may resize and place the representations in ways that are representative of the power, meaning, and/or impact that the cognition holds for them. If these options are available on the selected sand tray platform, clients can utilize color in the sky, under the sand, and in camera filters to communicate and amplify emotions based on what is chosen. The following questions may be used to guide this process:

   • How would you like to represent [negative cognitions] in the tray? What objects or symbols do you think best represent them?

   • How would you like to symbolize [positive cognitions] in the tray? What objects or symbols do you think best represent them?

   • What colors or visual effects would you like to use to convey the emotions and/or mood associated with these cognitions?

7. ***Represent emotions.*** Prompt clients to make any changes in their tray that may help to represent the impact of their cognitions on their emotions. The following questions may be used to guide this process:

   • How might the tray help you express the emotions that are associated with these cognitions? Are there any changes that you might make to the tray to represent these feelings?

   • If you could use colors or weather effects to represent your emotional state related to these cognitions, what would they look like?

   • How do you imagine using camera filters to convey the emotional journey you are experiencing in the tray?

8. ***Make changes.*** As clients become ready to process the negative and positive cognitions, the size and position of the items can be changed to represent what has been processed. For instance, if an item represented something that is feared, it may initially be placed as a large, looming item. It could later be made smaller and even knocked over to signify a reduction in its power over the client/situation. Something that is defined as a positive cognition could then be made larger or levitated into the sky to depict an increase in power and importance. The following questions may be used to guide this process:

   • As we work through these cognitions, how do you envision changing the size or position of the representations to signify shifts in their impact on you?

- Can you describe how you would like to visually depict the transformation of a negative belief into a positive one within the tray?

- What effects or changes in the tray's elements symbolize your progress in managing these cognitions?

9. **Save the sand tray.** Some digital sand tray applications allow created sand trays to be saved for future use. If the application that you are using allows this, save the sand tray in case clients would like to continue working on the same world in future sessions. Rather than saving just one tray for each client, save trays with unique names after the completion of each one so clients can revisit any tray that they have created at any point in therapy. You can also review saved trays for progression, regression, and theme changes throughout treatment. If the application does not allow the sand tray to be saved, take a screenshot of the final sand tray so clients can revisit the image and process changes between sand trays in future sessions.

Virtual Sandtray®© Underworld Technique

The Virtual Sandtray®© Underworld Technique is a unique intervention available through the Virtual Sandtray®© App. It allows clients to create a multilayered, multidimensional depiction of their world. One world layer is easily visible; it is created on top of the sand, as is done in traditional sand therapy work. The other layer is built underneath the visible sand layer. To see this second layer, one has to tilt the view and zoom in deliberately to see the world beneath.

This multilayered world can be used in therapy settings in various ways. One common use is that clients may create a tray on the top layer of the sand to represent the parts of themselves they share with others and another tray in the underworld to represent portions they do not share. Clients who are familiar with the show *Stranger Things* (2016, 2023) may use the show's premise of the upside-down (Gemmill, 2019) to create the worlds.

The following offers step-by-step instructions on using the underworld technique in teletherapy using the Virtual Sandtray®© App.

1. **Access the Virtual Sandtray®© App.** Provide login credentials to clients. The therapist's and client's apps will join with an encrypted connection.

2. **Provide general instructions on features of the Virtual Sandtray®© App.** Some clients may intuitively explore the application and may not need specific instructions. Others may need more guidance. Provide instructions and demonstrate features of the Virtual Sandtray®© App as needed.

3. **Introduce the underworld technique.** Introduce this technique by explaining that the client may create a world above and below the sand.

4. **Activate the excavator tool.** Prompt clients to activate the dirt excavator tool and remove all the sand. This sets clients up for the next steps to customize the liquid layer and build the underworld.

5. **Customize the liquid layer.** The liquid layer lies under three layers of sand. By default, the liquid is blue, like traditional blue-bottom sand trays. Clients may customize the properties of the liquid layer to match their emotional or symbolic representation. Instruct clients that they may change the color of the liquid layer if they would like. For example, clients might choose poison or lava to represent various emotions or experiences. This allows for further customization and depiction of the mood and environment clients seek.

6. ***Build the underworld.*** Prompt clients to build the underworld using any tools available through the Virtual Sandtray®© App. A key is to make the items small enough to fit under the sand line. The following questions may be used to guide this process:

   - What aspects or feelings would you like to explore in the underworld layer?

   - Can you identify items or symbols that represent hidden aspects of yourself or experiences you haven't shared openly?

   - How do you envision customizing the liquid layer and color of the underworld to match the mood and symbolism you want to convey?

7. ***Activate the dirt-mover truck.*** After the underworld is created to satisfaction, the dirt-mover truck must be activated to replace the sand over the underworld. If any items are too tall, they may poke through the sand. Any items clients desire to fit under the sand can be made smaller.

8. ***Build the top layer.*** Instruct clients to create a world on top of the sand using any tools available through the Virtual Sandtray®© App. The following questions may be used to guide this process:

   - What elements, colors, and scenes would you like to create on the top layer that represent what you share with others or what is visible to the world?

   - How can you use the available items/objects to construct a meaningful representation of your public self?

   - What do you think the top layer communicates about your outer world and relationships?

9. ***Reveal both worlds.*** Once the top layer has been finished, instruct clients to tilt the tray using the right-hand joystick button. Then, instruct clients to zoom in until the underworld is revealed. Clients can toggle between the two worlds by tilting the tray up or down as desired. The following questions may be used to guide this process:

   - When you tilt the tray to reveal the underworld, what emotions or thoughts come up for you as you see what's hidden?

   - How might switching between the layers help you explore the relationship between your hidden self and your outward presentation?

   - Can you describe what you hope to discover or process by navigating between these two layers?

   - How do the two layers reflect your inner world and your external self-concept?

   - Who do you choose to reveal the top layer to? How do you decide this?

   - Who do you choose to reveal the underworld to? How do you decide this?

   - What insights have you gained about the parts of yourself that you conceal or reveal to others through this multilayered process?

   - How might you apply the understanding gained from the underworld technique to your daily life and relationships?

Vignette

Jared (9) presented for telemental health treatment due to behavioral difficulties at home and school, as reported by his mother. Jared lived with his mother and three younger brothers. His father moved to another state following an acrimonious divorce and ceased contact with his children. Concerning behaviors included anger toward mother, brothers, and staff at his school. He would yell, scream, throw items at people, and look at people with an extremely angry and unnerving stare when upset.

Jared was familiar with the Virtual Sandtray®© and had created several trays over the previous 12 sessions. Other play (e.g., Super Smash Bros) revealed that Jared felt he had two sides, and sometimes, one of the sides frightened him. He stated he worked hard to conceal the scary side, but sometimes, it became too much. He worried about which side would prevail as he got older.

The therapist described underworld technique as a way to create a depiction of these two sides of himself; one on top of the sand and one underneath. Jared stated that he wanted to try this creation.

The therapist initiated a remote connection with Jared via the Virtual Sandtray®© and provided instructions on how to activate the excavator tool to create an underworld and then how to activate the dirt-mover truck to create the top layer.

Jared created two trays in the session. The first tray depicted the way he wanted to present himself on the top layer of the sand (see Figure 13.1). He described the top layer as happy and helpful, someone others wanted to be around. The underworld was dark and frightening. It included a black layer with dead trees and animals strewn about.

Once he was finished with this first tray, he initiated the creation of a second by his own prompting (see Figure 13.2). The second tray depicted the frightening self on top of the sand and the happy, helpful self in the underworld. He said he can present in either way, depending on what happens in the day or week, at home or school.

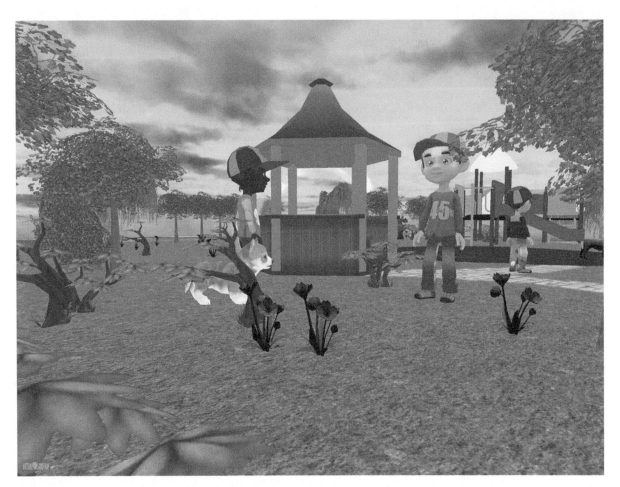

Figure 13.1 Jared's happy world above the sand, created with the Virtual Sandtray App®© using the underworld technique.

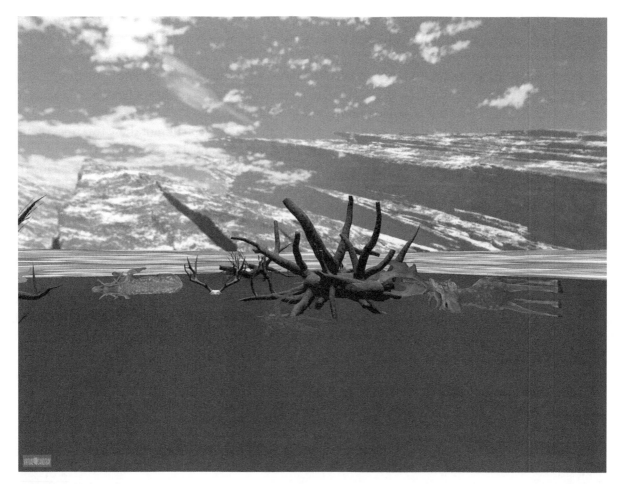

Figure 13.2 Jared's scary underworld, created with the Virtual Sandtray App®© using the underworld technique.

Jared shared a narrative of his tray that included a significant amount of pressure and stress he felt due to his father's absence from the home. He said he felt he had to be a pseudo-parent in the household, and he had mixed feelings about this.

The underworld technique was critical in Jared's ability to depict feelings and experiences that contributed to his behaviors. Having the ability to create, hide, and reveal these parts as Jared felt appropriate allowed him to express himself in ways that created a neuroception of safety, thus allowing him to move forward in his therapeutic process.

Future sessions focused on communication with his mother regarding his stresses, ways to reduce these, and alternative ways to express his anger and sadness.

Suggestions for Follow-Up

An advantage of digital sand work is that it can be saved for further review by the therapist, client, caregivers, or any combination of people involved. Comparison of tray creation both within and between sessions allows for detailed and nuanced understandings, insight, and discussion.

For the positive/negative cognitions intervention, schedule sessions to review and reflect on the client's tray creations, monitor changes in cognitions, and encourage the application of insights to daily life. For the underworld technique, debrief after initial exploration, process hidden aspects revealed in the underworld layer, and connect these discoveries with the client's narrative and experiences. Continued exploration, application to real-life scenarios, and emotional support are key components of effective follow-up. In both interventions, ongoing communication and adjustments in the therapeutic approach are essential to support the client's journey toward self-discovery and healing.

Contraindications

Seek training and supervision when incorporating sandtray therapy into clinical practice. In addition, carefully consider if digital sandtray therapy is appropriate for each specific client. Some individuals might feel overwhelmed or anxious when introduced to a digital form of sand tray. It is essential to assess the client's digital literacy and comfort level with technology before incorporating it into therapy. These interventions may also reveal information that clients may not be ready to express or process. In digital sandtray therapy, adhere to your theoretical foundation and only encourage clients to create, explain, or discuss content to the extent that they are comfortable doing so.

References

Akimoto, M., Furukawa, K., & Ito, J. (2018). Exploring the sandplayer's brain: A single case study. *Archives of Sandplay Therapy, 30*, 73–84.

Andreas, C. (2021). *EMDR, EMI, and wingwave.* www.nlp.ch/pdfdocs/Historie_EMDR_Wingwave.pdf

Ayres, K. (2016). *Indicators of trauma in a single sand tray scene of a rural school youth.* [Unpublished master's thesis]. University of Pretoria.

Cunningham, C., Fill, K., & Al-Jaime, L. (2000). Sandtray play with traumatized children. *Journal of Aggression, Maltreatment & Trauma, 2*(2), 195–205. https://doi.org/10.1300/j146v02n02_09

Foo, M., Freedle, L., Sai, R., & Fonda, G. (2020). The effect of sandplay therapy on the thalamus in the treatment of generalized anxiety disorder: A case report. *International Journal of Play Therapy, 29*(4), 191–200. https://doi.org/10.1037/pla0000137

Gemmill, A. (2019). Stranger Things' upside-down explained. *Screenrant.* https://screenrant.com/stranger-things-upside-down-explained/

Homeyer, L., & Lyles, M. (2022). *Advanced sandtray therapy: Digging deeper into clinical practice.* Routledge.

Homeyer, L., & Sweeney, D. (2011). *Sandtray therapy: A practical manual.* Routledge.

Ismail, M. R., Amat, S., Johari, K. S. K., & Mahmud, Z. (2019). Sandtray therapy for young girls in a shelter home. *Advances in Social Science, Education and Humanities Research, 464*, 666–670. https://doi.org/10.2991/assehr.k.200824.151

Lowenfeld, M. (1993). *Understanding children's sandplay: Lowenfeld's world technique.* Sussex Academic Press.

Lu, L., Peterson, F., Lacroix, L., & Rousseau, C. (2010). Stimulating creative play in children with autism through sandplay. *The Arts in Psychotherapy, 37*(1), 56–64. https://doi.org/10.1016/j.aip.2009.09.003

Maharjan, C. L. (2019). *Sandplay therapy for children with trauma living in a residential facility in Nepal: A multiple case study* (Publication No. 27669449) [Doctoral dissertation, California Institute of Integral Studies]. ProQuest.

Marques, D. (2023). These 4 NLP techniques will change how you think. *Happiness.com.* www.happiness.com/magazine/personal-growth/nlp-happiness-techniques/

Parker, N., & O'Brien, P. (2011). Play therapy – Reaching the child with autism. *International Journal of Special Education, 26*(1), 80–87.

Popejoy, E. K., Perryman, K., & Broadwater, A. (2020). Processing military combat trauma through sandtray therapy: A phenomenological study. *Journal of Creativity in Mental Health, 16*(2), 196–211. https://doi.org/10.1080/15401383.2020.1761499

Rosen, G. M. (2023). Revisiting the origins of EMDR. *Journal of Contemporary Psychotherapy, 53*(4), 289–296. https://doi.org/10.1007/s10879-023-09582-x

Stone, J. (2020). *Virtual Sandtray®© underworld.* Jessica Stone, Ph.D. https://jessicastonephd.com/blog/

Stranger Things. (2016). *Stranger things.* IMDB. www.imdb.com/title/tt4574334/

Stranger Things. (2023). *Stranger things.* Netflix. www.netflix.com/title/80057281

CHAPTER 14

VIRTUAL PUPPET PLAY THERAPY

Karen Fried

Materials for Therapists: None.

Materials for Clients: Internet-connected desktop or laptop computer with a screen at least 13" for an individual and larger for a family or group sharing it.

Objective

Puppet play is a widely accepted instrument for therapeutic assessment and intervention (Bernier, 2005; Measelle et al., 1998). This chapter describes how to conduct this traditionally in-person technique via an online therapy platform.

Rationale for Use

Puppet play allows people of all ages to enact past, current, or future experiences, relationships, and emotions. Thus, it provides therapists insight into client history and feelings through symbolic projection (Oaklander, 1978). In allowing children and adolescents to project and process their internal reality, it offers a means of both evaluation and healing as clients access, depict, and reflect on themselves in a playful dance between the unconscious and the articulated. Projecting thoughts, emotions, and words onto a puppet can also feel safer than direct speech (Oaklander, 1978). Puppet play thereby reveals and heals by drawing clients to discover, enact, describe, and integrate feelings.

To enable clients to engage with puppet play via an online platform, the author's office-dwelling puppets were photographed in varied poses to mimic animation. The collection of puppets includes diverse people, animals, and objects. These photos were then used in the creation of a website (i.e., onlinepuppets.org), where anyone can now engage in online puppet play. Here, a background can be selected to set the scene, and puppets can be selected, placed, moved, duplicated, shrunk, enlarged, and made to speak, jump, hug, and hit on command. This digitized version allows therapists to offer clients in online sessions a self-affirming choice and client-led activity similar to puppet play activities available at an in-person therapy office. Therapists in more than 100 countries have used onlinepuppets.org (Fried, 2023). It is appropriate for all ages and can be used to engage individuals, families, or groups participating in therapy using the same or separate devices.

DOI: 10.4324/9781003289920-17

Setup

The following specifies setup required to engage in virtual puppet play for online assessment and intervention.

1. ***Familiarize yourself with the online platform.*** Therapists should familiarize themselves with the online tools available at onlinepuppets.org prior to introducing them to clients for the first time. Intimate knowledge of the website and its functions allows the therapist to guide clients during the intervention as needed.

2. ***Offer options.*** When offering the activity, suggest puppet play among other activities and explore each option with clients. This initial choice-making affirms clients' sense of self.

3. ***Share the link.*** If puppet play is chosen, access the online platform at onlinepuppets.org and share the website with clients utilizing the chat function in your HIPAA-consistent therapy platform. Sharing a direct link allows clients to go to the website at the same time as the therapist without needing to spell or type out the name of the website, which may be more difficult for younger clients.

4. ***Share your screen.*** Allow screen sharing on your device. Only share the browser, not the entire computer screen, which may contain confidential data.

5. ***Provide a visual tour.*** Show clients the website and how it works. For example, display all puppets and backdrops (see Figure 14.1 for a selection of available puppets displayed on one of numerous available backdrops). Explain, "You may choose any of the puppets to play with and you may select any of the backdrops for your scene. You may change characters and backdrops any time you like. You can change the size and position of puppets. You can move them in front of or behind other puppets. You can make them hug, hit, jump, and speak."

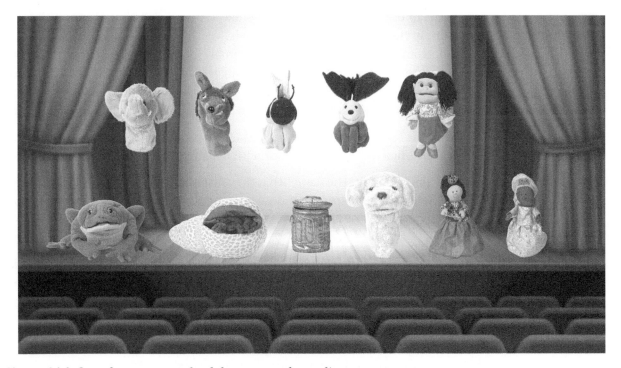

Figure 14.1 Sample puppets on backdrop, created at onlinepuppets.org.

6. ***Discuss options to save scenes.*** Explain that the online platform allows them to save the scene as a file on their device at any point and that this can be used to reengage in the same scene in future sessions. Also discuss that the therapist has the option of taking screenshots of the puppet play during and/or at the end of their puppet play. These can be used to talk about the puppets after they're done playing or to help them remember where they left off if they forget to save the scene or lose access to it. Discuss with clients their preferences about saving scenes and taking screenshots. If it appears that either of these options may inhibit clients in their play or if clients express discomfort with this, avoid saving scenes or taking screenshots.

7. ***Share the clients' screen.*** Request that clients share their screen(s). If family or group members are participating in therapy from different locations, discuss with them who will share their screen, or strategically ask someone to share their screen based on family or group dynamics (e.g., engage someone who may not normally be as likely to participate).

8. ***Practice.*** Invite clients to practice using the platform. Have them try selecting different backdrops and puppets, drag puppet images across a backdrop, adjust their sizes and positions, and animate them.

Instructions

The following offers step-by-step instructions on engaging in the virtual puppet play intervention.

1. ***Select puppet(s).*** Playfully select a puppet and move it around your own screen. Then, prompt clients to pick one or more puppets of their own. You may leave this an open-ended prompt or provide a specific prompt that relates to a presenting problem. For example, you might say, "Pick puppets for your sad and happy feelings" or "Pick puppets that remind you of you and your parents."

2. ***Choose a scene.*** Ask clients to think of a scene. You may take a more nondirective approach with this by asking clients to simply "tell a story with your puppets." With families or groups, invite each member to "choose a puppet and introduce yourselves" or "make a story together." If clients have difficulty choosing a scene, support them as they decide or suggest a theme relevant to the goals of therapy. Alternatively, you may take a more directive approach at the onset of the scene selection by asking clients to think of a scene such as "your best day at school," "your worst day at school," or "your past, present, and future."

3. ***Imagine the scene.*** Ask clients first to "imagine the scene" in their mind as vividly as possible.

4. ***Make the scene.*** Prompt clients to "make the scene" that they just imagined. If working with clients on different devices, each client can take turns, or choose one puppeteer to enact the show they collaboratively direct. Some clients may choose to have the therapist be the puppeteer, which is also a good option.

5. ***Be it.*** Have clients choose one or more puppets or objects depicted in their scene to be, or enact, whether in speech (e.g., "What does the _____ say?") or action (e.g., "What does the _____ do?"). You may have the client's chosen puppet(s) be in dialogue with yours. If requested by a client, you may also have your puppet(s) join the puppet show or collaborate on a story.

6. ***Own it.*** Ask clients to reflect on ways in which the puppets or the story might align with components of their own lives and/or relationships. For example, when working with a family, you might

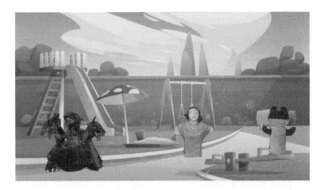

Figure 14.2 Completed playground scene, created at onlinepuppets.org.

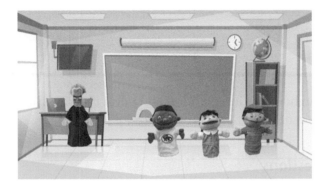

Figure 14.3 Completed classroom scene, created at onlinepuppets.org.

ask, "Did the ways that the characters relate to one another in the story look like the ways that you interact with one another in real life in any way?"

7. ***Make changes.*** Ask if the client(s) would like to add or change anything in the scene. If so, let them add, delete, move, or resize images. If family or group members display signs of uncertainty and/or conflicts regarding their decision-making process, you may explore this with them by asking what each person wants, how their desires differ, and how they might come to a consensus.

8. ***Save the show.*** If clients consent and express interest in saving their show, they can save the show on their desktop and use it again in future sessions. If they have consented to taking screenshots of the show, screenshots may also be taken at this point in time (see Figures 14.2 and 14.3 for examples of created scenes).

9. ***Assess.*** While clients learn about themselves and others, therapists learn about clients and their relationships from their manner of play and interactions with one another during the process. As you observe, make note of the following:

- Puppet choice
- Backdrop choice
- Puppet positioning, sizing, actions, silence, or speech
- Plot and theme

- If clients can "own" their projections (i.e., apply the work to their own lives)

- Comments made by clients about their show (e.g., good, bad, desired improvements)

- Interactions between clients

  - Did family or group members collaborate?

  - Did anyone take charge?

  - If members disagreed, how did their disagreement(s) come to resolution?

Throughout the activity, the therapist's enthusiasm and spirit of fun and playfulness is critical, especially when working with teenagers (Gallo-Lopez, 2005). Yet since some clients may lose interest from weak attention or a healthy resistance to painful emotions, be ready to save an unfinished show and offer another activity.

Processing

Processing may occur throughout the intervention and upon its conclusion. The following processing questions address puppets, scenes, and families or groups.

Puppet Processing Questions

Ask about particular puppets by inserting the names chosen by clients for their characters.

- What would _____ say to _____? How might _____ respond?

- How did _____ feel when [action that occurred between puppets]?

- What's it like for _____ to know that _____ is [happy with/angry with/afraid of] them?

Scene Processing Questions

- What do you like about this scene?

- Is there anything about this scene you'd like to change? What?

- Is there anyone or anything else that should be in this scene? Who or what?

- Is there anyone or anything you'd like to take out of the scene? Who or what?

- What's your ideal scene? What's special about it?

- What would you change about this scene to make it more like your ideal scene?

Family or Group Processing Questions

- How does your scene compare with _____'s scene?

- How did your characters get along with _____'s characters?

- How did your characters feel toward _____'s characters during the play?

- What did you learn about one another through the puppet play?

Vignette

Maya (9) identifies as a female Caucasian American. Maya lives with her parents, both of whom hold advanced degrees, and an older brother and sister. She has the position as "the baby of the family." Maya had early childhood speech and motor delays and, while now presenting as a neurotypical learner, uses a less-mature voice when discussing difficult subjects. Nonetheless, she connects well with her therapist and others. Early in therapy, Maya discussed anxiety around the time of her paternal grandfather's death and again when her grandmother died. Her grandparents, both Holocaust survivors, were significant in her family. After a several-month hiatus from therapy, Maya returned to address obsessive symptoms (e.g., hand-washing and masking) at the onset of the COVID-19 pandemic.

To assist her in processing her anxiety, the therapist had Maya go through the four-part Oaklander process in puppet play: (1) "Imagine your past before the pandemic, the present, and what the future will look like for you after the pandemic," (2) "Make it. Choose a puppet for each phase," (3) "Be it. Describe yourself as each puppet," and (4) "Own it. Does this scene fit for you in your life?"

The following highlights key components of their dialogue during this process.

Therapist: Imagine your past, present, and future. Then pick three puppets. Choose one for before the pandemic, one for during it, and one for after. You can also choose the backdrop.

Maya: Can I pick two for one of them?

Therapist: Of course!

Maya chose two girl puppets for the past, a spider hiding in a trash can for the present, a big-eyed Grandfather Smurf for the future, and the puppet stage backdrop.

Maya: For the past I chose two girls together because they could still be together. For the present I chose Oscar the Grouch hiding in a trash can to jump out at people. For the future, people will have wide eyes when they see things they couldn't see when Corona was showing, and they're so amazed.

Therapist: Next, I'd like you to 'be' the future puppet. How is it to be you, as the future?

Maya: I wish it was the future already.

Therapist: What would you say to Grandfather Smurf?

Maya: I would say, 'You're lucky you already got the vaccine.' He's over 75.

Therapist: What would he say to you?

Maya: He would say, 'Well, everybody will get the vaccine in a few months.'

Therapist: Next, I'd like you to imagine what the future would say to you.

Maya: Maybe the future would say to me, 'There's always light at the end of the tunnel. There's a bunch of bad things but at the end you'll feel more happy than you did before Corona because you'll feel free. If it was always like before, you wouldn't know what it was like for it to be over.'

Therapist: Now, what would you say to your past after knowing what your future is like?

Maya: I'm the past, and I don't know what the heck these people are talking about. What the heck is Corona?

Therapist: What's it like to not know?

Maya: I just want to sleep over at my friend's and eat a bunch of dessert.

Therapist: What would your past puppets say to your future puppet?

Maya: 'I don't even know what you're talking about. You're crazy.'

Then, Maya had that puppet hit the future puppet. The therapist processed and encouraged the anger.

Therapist: Ooh – it seems like that puppet is angry at the future! Do you want to do that again? Or did you do it enough?

Maya: I did.

Therapist: Can you describe the present puppet?

Maya: I'm the present. I'm hiding in this trash can. I'm not scared. It's fun scaring people because they think I'm a disgusting animal thing and I just hide there and they come to throw something away, and then, boom!

Therapist: You scare people! You like seeing their reaction.

Maya: Because Maya likes to just have fun, I guess. She likes to do things that are funny and sneak up on her brother and sister.

Therapist: Which puppet, past, present, or future, do you connect with the most?

Maya: I connect with the present. It's more funny. Except I don't like being in a trash can because nobody's going to see me if I don't pop up.

Therapist: Is there anything you'd add or change in this scene?

Maya: No.

Finally, the therapist assessed whether Maya could own the projections by asking if the scene fit for her in her life.

Therapist: Does the way you worked with these puppets fit for you?

Maya: Yes. I'm more funny and not that annoying and weird. And I like to stay safe.

A later session focused on Maya's argument with her siblings, who did not want to wear masks at home and thus exacerbated Maya's anxiety. As before, Maya "imagined" a scene and then "made it." She chose the frog for herself, the three-headed dragon for her siblings, and the bedroom backdrop.

Therapist: Which puppet would you like to be first?

Maya: I'll be the frog, which is me. I'm the frog and I hate this dragon here.

Therapist: Oh, you hate the dragon? Why?

Maya: Because they're always mean to me and they don't wear masks enough, so we're never safe at home.

Therapist: And do you, the frog, want to tell them that?

Maya: Why don't you wear masks?! I keep telling you and you don't listen!

Therapist: How does it feel to tell them that?

Maya: Frustrating!

Maya clicked the hit button.

> **Therapist:** What would you, the frog, like to say to the dragon?
>
> **Maya:** I'm stuck with you as one of the heads! I hate having to be stuck with you! Wear your masks!

Maya had the frog hit the dragon repeatedly, then stopped.

> **Therapist:** How does it feel in your body after you said that to the dragon?
>
> **Maya:** A little calmer.
>
> **Therapist:** Okay. Do you still have anything you'd like to say or do?
>
> **Maya:** No.
>
> **Therapist:** Is there anything you'd like to add, take out, or change in the scene?

Wordlessly, Maya shrank the dragon.

> **Therapist:** Aha. What did you do?
>
> **Maya:** I made the dragon smaller because I'm not as upset.
>
> **Therapist:** Okay. So, Maya, is there anything that fits for you in your life that you made in this scene?
>
> **Maya:** Yes; that's me as part of the 3-headed dragon. Because I can catch COVID from my brother and sister. I'm stuck with them.
>
> **Therapist:** Is this a good place to stop?
>
> **Maya:** Yes.

Maya's puppet work indicated mourning for her sociable past, fear of the present, and anger at the pandemic. The therapist allowed her to grieve for lost connections (e.g., grandparents, friends, activities, perhaps being "the baby of the family"), be angry with COVID, and revisit the security she depicted as hiding to have fun safely.

Using puppets, Maya projected, accessed, and processed feelings by imagining and enacting times she felt safe, angry, sad, and hopeful. While difficult topics often made her talk in a younger-sounding voice, she described puppet work as "relaxing" and "fun" and conveyed surprisingly profound points.

If this session had not relieved some tension with siblings over masking, and if Maya had agreed, a later session might include them and/or her parents. This technique readily accommodates family work. A suitable prompt for Maya's family could be "Pick a puppet for how each of you is feeling about wearing masks in the house." Each could take turns "being" their chosen puppet, and the puppets could engage in dialogue. Each member of the family would likely feel safer sharing their points of view as puppets rather than as themselves.

Suggestions for Follow-Up

Therapists may take screenshots or record evolving puppet shows for use in future sessions. Clients may review work done in previous sessions, continue processing, add to the story or scene, or alter it in ways that may represent change in their own narratives.

Contraindications

Though therapy must take place on a HIPAA-consistent platform, onlinepuppets.org is not HIPAA consistent, which may leave created scenes accessible to others. While the scene itself does not contain verbal information, it may show private content, and some clients may be uncomfortable using an online platform that is not HIPAA consistent. This activity may also be inappropriate for clients in unsafe households (Smith et al., 2021).

References

Bernier, M. (2005). Introduction to puppetry in therapy. In M. Bernier & J. O'Hare (Eds.), *Puppetry in education and therapy: Unlocking doors to the mind and heart* (pp. 127–134). Authorhouse.

Fried, K. (2023). How the Oaklander model sparked a global community of therapists in a pandemic, and enriched training and treatment. *Psychotherapie-Wissenschaft, 13*(1), 59–69. https://doi.org/10.30820/1664-9583-2023-1-59

Gallo-Lopez, L. (2005). Drama therapy with adolescents. In L. Gallo-Lopez & C. E. Schaefer (Eds.), *Play therapy with adolescents* (pp. 81–95). Jason Aronson.

Measelle, J. R., Ablow, J. C., Cowan, P. A., & Cowan, C. P. (1998). Assessing young children's views of their academic, social, and emotional lives: An evaluation of the self-perception scales of the Berkeley puppet interview. *Child Development, 69*(6), 1556–1576. https://doi.org/10.2307/1132132

Oaklander, V. (1978). *Windows to our children: A Gestalt therapy approach to children and adolescents*. Real People Press.

Smith, T., Norton, A. M., & Marroquin, L. (2021). Virtual family play therapy: A clinician's guide to using directed family play therapy in telemental health. *Contemporary Family Therapy, 45*(1), 106–116. https://doi.org/10.1007/s10591-021-09612-7

CHAPTER 15

CHESS AND TELEMENTAL HEALTH

A STRUCTURAL THERAPY APPROACH

Amy Marschall

Materials for Therapists and Clients: Device connected to the internet with a screen large enough to play digital chess and access to the LiChess website. Laptop or desktop computer preferred.

Objective

Chess is a popular intervention for therapists who want to incorporate play-based therapy interventions because it has a set structure, adheres to a specific set of rules, and requires the use of skills that fit with many clients' treatment goals. For example, chess requires focus, planning, impulse control, decision-making, problem solving, patience, taking turns, and managing frustration. The following describes ways in which to implement chess into teletherapy sessions utilizing a structural therapy approach.

Rationale for Use

Structural therapy is considered an evidence-based approach to treatment, particularly in family therapy. It emphasizes viewing the family as a structured system, consisting of interacting relationships and patterns, power hierarchies, values, and boundaries. These structures can be healthy or unhealthy, and even healthy structures can be disrupted by transitions and changes (Minuchin, 2012). Structural family therapy helps families to change structures that no longer work for them into ones in which they no longer experience presenting problems. Through the process of restructuring, therapists help clarify boundaries, redistribute power, and realign hierarchical structures within the family (Minuchin, 1974). Though this approach is best suited for working with an entire family, its goals may be applied to working with individuals, children, and adolescents.

Chess is an excellent therapeutic intervention for individual clients ages six and up because it has a specific and predictable set of rules. Players are expected to take turns, move pieces in specific ways, and try to capture the king. Chess aligns well with the goals of structural therapy as it relates to working with an individual. Chess requires clear rules and boundaries. By playing the game of chess within the context of therapy with children and adolescents, the therapist supports them in identifying the rules and boundaries of the game and then abiding by them. Playing chess over telehealth is even more effective in this endeavor than

DOI: 10.4324/9781003289920-18

playing chess in person because diffuse boundaries are obsolete in the online implementation of the game. When playing chess in person, clients might attempt to change the hierarchical order of chess pieces and move them in ways that are against the rules of the game. When playing via an online platform, players can only move pieces in ways that follow clear boundaries or set rules, and they must wait until the other person takes their turn before moving another piece. Instead of the therapist needing to impose structure as an authority figure, they can focus on joining with clients and attending to their emotional experience while simply allowing the online platform to implement the boundaries and structure (Marschall, 2022).

Setup

There are a multitude of online platforms available for playing chess over the internet. You may use any trusted source for this activity. However, LiChess is recommended because it offers variations of traditional chess rules to keep clients engaged. Clients can also customize their board and pieces, which they often enjoy doing. The rules are coded into the platform, allowing for a clearly structured approach to the activity, and it has an undo feature that lets clients take back mistakes.

This activity works best if both the therapist and client are on laptop or desktop computers. Some telehealth platforms will pause the video function on tablets or smartphones while clients have a web browser open. Computers typically allow users to keep the video screen from teletherapy platforms visible while simultaneously seeing the web browser with the chess game on it. It is possible to use this intervention if the client is not visible and rely on verbal communication during game play. However, use your own discretion when determining if it is appropriate to conduct the intervention without being able to see the client throughout the game.

There are several variations of chess games to choose from using LiChess. Use your clinical judgment to determine whether the client chooses, you choose, or you work together to come to a mutual decision. Early in therapy, it may benefit rapport to let the client decide. On the other hand, clients who are working on issues like accepting "no" or regulating when they do not get what they want may benefit from the therapist making this decision and working through their emotional response with the therapist.

Regardless of the variation, decide whether the game will have a time limit or not. Again, you can decide on a case-by-case basis what is most appropriate. Some clients benefit from not having to adhere to a time limit. Others might need to work through anxiety about timed tasks such as scholastic testing. Imposing a time limit can create an opportunity to work through anxiety about timed tasks through in vivo exposure. However, eliminating the time limit can allow therapists to encourage clients to stop and think before making moves, creating space to practice appropriate impulse control. These choices should be informed by each client's unique needs and treatment goals. It is typically helpful to explain your reasoning to clients so that they understand and can actively participate in working toward their treatment goals.

Instructions

The following instructions provide detailed guidance in implementing the intervention.

1. ***Establish boundaries for communication during the game.*** Since the platform itself is not HIPAA consistent, clients need to understand that all communication must be through the encrypted telehealth platform and not through the chat feature on the website.

2. ***Establish rules for the game.*** The online platform will automatically establish and enforce basic rules for the game (e.g., how each piece is permitted to move). Additional rules may also be established depending on the needs of each client. The therapist can either set rules for the game by themselves

or they can work collaboratively to decide on them together. For example, if a client wants to work on their anxiety response when faced with timed tasks, the therapist might decide that turns should have a time limit. If a client is working on impulse control, the therapist might limit how many take-backs they can use to practice stopping to think before making a move. Rules should be set in ways that are both developmentally appropriate and in support of client goals. The rules set in the game create boundaries that promote clients working toward their individualized treatment goals. The following questions should be considered in determining additional rules for game play:

- What version of chess will you play?

- Will players be allowed to use takebacks? If so, how many takebacks will each player be allowed to use each game?

- Will you use a time limit? If so, what will the time limit be?

- Are players allowed to offer a draw, and under what circumstances?

- How will the client ask for help if they are feeling frustrated or need a break?

3. **Create the game.** Go to lichess.org. Click "play with a friend." Select the variation of the game that the therapist and/or client have chosen to play. Decide who will be black and who will be white or indicate that this should be randomly assigned. If you are early in treatment and want to focus on rapport, you might let the client decide. If you are working on social skills, you might have the game randomly decide to promote taking turns and coping with not always getting what you want.

4. **Send link.** Once the game has been created, copy the link provided on the website and send the link to clients using the chat function available in the HIPAA-consistent teletherapy platform. The link can also be emailed to clients at the start of the session if clients have consented to email communication.

5. **Start the game.** Upon receipt of the link, the therapist and client should enter a private game room from each of their respective devices that are concurrently being used for the therapy session. When clients enter the game room on their browser, the game starts automatically.

6. **Play the game.** Play by the rules established by the platform based on the variation you chose. The platform has rules coded in, and you can view your options for any piece by clicking on it. It will only allow you to choose "legal" moves within the game, so the therapist does not have to teach clients how to play the game. Process emotions and themes as they come up, narrate the client's problem solving and emotional reactions, and check in on how they are processing the game in real time.

7. **Replay the game.** If the game finishes before session time is up, the game can be played again either in the same format or by playing a different variation of the game. Clients who need novelty to sustain attention might benefit from changing the version after each round to keep them interested, but clients working on building problem-solving skills might benefit from doing the same version multiple times so they can practice this skill.

Processing

Because this intervention can be used with a variety of presenting symptoms, specific reflections and processing questions will vary depending on the client's specific needs. In general, monitor clients' emotional responses throughout game play and bring them to their attention for processing.

Emotion processing questions can include:

- How are you feeling right now?

- It looks to me like you might feel [anger/sadness/frustration/excitement/nervousness] based on your [facial expression/tone of voice/hand gestures/word choice]. Is that accurate?

- What happened for you when I captured your piece?

- What happened for you when you captured my piece?

- What are you focusing on as we play? What feelings come up for you as you focus on that area?

If clients express big feelings in response to losing, you can ask the following questions:

- How are you feeling right now?

- What comes into your mind when you lose?

- What does it mean for you when you lose the game?

- What's another time you can think of that you have felt this way?

You can narrate client problem solving by pointing out when they are stopping to think before taking a turn or pointing out that they are fixing a mistake when they propose a takeback. Below are possible questions to parallel the skills learned in the game with the client's life outside of session:

- Can you think of a time you made a mistake and had to fix it?

- What is another problem you solved recently?

When you use a takeback, you might reflect or ask:

- I think I made a mistake. I'd like to try to fix it.

- When was a time someone else made a mistake and you helped them?

- How does it feel to see an adult make a mistake and then fix it?

When applying structural theory, the following questions might be asked by applying the game of chess as a metaphor for the family:

- In the game of chess, there are clear rules. What rules do you have in your family? What happens if you break a rule?

- Are takebacks allowed in your family? What happens if you or someone else makes a mistake?

- The queen is the most powerful piece in the game of chess. Who in your family is most like the queen?

- Pawns can sometimes be promoted to a queen. Have you ever changed roles in your family? How did that happen?

- Everyone is always trying to catch the king. Who in your family is most like the king?

Vignette

Matt is a seven-year-old Native American boy who entered foster care at six months of age and was adopted at age one. He was born on his tribe's reservation and has lived in a small town outside of Sioux Falls, South Dakota, since he was taken into care. Matt's adoptive parents are both White but have kept in contact with extended biological family so that Matt is exposed to his culture, knows some words in his tribal language, and is able to participate in his tribal religion.

At approximately age four or five, Matt was diagnosed with oppositional defiant disorder (ODD). When he presented for therapy services, the therapist conducted a reevaluation considering Matt's early developmental trauma and the prevalence of children of color being misdiagnosed with ODD by White providers (Potter et al., 2014). Reevaluation was not consistent with ODD, so Matt was evaluated for depression, anxiety, and possible trauma.

Structural therapy is effective with many populations and presenting problems, including families undergoing transitions and changes (e.g., adoption), making it an appropriate approach for Matt's therapy (Jiménez et al., 2019).

Matt was slow to build trust with his therapist and exhibited a strong need for control in sessions. The therapist used nondirective play to empower him and build trust. However, he continued to struggle with severe meltdowns both at home and at school several times per week, and he was not able to engage in skill practice due to this need for control. Meltdowns included yelling, throwing toys, sometimes breaking them, making statements including, "I hate you," and curling up in the corner for up to two hours.

Matt was receptive to directive play interventions in the form of online games, and so the therapist introduced the game of chess. While he sometimes struggled to talk directly about emotions and challenges, he engaged in play activities with set rules and explored boundaries and emotions in this way. Games created a low-stress environment that allowed Matt to have fun and play in his therapy sessions while exploring triggers for frustration.

Though Matt had not played chess before using it in his telehealth sessions, the game's built-in rules allowed him to quickly learn how each piece moved and how to play the game. At first, he lost several games, creating an opportunity to process his frustration with the game and with the therapist in real time. He made moves quickly and sometimes did not pause to see where the therapist moved before choosing his piece.

For example, after Matt made quick, impulsive moves, the therapist would pause and reflect the move verbally (i.e., "I see you moved the pawn"). This cued Matt to notice and reflect on his choice. Sometimes, he would say, "Oh, I didn't mean to," and request a takeback. In this way, the activity helped him stop, think, and regulate impulses.

Matt's impulsive choices in the game mirrored impulsivity seen by his parents and teachers. Additionally, the boundaries in the game reflected boundaries his parents set in their household. As Matt learned to regulate, he used this skill outside of therapy sessions, allowing him to recognize and respect boundaries in the household and self-correct behaviors.

Over time, Matt slowed down. He used the takeback feature to see where he had made mistakes and to try something else. He and the therapist processed how it felt for him when he made a mistake versus how it felt for him knowing he had the option to fix it. For example, if the therapist captured Matt's queen, he would take back a few moves and explore the choices he made that left the queen vulnerable and tried different strategies to better protect that piece.

Matt shared that he enjoyed playing chess with the therapist, which kept him connected and focused in the session and allowed him to process emotion and adhere to structure in a way that felt safe and comfortable for him. He built skills that his adoptive parents reported observing between sessions, including waiting his turn, thinking before acting, and accepting gentle corrections without having a meltdown. For example, he was able to take turns with a sibling in play rather than directing the sibling's choices in their games, and he would take breaks with prompting from his parent rather than becoming agitated, yelling, and throwing things.

In this way, the directive, rules-based chess activity in therapy sessions taught Matt to adjust his behaviors and change family dynamics outside of the online therapy space. He was able to honor appropriate boundaries and better express when he needed clarification and support.

After several sessions focused on playing chess, Matt won several games. He was able to compare this to learning to read, which had been a struggle for him. He noted that a certain book that was difficult for him at first got easier after he practiced several times, much like he was able to win the chess game after several games. This showed Matt that he could do difficult things with perseverance, practice, and support, which he was able to apply elsewhere in his life.

The LiChess platform allowed Matt's therapist to implement structural therapy in his sessions without triggering a power struggle or taking away Matt's need for control. He was able to experience clear rules and boundaries and understand his place in the structure. This allowed him to practice skills in real time and work through strong emotions in a safe and fun environment.

Suggestions for Follow-Up

Because the LiChess platform has several variations of traditional chess games, clients can play the same game in new ways over several sessions. This helps clients sharpen the skills they are working on in new ways and keeps the activity exciting for long-term clients.

Chess is a difficult game that takes a lot of practice. If clients are engaged in the game over several sessions, let them know that you have noticed the progress that they are making and point out if they show improved strategy or problem-solving skills. For example, you might tell clients that you see them doing something challenging and getting better at it and ask them about other hard things they have been able to figure out with practice.

Possible follow-up questions could include:

- Can you think of another time that something was very difficult for you, but with hard work, you got better at it?

- What is something that is difficult for you now that it has been hard to work on to improve?

- How does it feel when it seems like the hard thing will never seem easier?

- How does it feel when the hard thing gets easier with practice?

- What helped you when you were struggling with the game that allowed you to keep trying?

- How could we implement those things in other parts of your life?

Therapists may also follow up by collaborating with other members of the family and discussing parallels between the game of chess and structure within the family. For example, the therapist might engage in the structural intervention of family mapping to identify hierarchies, roles, and relationships within the family by asking "If each member of the family was a chess piece, what piece would they be (i.e., pawn, rook, knight, bishop, queen, king) and why?" Family rules could be discussed by explaining, "In the game of chess, there are clear rules. What rules in your family are clear? What rules might not be so clear?"

Contraindications

The LiChess platform for chess is not HIPAA consistent. Although rooms are private, they are not encrypted. In theory, this means that a third party could join the room and observe the game. If the therapist and client communicate through a HIPAA-consistent platform, the observer would only see that two people are playing chess together and would not know that it was a therapy session, the identity of either player, or the nature of any discussion. Because of this, make sure that clients understand to keep all conversations in the telehealth platform and do not use chat functions available on any external website, such as the LiChess platform. Additionally, let legal guardians know you are using this activity for therapy.

If clients join session from school or another setting with internet filters, the LiChess platform might be blocked. In this case, if your teletherapy platform allows screen sharing, search for "two-player chess" through a search engine and find a version of the game that allows both players to join from the same device. You can then share your screen and move the client's pieces for them.

Since the LiChess platform shows the options for how each piece can move, extensive knowledge of the game is not necessary. However, it helps for the therapist to have at least a basic knowledge of the chess game. You can teach clients how to play as part of their session. As long as they can grasp the rules of the game, they do not need to come to the session already knowing how to play chess.

Chess involves complex and specific rules for play. Clients who are developmentally unable to comprehend and follow these rules are not appropriate for this activity. This is a two-player game, so it will usually not work for family or group settings. However, you could observe while the client plays chess with a parent or sibling and narrate themes, process emotions, and guide communication between the two players without directly playing the game. Alternatively, families could create a team to play against the therapist and collaboratively decide which moves to make.

References

Jiménez, L., Hidalgo, V., Baena, S., León, A., & Lorence, B. (2019). Effectiveness of structural-strategic family therapy in the treatment of adolescents with mental health problems and their families. *International Journal of Environmental Research and Public Health, 16*(7), 1255. https://doi.org/10.3390/ijerph16071255

Marschall, A. (2022). *Telemental health with kids toolbox: 102 games, play and art activities, sensory and movement exercises, and talk therapy interventions*. PESI Publishing.

Minuchin, S. (1974). *Families and family therapy*. Harvard University Press.

Minuchin, S. (2012). *Structural family therapy*. Routledge.

Potter, N. N., Kincaid, H., & Sullivan, J. A. (2014). Oppositional defiant disorder: Cultural factors that influence interpretations of defiant behavior and their social and scientific consequences. In H. Kincaid & J. Sullivan (Eds.), *Classifying psychopathology: Mental kinds and natural kinds*. MIT Press. https://doi.org/10.7551/mitpress/8942.003.0010

CHAPTER 16

THE SOLUTION-FOCUSED SCAVENGER HUNT

Jacob Priest

Materials for Therapists and Clients: None.

Objective

This chapter describes a therapeutic activity aimed to help children, adolescents, and families find solutions that are already available to them in their home. Through this activity, clients can begin to envision a future in which the problem that brought them to therapy is less prominent or no longer present. If the therapist guides clients through a scavenger hunt, they can begin to realize that the solutions they need are already present; they just need to discover them.

Rationale for Use

Solution-focused therapy is a postmodern psychotherapy model that is practical, positive, and empowering. The goal of this model is to help clients identify their strengths and resources to create meaningful solutions to their problems. This is done by recognizing and amplifying solutions that are already present in their life (De Shazer et al., 2021). There is evidence for the effectiveness of this model (e.g., Gingerich & Peterson, 2013; Kim, 2008), and its application to telehealth is beginning to be explored (Finlayson et al., 2023; Hurford, 2021). One of the most common interventions used in solution-focused therapy is the miracle question. Like the model, this intervention has evidence to support its use (e.g., Nau & Shilts, 2000; Weatherall & Gibson, 2015). With a few changes to the typical approach of the miracle question, this intervention can be effective via telehealth. One possible adaptation that therapists can use is the solution-focused scavenger hunt.

The solution-focused scavenger hunt is a variation of the miracle question that allows therapists and clients to explore solutions that are already present within the home, bring them into the teletherapy session, and discuss ways in which they are possible solutions. In implementing this intervention, the therapist asks some form of the miracle question, but instead of asking clients what they would notice in response to a miracle that occurred overnight, they are encouraged to explore their home to find something that would represent the change that occurred. The therapist provides time for them to go throughout their home to find things that represent the miracle and invites them to bring any tangible items that they find into the

DOI: 10.4324/9781003289920-19

virtual therapy room to discuss them. This activity helps clients refocus on solutions to problems that they may be overlooking and presents them with the opportunity to shift from problem-focused talk to solution-focused talk.

Setup

No setup is necessary for this intervention.

Instructions

The solution-focused scavenger hunt takes place in three steps: (1) introduction, (2) scavenger hunt, and (3) encouraging exploration and change.

1. ***Introduce the activity.*** Before asking the miracle question, it is important to get buy-in from the client(s). This can be done by asking something like, "Would it be okay if I asked you a bit of a silly question?" This allows them to consider their willingness to try something different and helps to assess whether it is an appropriate time to ask the miracle question. If they agree, you can ask the miracle question. This may sound something like, "Imagine that tonight, while you are asleep, a miracle occurs, and [the issue that brought them to therapy] has been solved completely. But nobody knows that this miracle has occurred. What things would you notice that would help you realize that this miracle occurred? What might you notice around your home that clues you into the fact that this miracle occurred?" Then, provide time for each person to discuss and respond to this question. Encourage more details and richer descriptions of those things that would tip them off to the fact that the miracle occurred.

2. ***Hunt for solutions.*** Using the discussion of the miracle as a jumping-off point, you may say something like, "Would it be okay to take this silly question a bit further?" If they agree, then introduce the scavenger hunt by saying something like, "I'd like you to stand up and begin to search around your home for objects that you think would help you realize that this miracle occurred. I want you to take five or ten minutes and find at least one but maybe two or three items around your home that you think would help you realize that this miracle occurred." When working with more than one person, help them to identify a timekeeper, and ask this person to set an alarm to notify them when it is time to return to the device that is being used for teletherapy. If clients are using a mobile device, they may even take you with them during the hunt. Then, allow time for them to explore and find objects around their home.

3. ***Encourage change and exploration.*** Once clients have returned with their objects, ask them to describe what they found and how this links to the indication that the miracle had occurred overnight. Ask follow-up questions about these items and extract more details about each one. Then ask them to discuss how these items relate to what they discussed in the introduction step of this intervention. The goal is to help clients see the connection between what they might notice in their relationships and how that relates to the objects that they found. With this information, the therapist and clients set small goals that use the objects that were found to help them reach these goals.

Processing

The following questions can be used to help clients process this activity and work toward making tangible steps in achieving their miracle:

- When you look at the object that [you/name of another person] found, what surprised you about the object? How would you see this object as part of the miracle that occurred?

- Do you see any connection between the object you found and the object [name of another family member] found? How might this connection help you realize that the miracle occurred?

- If this miracle had occurred, how would you use the object you found in unique ways? How would your day-to-day use of this object change? How would you feel about this change?

- On a scale from 1 to 10, with 1 meaning you have no clue that the miracle happened and 10 being you are 100% certain the miracle happened, how much of a clue is the object you found? How about the object that [name of another person] found? What would need to happen to make this object change from a [the number provided] to a [a number a half a point or full point higher than the number provided]? How would other people's objects help make that happen?

Vignette

Tyrone (38), Molly (38), and their son, Daniel (11), came to therapy because Daniel had been refusing to go to school. During the COVID-19 pandemic, Daniel had done school online, but when classes began in person again, Daniel started to have anxiety about attending school. In his first year back in the classroom, the anxiety was present but manageable. Daniel would go to class but would complain or get upset every morning before school. After summer break, the refusals really began. Daniel would scream and yell and refuse to get on the bus or out of the car when his parents tried to drop him off. Tyrone and Molly shared that they felt totally defeated and like they had tried everything to get Daniel to school.

During the second teletherapy session, the therapist said, "I have a rather weird question to ask you all. Is it okay if I ask a weird question? Let's say that tonight, when you go to sleep, a miracle happens. All of the fear, stress, and anxiety about going to school magically disappears. But nobody knows that this miracle has happened. When you wake up the next morning, the stress of going to school is gone, but nobody knows that yet. What would be one thing that you notice that would start to tip you off that this miracle occurred? What would be something that you would notice that would get you saying, 'something is different now'?"

Molly was the first to reply, saying that getting Daniel up and to breakfast would be easy. She shared that when she woke him up, they would both feel relaxed, and she might even lie down next to him and talk a bit about what he was excited about. Tyrone said that he would notice that his stress level was down. He would be calmer and not be preparing for Daniel to get upset. Daniel said that he didn't know, and when the therapist tried to prompt him, he didn't engage any further.

The therapist then asked Daniel, "I wonder if there is a different way we could all answer this question. Daniel, do you think you could find an object in your house – anything really – that would help you know that this miracle happened? Do you think you could walk around the house with your mom and dad and find things that might give you a clue that this miracle took away all the stress?" Daniel agreed. The therapist and the family worked together to determine who would be the timekeeper and settled on Daniel. Then, Daniel, Molly, and Tyrone all got up and began searching. After five minutes were up, Daniel came back with a soccer ball and his backpack; Molly brought a box of cereal; and Tyrone brought his car keys.

The therapist and the family talked about each of the items and what they represented. Daniel talked about how the only thing he liked about school was playing soccer. When he played soccer, he had a lot of fun and didn't feel worried. Daniel also said that typically, when he packed his backpack, that was when he started to feel scared. He said that if the miracle really did happen, he wouldn't be scared when he started packing his backpack. Molly tied her object into what she had discussed before. She talked about if the miracle occurred, she and Daniel would have more fun around breakfast. Instead of it being a time when everyone was on edge, she would enjoy her morning coffee and be able to talk with Daniel about school while he ate his cereal. Tyrone talked about the keys and said that he is typically the one who drives Daniel to school. He talked about how if the miracle occurred, he would feel relaxed and excited to take Daniel to school, knowing that they would have time for just the two of them to talk. The therapist then asked the family to make connections between the objects and how they might work together to clue the family in even more that the miracle had occurred. As the conversation switched from problems to solutions, the therapist and the family set small goals together that focused on making the mornings more about connection than stress.

Suggestions for Follow-Up

The solution-focused scavenger hunt may be best used during the beginning of therapy as a way to shift clients' perspectives from a problem focus to a solution focus. Therapists may find it useful when clients get stuck to go back to the miracle question and scavenger hunt and ask them to find additional items that might represent clues of the miracle. The therapist may also tie the objects that are found at different times together in ways that produce potentially even more solutions. For example, if Daniel found a soccer ball the first time and his soccer cleats the second time, the therapist and the family may talk about how these objects might work together to tell us more about the miracle.

Contraindications

Assess the safety of all members involved before doing the solution-focused scavenger hunt. To focus only on solutions when there may be current or past emotional, verbal, or physical abuse or neglect may feed into a pattern of avoiding discussion of these issues. What's more, if clients have identified a pattern of abuse or neglect, and if this is occurring in the home, it may not be appropriate to ask clients to do a scavenger hunt in the home.

The miracle question can be difficult when clients aren't ready to move to solutions. In this case, it may be better to view the miracle question as an assessment tool. For example, if you ask the miracle question and most or all members of the client system seem unwilling or unable to engage in the question, you may want to discuss with them what makes it so difficult to come up with the things that would let them know that a miracle occurred. You may return to the miracle question later to reassess if they are ready to move toward solutions.

Finally, it is important to be aware of the developmental and cognitive abilities of each client. If age or other factors make it difficult to engage with the miracle question, this intervention may not be appropriate in this context.

References

De Shazer, S., Dolan, Y., Korman, H., Trepper, T., McCollum, E., & Berg, I. K. (2021). *More than miracles: The state of the art of solution-focused brief therapy*. Routledge.

Finlayson, B. T., Jones, E., & Pickens, J. C. (2023). Solution focused brief therapy telemental health suicide intervention. *Contemporary Family Therapy, 45*(1), 49–60. https://doi.org/10.1007/s10591-021-09599-1

Gingerich, W. J., & Peterson, L. T. (2013). Effectiveness of solution-focused brief therapy: A systematic qualitative review of controlled outcome studies. *Research on Social Work Practice, 23*(3), 266–283. https://doi.org/10.1177/1049731512470859

Hurford, D. K. (2021). Creative approaches in solution-focused teletherapy: A COVID-19 renaissance man. *Journal of Systemic Therapies, 40*(1), 21–35. https://doi.org/10.1521/jsyt.2021.40.1.21

Kim, J. S. (2008). Examining the effectiveness of solution-focused brief therapy: A meta-analysis. *Research on Social Work Practice, 18*(2), 107–116. https://doi.org/10.1177/1049731507307807

Nau, D. S., & Shilts, L. (2000). When to use the miracle question: Clues from a qualitative study of four SFBT practitioners. *Journal of Systemic Therapies, 19*(1), 129–135. https://doi.org/10.1521/jsyt.2000.19.1.129

Weatherall, A., & Gibson, M. (2015). "I'm going to ask you a very strange question": A conversation analytic case study of the miracle technique in solution-based therapy. *Qualitative Research in Psychology, 12*(2), 162–181. https://doi.org/10.26686/wgtn.14344025.v1

CHAPTER 17

TELETHERAPY POETRY

Tiffany Alexis Leal, Molly P. Downes, and Rebecca A. Cobb

Materials for Therapists and Clients: A collaborative whiteboard function on a HIPAA-consistent teletherapy platform, PowerPoint, or another program that allows for the creation of text boxes that can be saved and then rearranged.

Objective

Poetry has been used in therapeutic settings to help children and adolescents identify and express a full range of thoughts, feelings, and experiences. The following offers instructions on how to conduct a poetry intervention via teletherapy to support younger clients who may lack the structural, organizational, and verbal skills to compose a poem by themselves. The intervention supports clients in creating poetry by supplying them with words that they can then simply select and arrange into a poem in support of externalizing presenting problems. This alleviates the need for clients to come up with words on their own while still allowing them to express themselves through written word in a teletherapy setting.

Rationale for Use

Narrative therapy is grounded in the idea that the stories we tell about ourselves and that others tell about us shape the way we make meaning in our lives. It also influences the way individuals and families organize their experiences and memories of their lives in narrative form (Corey, 2013; Mehl-Madrona & Mainguy, 2015). Narrative therapists aim to assist clients in creating meaning from stories they share and assist clients with identifying painful, problematic narratives. Using a posture of curiosity and open-mindedness, the therapist supports clients in deconstructing a problem-saturated narrative and guides clients to create an alternative narrative that aligns with their preferred outcome. One narrative therapy technique that helps in meeting this objective is to externalize the problem. Externalization allows clients to differentiate and separate themselves from the problem (Gehart, 2016). This affords clients the objectivity to retell or reexamine the dominant story that has caused them pain or distress, fight against it, and create a new, preferred story in which the externalized problem is no longer the main character in charge of their life (Gehart, 2016). The fruit of this process is that the client emerges as a victor, with vivid and important stories to tell (Corey, 2013).

DOI: 10.4324/9781003289920-20

As development progresses, children become more inclined to use verbal metaphors and spoken language to create these analogies. Young children frequently express their feelings or thoughts using age-appropriate metaphors because they struggle to find a more accurate way to express deep thoughts and feelings (Mehl-Madrona & Mainguy, 2015). For example, a young child is probably more likely to say, "I feel scared, like Piglet" instead of saying, "I feel anxious, and I don't know why." Actor Patton Oswalt noted that while his daughter was processing the death of her mother, she reported to her father, "I think Sadness is doing her job right now" (Zinoman, 2016), in reference to the Disney film *Inside Out* (Docter & Del Carmen, 2015; Mehl-Madrona & Mainguy, 2015).

The use of poetry with children and adolescents in therapy has been used to promote personal growth and healing while giving voice to the meaning and transformation of client narratives (Holman, 1996; Ramsey-Wade & Devine, 2017). Poetry therapy differs from bibliotherapy and creative writing, as clients work collaboratively with the therapist in reflecting on their own writing or a published poem while therapeutically processing the material and its significance (Ramsey-Wade & Devine, 2017). In addition, a key piece to poetry therapy is the recitation of the poem through means of storytelling (Ramsey-Wade & Devine, 2017). Through the integration of poetry and narrative therapies, child and adolescent clients can express overwhelming feelings and emotions by writing poems while processing difficult narratives and externalized problems (Ramsey-Wade & Devine, 2017). In collaboratively writing poetry in therapy, child and adolescent clients are empowered to co-create new narratives and find meaning and healing through storytelling (Holman, 1996; Seiden, 2007).

Encouraging children and adolescents to create a poem about an externalized problem is a creative intervention that allows them to create their own narrative of their problems. It empowers them to take charge of the narrative and allows creative freedom to articulate their lived experience. Clients reclaim their voice when they describe their own narrative. However, some clients, especially children and adolescents, may be hesitant or feel less capable of creating their own verbal stories or poems. By helping clients to simply brainstorm words associated with their presenting problem or externalized problem and then creating text boxes using those words that clients can rearrange, verbal expression and the creation of poetry can feel easier and less intimidating to many clients. Further, therapists may select words and create prompts specifically tailored to presenting problems, developmental needs, culture, and other details that are unique to each client. Collaboration between the therapist and client's family may also allow children and adolescents to discern an alternative narrative that enriches their self-image, family relationships, and place in the world (Simons & Freedman, 2005).

This activity may be conducted with individual children and adolescents, siblings, families, or groups. It takes two sessions to prepare for and conduct the activity.

Setup

1. ***Externalize the problem.*** Work with clients to externalize their presenting problem by helping them verbally separate the presenting problem from themselves. By separating the client from the problem, you help shift the client's current narrative and perspective to see that they are not the problem. The problem is the problem.

2. ***Introduce the idea of collaboratively creating a poem about their externalized problem.*** If clients are hesitant about the idea, explain that you will help them to write the poem and that they don't need to do it on their own. Yet, poetry may not be a fitting intervention for all clients. If clients do not express interest, provide other activities as options for intervention. If clients enjoy poetry and have a history of poetry writing, they may prefer to simply write their own poem. However, even

clients who have prior experience with writing poetry may enjoy creating a poem in a new way and may be open to the activity.

3. ***Assist clients with brainstorming words and images related to the externalized problem.*** As clients share their ideas, create a written list. Prompts for this portion of the intervention may include the following:

   • What images come into your head when you think of [externalized problem]? Say anything and everything that comes to mind.

   • Engage your senses. What adjectives describe [externalized problem]? What does it look, feel, sound, taste, and smell like?

   • How do you feel when you think about [externalized problem]?

   • What happens in your body as you think about [externalized problem]?

   • What action words and verbs might be related to [externalized problem]?

   • How do you and other people respond to [externalized problem]?

   • How would you like to respond to [externalized problem]? How would you like others to respond to [externalized problem]?

   • What do you like about [externalized problem]?

   • What do you not like about [externalized problem]?

   • Does anything else come to mind as you think about [externalized problem]?

   • Are there any other words that you want to add to this list?

4. ***Transfer words to a collaborative whiteboard, PowerPoint, or another program that allows for the compilation of text boxes and images.*** Each word should be added as a separate text box so that clients can move the text around as desired. Depending on the number of words that have been listed, you may need to select the most relevant words or may need to add to the list. Additional words such as "the," "it," and "I" should also be included. You should add enough words for clients to have choices in creating their poem. Avoid including so many words that the activity feels overwhelming.

   You may also search the internet for clip art images that appear representative of key words that the client has said to include on the slide. For example, if a client were to externalize "anxiety" by calling it the "anxiety monster," you may include the words "anxiety" and "monster" on the slide. You may also include several clip art images of monsters – happy monsters, scary monsters, silly monsters, etc. This may be especially relevant for younger children and children or adolescents who are more visual processors. This step is usually best completed between sessions so you can take time to thoughtfully compose the materials.

Instructions

In the next session, do the following:

1. ***Share your screen.*** Open the document created and share your screen so that clients can see it.

2. ***Explain the activity.*** Tell clients that you have created a word bank for them. On it, they will find words that they shared in the previous session. If appropriate, also explain that you added some

additional words and/or images for use in the creation of their poem. Tell them that they may arrange the words in any order that they prefer. They can set aside any words and images that they don't want to use. They can also copy any words and images that they would like to use more than once. They can change the font, size, and color of words (if allowed by the platform being used). If images have been included, they may also arrange any images as they see fit. The poem doesn't need to take any particular shape or form unless they have something in particular that they would like to create. If, during the process, clients would like to add additional words, they may do so.

3. ***Send the clients the file or allow for collaboration on the whiteboard.*** When working with younger children, this step may be skipped if it's more appropriate for children to verbally guide you in arranging the words and images.

4. ***Introduce a prompt if desired.*** You may leave the invitation to create a poem open-ended. You may also provide a more specific prompt if you think it would be helpful. For example, you may ask clients to:

   • "Create a poem about [externalized problem]."

   • "Create a poem about when [externalized problem] comes to visit."

5. ***Invite clients to create their poem.*** Provide additional guidance as needed. Allow silence and reflections as appropriate.

6. ***Save the poem.*** Once clients have finished their poem, ask them to save it to their device. Also ask if they would be willing to share the file with you so you can save it to their file for use in future sessions. If the poem was created on your own device or via a collaborative whiteboard, save the poem to the client's file and ask if the clients would like you to share it with them. Share the file with them if requested.

7. ***Read the poem.*** Ask clients if they would like to read the poem aloud or if they would prefer that you read the poem either silently or out loud. Proceed according to the client's request. Listen with a posture of curiosity and wonder.

Processing

Once the poem has been read, you may discuss it using the following questions:

• What story does this poem tell?

• How is that story different from the story you tell yourself about the subject of the poem?

• Is there anything about the poem that you would like to change? If so, what?

• How did it feel to create the poem?

• What did it feel like to hear the poem read aloud?

• How did it feel to share the poem with someone else?

• What do you think your [family/teachers/parents/friends] would think of this poem?

• Would they learn something new about you if they read it?

• Is there anyone you would like to share the poem with?

Vignette

Anastasia (10) was in the fourth grade and presented to therapy due to difficulty transitioning to a new school. She came from a first-generation multiracial family and identified as Catholic. Her family consisted of her mother, Alessia (44), father, Kevin (43), and brother, Sebastian (14). Anastasia had been struggling with her ability to express her experience, thoughts, and emotions to her teachers and parents surrounding this new transition. As a result, Anastasia had been having difficulty at school and home with expressing and regulating emotions. Her parents reported that she had been acting out at home, not wanting to go to school, and struggling to pay attention in class. Anastasia was referred to therapy by her school. Anastasia's teachers and parents both corroborated her presenting concerns and agreed with a referral for therapy.

Anastasia presented to therapy via telehealth. In the first session, the therapist worked with Anastasia to externalize her presenting problem. Anastasia shared that she struggled to regulate her emotions at home and described frequent outbursts with her parents and brother. She expressed having frequent tummy aches and struggling in the morning to go to school due to feeling worried and nervous. The therapist externalized Anastasia's anxiety and presenting symptoms associated with it to help her separate the anxiety from herself and to fight against it. Anastasia liked the idea of referring to her anxiety as the "anxiety monster."

The therapist introduced the idea of a poetry activity in the first session after learning that Anastasia's favorite subject in school was English. The therapist introduced the idea of collaboratively creating a poem about the anxiety monster. When Anastasia expressed interest in this activity, the therapist assisted Anastasia in brainstorming words and images related to anxiety and the anxiety monster. The therapist asked Anastasia, "What images come into your head when you think of the anxiety monster? Say anything and everything that comes to mind. What does it look, feel, sound, taste, and smell like? How do you feel when you think about the anxiety monster?" At this point, Anastasia had already come up with a substantial number of words that could be used in their poem. The therapist added, "Are there any other words you want to add to this list?" Anastasia added, "rainbow," "tiger," "dinosaur," and "unicorn," which were some of her favorite things. The therapist then created a written list via the whiteboard function on Zoom, which Anastasia could view on the shared screen. This allowed Anastasia to add words and images to the whiteboard as well, though she reported being happy with the list and decided to leave it as it was. The therapist structured the words in a word bank (see Figure 17.1).

Word Bank

Anxiety	Worry	Fear	Rainbow	Life	Colors	Nervous	Stress	Tired	Lucky Charm
The	It	I	A	Hide	Tummy Ache	Monster	Big	Happy	Potion
Scary	Scared	Run away	Jittery	Cry	Yell	Hug	Love	Comfort	Magic
Unicorn	Sunshine	Bloom	Joy	Stardust	Tiger	Mouse	Small	Fairy	Pixiedust
Brave	Magical	Strong	Rocketship	Dinosaur	Pirate	Peace	Hope	Caring	Inspire

Figure 17.1 Word bank.

Anastasia's Poem

The Small Mouse was Scared and Ran Away.

It had A Tummy Ache and Jitters that didn't want to go away.

The Small Mouse was Nervous and Worried and Hid in Fear.

The Small Mouse said The Anxiety Monster is here.

One day the Small Mouse meets a Fairy.

She offers her Magic Stardust to help her become Brave and merry.

The Small Mouse uses it to become Big and Strong.

The Mouse is able to overcome the Monster and call it out when it's wrong.

The Mouse was Happy to find Magical Stardust to use if the Monster ever comes along.

Figure 17.2 Example poem.

In the next session, the therapist shared their screen, displaying the word bank created on the Zoom whiteboard from the last session. The therapist explained the activity to Anastasia and invited her to write a poem about her anxiety and the symptoms she experienced as a result. The therapist explained that she could drag the words down from the word bank to make the poem below. She could use any words in the creation of her poem as she saw fit. She could even add new words or edit existing ones. She could also copy words and paste them if she wanted to use the same word more than once. The therapist allowed Anastasia time to write her poem and provided support and guidance as needed, though Anastasia took well to the activity and didn't need much help.

Once Anastasia finished her poem (see Figure 17.2), the therapist asked her if she would like to read it out loud or if she preferred for the therapist to read it quietly or out loud. Anastasia said that she wanted to read it out loud to the therapist, and she did so enthusiastically.

Then, the therapist processed the poem and its creation with Anastasia. The therapist asked Anastasia to share what story this poem tells. Anastasia shared that the story was about how she feels when the "anxiety monster" comes to visit her. The therapist worked with Anastasia on processing the emotions the small mouse felt when the "anxiety monster" was near. Anastasia was effectively able to reflect on these emotions and identified how they showed up for her at school and home.

The therapist invited Anastasia to share this poem with her family. Anastasia agreed, and her family was invited to join the next session. Anastasia shared the poem with her family in session, with the support of the therapist. The therapist invited Anastasia and her family into a conversation about how this activity helped Anastasia in identifying and processing her emotions related to anxiety. The therapist then supported the family in making a plan on what to do when the "anxiety monster" appears again.

Suggestions for Follow-Up

In future sessions, clients can create a new poem using the same list of words but with a new prompt. For example, if the initial prompt was to "Create a poem about when [externalized problem] comes to visit," a prompt in a subsequent session may be to "Create a poem about the defeat of [externalized problem]." Alternatively, a new list of words may be created in a subsequent session, and the two poems may be compared to examine changes in the client's narrative.

Contraindications

If you think this intervention might be a good fit for a client who cannot read, you can still do the activity but would need to read the words for the client and support them more directly in the creation of the poem. You may also do a different activity while integrating the same concepts. For example, the child could engage in drawing, acting, or telling their poem/story, and you could still utilize the same processing questions and methods to reach similar results. The goal is to get the child to creatively express themselves while sharing their story and experience of the externalized problem.

By externalizing the problem-saturated narrative apart from the self of the client, the external narrative of the client's extemporaneous poetry becomes explicit. Due to this, use caution when creating poetry with clients who are processing trauma. In this case, you must support clients in developing coping mechanisms first and monitor client responses while focusing on grounding as needed. Once this step is established and an assessment of the client's responses is complete, you can proceed with attempting this intervention.

References

Corey, G. (2013). *Theory & practice of counseling & psychotherapy* (10th ed.). Brooks/Cole.

Docter, P., & Del Carmen, R. (Directors). (2015). *Inside Out* [Film]. Walt Disney Studios Motion Pictures.

Gehart, D. R. (2016). *Theory and treatment planning in family therapy: A competency-based approach*. Cengage Learning.

Holman, W. D. (1996). The power of poetry: Validating ethnic identity through a bibliotherapeutic intervention with a Puerto Rican adolescent. *Child and Adolescent Social Work Journal, 13*(5), 371–383. https://doi.org/10.1007/bf01875855

Mehl-Madrona, L., & Mainguy, B. (2015). *Remapping your mind: The neuroscience of self-transformation through story*. Bear & Company.

Ramsey-Wade, C. E., & Devine, E. (2017). Is poetry therapy an appropriate intervention for clients recovering from anorexia? A critical review of the literature and client report. *British Journal of Guidance & Counselling, 46*(3), 282–292. https://doi.org/10.1080/03069885.2017.1379595

Seiden, H. M. (2007). Using collaborative poetry in child psychotherapy: The tale of the terrible rabbit. *International Journal of Applied Psychoanalytic Studies, 4*(2), 170–184. https://doi.org/10.1002/aps.138

Simons, V. A., & Freedman, J. (2005). Witnessing bravery: Narrative ideas for working with children and families. In C. E. Bailey (Ed.), *Children in therapy: Using the family as a resource* (pp. 20–45). W. W. Norton.

Zinoman, J. (2016, October 26). Patton Oswalt: "I'll never be at 100 percent again." *The New York Times*. https://www.nytimes.com/2016/10/30/arts/patton-oswalt-ill-never-be-at-100-percent-again.html

Part 4

Adults

CHAPTER 18

TRANSFORMATIONAL TELETHERAPY CHAIRS

George A. Garcia III

Materials for Therapists: Digital images depicting chair(s) in various positions (included as supplemental materials to this book).

Materials for Clients: Chair(s) and various objects for concretization (optional).

Objective

The empty-chair technique, a hallmark of Gestalt therapy traditionally used for in-person sessions, externalizes interpersonal and internal conflict to provide clients and therapists with new perspectives and unique opportunities for growth and healing (Corey, 2012; Giacomucci, 2021). This chapter will present two different ways to conduct the empty-chair intervention via teletherapy.

Rationale for Use

The empty-chair technique is a process in which clients are invited to sit across from an empty chair and have an imaginal encounter with someone or something from the past, present, or future (Kellogg & Garcia Torres, 2021). This technique allows clients to externalize the introject, playing out all necessary parts in a dialogue to allow for more complete conflicts, acceptance, and integration (Corey, 2012). The empty chair allows people to explore themselves, both intrapersonally and interpersonally, and bring resolution to conflicts and incomplete narratives in the present moment. By becoming more fully aware of problems in the here-and-now, clients' emotional distress can be brought to resolution (Pugh, 2017). Research shows that this technique can be successfully applied across disciplines and is clinically effective in treating emotional disorders and problematic psychological processes (Greenberg & Watson, 1998; Neff et al., 2007; Pugh, 2017; Shahar et al., 2012).

Setup

The following specifies setup required of the therapist and clients to conduct two different variations of this activity. Discuss each option with clients prior to conducting the intervention to determine

DOI: 10.4324/9781003289920-22

the best fit. The first variation requires the use of an actual chair in the client's physical location. The second requires only the use of the teletherapy platform as a virtual representation of someone or something.

Physical Chairs

For the empty-chair technique using a chair in the client's physical location, instruct clients to bring an additional chair or chairs into the room where they will be during the teletherapy session. Clients can also be instructed to bring additional objects into the room that represent people, places, and things in a concrete and symbolic way (Giacomucci, 2021; Kellermann, 1992; Watersong, 2011).

Virtual Visual Representations

The teletherapy platform may also be used to display a virtual visual representation of someone or something for the activity. For this option, have pictures of chairs arranged in various positions to share with the client via the share screen function on the teletherapy platform. Several images of chairs that can be used for this activity are included with the supplemental materials that accompany this book (see Figure 18.1).

Alternatively, clients can send you a photo of the person or thing that they will be in dialogue with, and you can share this photo on their screen during the intervention. Pictures can be saved to a Word document or PowerPoint for easy access.

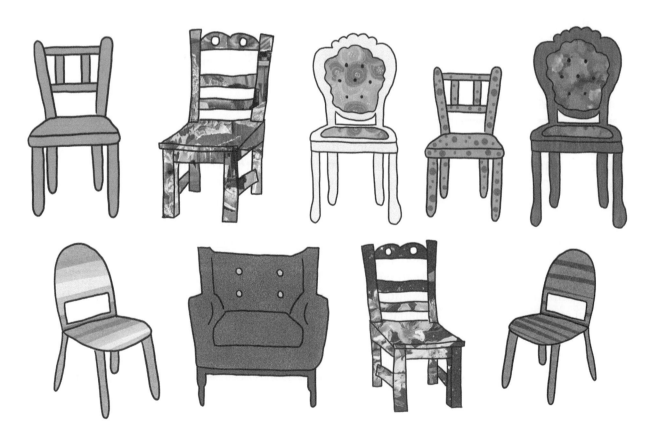

Figure 18.1 Virtual visual representations of chairs. Credit: Dr. Christine Borst.

Instructions

1. ***Introduce the intervention.*** Provide a brief description of the purpose of the empty-chair technique and its structure. It may be helpful to model parts of the exercise for the client (i.e., role reversal). The following is an example statement that can be used: "This technique helps create space for conversations to happen. Using your imagination, you will begin by placing a person or thing in the chair. Then I will help guide a conversation with you and the person or thing in the opposite chair. You may have the opportunity to role reverse and respond from the other's perspective."

2. ***Create goals.*** Collaboratively create goals for the empty-chair intervention to provide a roadmap for the exercise. Goals can be related to obstacles, people with whom they have conflict, various parts of a person, past, present, or future, and more.

3. ***Set the scene.*** If clients are using their own chairs, guide them in setting the scene by outlining the boundaries of the stage and conducting a sound check to ensure clear audio and a clear view of the client's face while they are in position to do the activity. Provide guidance as necessary to move chairs if the client's face is not visible. If the teletherapy platform is used to display a virtual representation of someone or something, support clients in choosing the image that they would like to use (i.e., chair, person, or thing) and share this image on the screen. If clients are using a physical chair and would benefit from further visualization, guide them in identifying objects to represent the person, place, or thing in the opposing chair.

4. ***Imagine a person, place, or thing.*** Instruct the client to imagine the opposing chair or image on the screen representing a person, place, or thing. For example, a client who is working to relieve themself of guilt may be told, "Imagine that heavy ball of guilt we've talked about sitting in the chair across from you."

5. ***Begin the conversation.*** Guide the client in beginning the conversation with the person, place, or thing. Encourage them to say whatever comes to mind.

6. ***Reverse roles.*** Provide the opportunity for clients to speak back to themselves as if they were the person, place, or thing with whom they were just talking. For example, the client speaking with guilt may be told, "Go ahead and switch places with guilt. As you switch, imagine that you are now guilt, thinking, feeling, acting, and speaking as guilt would." Clients using a virtual visual representation may wish to use a new image of a chair or a photograph of themselves to visually represent this change in roles.

7. ***Repeat the process.*** Guide clients in moving back and forth between chairs to reengage with the thoughts and feelings of each role.

Throughout the activity, pay attention to nonverbal cues. Changes in body language and breathing could be signs of potential dysregulation or flooding. Pause the activity if necessary. Be prepared with grounding and containment strategies and implement them as needed.

Processing

After the completion of the activity, ask process questions to discuss the client's experience. Process questions may include the following:

- Can you tell me about your overall experience of the exercise?

- What was it like to have this dialogue?

- What was it like to use different chairs to explore this inner dialogue with [person/place/thing]?

- What feelings came up for you as you spoke with [person/place/thing]?

- What was it like being [person/place/thing]? How did this feel different than when you were talking to [person/place/thing]?

- How has your experience during the exercise influenced the way you understand and relate to [person/place/thing]?

Vignette

Matt (27) and Arianna (30) are a married couple of seven years. Matt is a Hispanic, heterosexual male. Arianna is a Caucasian, heterosexual female. Matt comes from a Pentecostal background, and Arianna comes from a history rooted in Catholicism. Matt works as a medical doctor, and Arianna works as a dietician and fitness coach. The couple have struggled with male infertility for the last three years, resulting in two unsuccessful in-vitro fertilization treatments and involuntary childlessness. Matt sought treatment to address feelings of grief over their childlessness and the relational toll experienced with his wife. During early assessment, Matt identified guilt over the treatment process and childlessness that Arianna had to endure, resulting in withdrawal in his relationship and a sense of hopelessness contained by overworking himself.

The empty chair was chosen to assist Matt with his unresolved guilt. The following outlines the process that the therapist followed in conducting the empty-chair technique with Matt via a teletherapy session.

The therapist first explained the activity and offered various ways in which he could represent "guilt" (i.e., physical chair or an image). Due to space limitations in the room that he used to attend teletherapy, Matt chose to use an image of an empty chair.

The therapist discussed with Matt possible goals of the activity. Matt decided that he simply wanted to learn more about the guilt that he carried with him. He was skeptical about his ability or desire to tell it to go away.

The therapist shared an image of several empty chairs and asked Matt to choose the one that felt most fitting to him. Matt chose the image of a colorless gray-and-black chair. The scene was set by briefly introducing "guilt" sitting on the chair that had been selected.

Matt was invited to imagine "guilt," sitting in the chair depicted.

The therapist invited him to begin the conversation and observe his own response to guilt in the other chair, share about their relationship, and begin dialoguing with "guilt." The therapist helped Matt process the conversation thus far.

Therapist: What is it like to have guilt seated in this position?

Matt: It feels heavy. Like I'm holding my breath but can't exhale.

Therapist: Take a deep breath. What would you like to say to guilt, if anything?

Matt: I'm not sure.

Therapist: How does guilt make you feel?

Matt: Like I'm unworthy of Arianna. Like I'm a failure.

Therapist: Can you say that to guilt sitting there?

Matt: Sure. You make me feel so unworthy of Arianna. Like I'm the cause of all her pain. Like it's all my fault.

After this initial exchange, Matt was invited to imagine changing chairs and enact the part of guilt, connecting to its voice-tone, emotion, and motivation. Matt selected a different image of a chair to symbolize a switching of roles. This time, Matt selected a large, bluish-green, cushioned armchair. Sitting in guilt's chair, Matt was invited to respond to himself from the position of guilt and continue the inner dialogue that was now being externalized.

Therapist: Now imagine switching chairs and speaking from the position of guilt. Hearing Matt talk about feeling unworthy, how would you like to respond? What would you like Matt to know about your purpose?

Matt: That wasn't my intention. In fact, my hope was quite the opposite for you. I didn't want you to ignore your feelings and simply care for Arianna. I wanted to remind you of your feelings, hoping you would care for them as well.

Finally, Matt was invited to repeat this process, moving back and forth between the chairs to reengage with the thoughts and feelings of each role that arose during the dialogue.

Therapist: Switch chairs, returning to the role of Matt. What comes up in response for you, Matt?

Matt: I've never considered that before. I guess underneath it all, I'm just sad that we can't have the life that we wanted the way that we had originally imagined. I guess it's because of me, but it's not my fault.

Therapist: Now that you've been able to have this conversation, how would you rearrange the scene if at all?

Matt: I would move the chair to the side, maybe in back of me.

Therapist: What would you say to guilt now that you've moved it behind you?

Matt: You can coexist. You have a part in my journey. But you're not the whole story. Another one is emerging.

Suggestions for Follow-Up

In follow-up sessions, encourage continued conversation between clients and the other that they were in conversation with. Modify the pace, topic, or process as needed (Giacomucci, 2021).

Contraindications

Low ego strength and high emotional instability may lead to adverse effects as a result of conducting the empty-chair technique (Giacomucci, 2021). You must consider individual needs and abilities of clients prior to introducing the activity. This activity may also be contraindicated if you cannot maintain visuals of client nonverbal cues required to intervene in the event of flooding or dissociation.

References

Corey, G. (2012). *Theory and practice of counseling and psychotherapy*. Cengage Learning.

Giacomucci, S. (2021). *Social work, sociometry, and psychodrama: Experiential approaches for group therapists, community leaders, and social workers*. Springer Nature Singapore Pte Ltd. https://doi.org/10.1007/978-981-33-6342-7

Greenberg, L. S., & Watson, J. (1998). Experiential therapy of depression: Differential effects of client-centered relationship conditions and process experiential interventions. *Psychotherapy Research, 8*(2), 210–224. https://doi.org/10.1093/ptr/8.2.210

Kellermann, P. F. (1992). *Focus on psychodrama: The therapeutic aspects of psychodrama*. Jessica Kingsley.

Kellogg, S., & Garcia Torres, A. (2021). Toward a chairwork psychotherapy: Using the four dialogues for healing and transformation. *Practice Innovations, 6*(3), 171–180. https://doi.org/10.1037/pri0000149

Neff, K. D., Kirkpatrick, K. L., & Rude, S. S. (2007). Self-compassion and adaptive psychological functioning. *Journal of Research in Personality, 41*(1), 139–154. https://doi.org/10.1016/j.jrp.2006.03.004

Pugh, M. (2017). Chairwork in cognitive behavioural therapy: A narrative review. *Cognitive Therapy & Research, 41*(1), 16–30. https://doi.org/10.1007/s10608-016-9805-x

Shahar, B., Carlin, E. R., Engle, D. E., Hegde, J., Szepsenwol, O., & Arkowitz, H. (2012). A pilot investigation of emotion-focused two-chair dialogue intervention for self-criticism. *Clinical Psychology & Psychotherapy, 19*(6), 496–507. https://doi.org/10.1002/cpp.762

Watersong, A. (2011). Surplus reality: The magic ingredient in psychodrama. *Journal of the Australian and Aotearoa New Zealand Psychodrama Association, 20*, 18–27.

CHAPTER 19

CHANGING NARRATIVES WITH VIRTUAL VISION BOARDS

Deneisha S. Scott-Poe and Khushbu S. Patel

Materials for Therapists: PowerPoint or other software that can be used for compiling text and images, digital images (e.g., drawings, cartoons, pictures) relevant to the client's dominant story and preferred outcomes, and sample vision board (optional; included as supplemental materials to this book).

Materials for Clients: PowerPoint or other software that can be used for compiling text and images, digital images (e.g., drawings, cartoons, pictures), and/or quotes.

Objective

Vision boards have been used for in-person therapeutic assessment and intervention using physical materials available in the counselor's office (Burton & Lent, 2016). This chapter provides instructions for using virtual vision boards in teletherapy using narrative therapy as a guiding framework.

Rationale for Use

Vision boards have gained societal popularity for people of all ages and have been used as an effective intervention for children and adolescents in disciplines such as education and career counseling (Benedict, 2021; Conderman & Young, 2021; Waalkes et al., 2019). Burton and Lent (2016) describe a vision board as "a collage of images that represents the things an individual wants out of [their] life" (p. 53). In therapy, vision boards can be used to help clients identify, illustrate, and discuss concrete goals for the future (Burton & Lent, 2016; Gladding, 2008). Future goals might include what one wants to accomplish, personal changes/improvements, or skills one wants to master.

Narrative therapy (White & Epston, 1990) can be a useful model in helping clients process what they have included on vision boards. It can also help them better understand the problem-saturated narratives they have about themselves and the world around them.

Traditionally, vision boards are created using physical materials, such as paper or poster board, images from magazines, newspapers, and other sources, scissors, glue, and/or tape. Digital vision boards can also be created using computers and online resources as an invaluable therapeutic tool for teletherapy intervention.

DOI: 10.4324/9781003289920-23

Setup

To conduct this activity, ensure that clients have a computer program that allows access to PowerPoint or other software that can be used for compiling text and images.

Vision boards may be created in or between sessions. Discuss with clients their personal preference. Also consider any support that clients may need. For example, you may discuss only working on the board during sessions if the client needs extra support or is actively processing major trauma. In-session creation of vision boards can take several sessions (Burton & Lent, 2016). Though some clients may complete the task more quickly depending on their computer literacy and confidence in their goals/improvements, it is essential to allow each unique client the time and support that they need (Waalkes et al., 2019).

Instructions

1. ***Describe the therapeutic use of virtual vision boards.*** First, explain that vision boards can help clients identify and reach short- and long-term goals, such as life, career, or even vacation goals. Then explain that this is done by collecting images, words, or sayings representing their identified goal(s). These are then arranged in one place where they can be quickly referenced and viewed for inspiration as they aspire to meet those goals.

2. ***Provide an example.*** If clients are visual processors, provide a generic example to show them what a virtual vision board might look like. An example of a generic vision board might be to envision the goal of owning a llama farm, filled with images of llamas, items that might be found on a llama farm, and images of other things that might be required to achieve this goal. An example vision board related to this goal has been included with the supplemental materials that accompany this book (see Figure 19.1).

3. ***Identify goals.*** After the vision board activity has been introduced, discuss what goal(s) the clients would like their vision board to illustrate. If clients do not have a specific goal, instruct them to browse through images to see if anything inspires them. Explain that this is a future-oriented intervention and that they may use pictures from the past representing an aspect of life they want back; however, they must be prepared to discuss the connection.

4. ***Provide written instructions.*** It is helpful to have written instructions that include possible software or websites (e.g., Canva, Jamboard, PowerPoint) that clients can use to create their digital vision board. The following is an example set of instructions that can be provided to clients using Power-Point to create their vision board:

   a. Create a folder on your computer or your preferred data storage website to save images for your vision board.

   b. Search the internet for images representing your identified goal(s) using Google images, websites such as National Geographic, or relevant online magazines and newspapers. You may also take photos of things you see in real life or use images of pictures you have taken of things in the past.

   c. Save selected images by right clicking the image and selecting "save image."

   d. Open PowerPoint and select a blank presentation when prompted.

   e. Copy the images from your file folder, paste them onto your blank PowerPoint page, and arrange them however you want. You may need to resize images to make sure they can all fit.

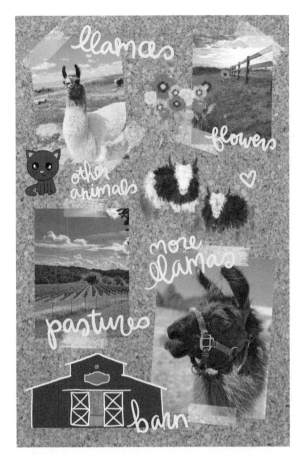

Figure 19.1 Sample vision board. Credit: Dr. Christine Borst.

    f. When you are finished, click the floppy disk icon at the top of the screen to save your vision board.

    g. Save the vision board under a name that will be easy to identify and put it in a location that can be easily accessed during the next therapy session.

5. ***Provide support as needed.*** Clients may require varying levels of support and guidance through the vision board–creation process. Comfortability can be based on factors such as familiarity with the software, experience navigating the internet, and the ability to process and complete new activities. Watch for signs that clients may be struggling with a step in creating their vision board. Client distress may require you to do the activity with the client. For example, a client might need support in determining what goal(s) they would like to illustrate on the vision board, or they may have difficulty finding pictures that connect to their goals. Offer any support needed by providing examples of goals relevant to the goals of treatment, sending links to pages with relevant images via the chat function in your teletherapy platform, or even having the client guide you in creating the vision board for them while using the share-screen function.

6. ***Discuss.*** Once a goal and associated images have been collected, begin a conversation by asking clients to discuss the images and any text that they might have included on their vision board. If this activity is completed in session, have clients arrange images and quotes on their virtual board as they discuss their thoughts and emotions related to their therapeutic problem.

7. ***Continue and/or complete the project as needed.*** Offer the opportunity for clients to complete any remaining details on their vision boards outside of therapy and share the finished product in a subsequent session.

Processing

Narrative therapy is a systemic therapeutic model that can be helpful as clients process their vision boards. Meaning making is one of the central concepts in narrative therapy, so a large part of the processing will be extending the foundational concepts of the theory. The use of language and the internalization of negative attributes are central to narrative therapy (White & Epston, 1990). In turn, clients use language to construct typically negative stories or problem-saturated narratives of themselves and the world (Etchison & Kleist, 2000). Through the lens of this therapy model, clients often see the continuation of their problems as personal failures or some personal flaw (Etchison & Kleist, 2000). When discussing client-presenting problems, "Problems may not be seen by [clients] as external events that affect and influence their lives and, thus, are maintained. Narrative therapy deals specifically with these stories as the loci of effective therapeutic goal setting" (Etchison & Kleist, 2000, p. 61). Using externalization, clients can create change in their lives because they begin to view the problem as separate from themselves. This way of processing helps to change the problem-saturated story to the preferred narrative, which are the images and quotes that clients place on their vision board.

While processing the activity, thicken the plot and identify unique outcomes by exploring how the images and quotes on the vision board relate to the client's goals for their life. This may also help clients as they work to construct their preferred narratives. Helping clients construct their preferred narratives is an opportunity to help the client combat their problem-saturated narrative and negative self-talk about their ability to achieve their goals. Ask about what meaning they draw from the vision board and how that meaning fits into the current narrative of their experiences. It is also helpful to ask about the differences between the current problem-saturated narrative and the person they envision having what is displayed on their vision board. Possible questions that may address these processes include the following.

Thickening the Plot

- What was it like for you to create this vision board?

- What is it like for you to look at your completed vision board?

- When choosing different images and/or quotes on your vision board, how did you decide what to include?

- When creating your board, what considerations did you make regarding your family, friends, co-workers, etc.?

- How might your family/loved ones respond to the images/quotes you included on your board?

Preferred Story and Unique Outcomes

- What timeframe of your life does your vision board represent?

- Tell me more about this specific image or saying. How does it relate to your goals?

- What does this image or saying represent to you?

- How do these images relate to you and your life story or to what you want for your future?

- I know that we've talked about _____ in the past. What impact does that problem/issue have on your relationships with others? How is that different from what you are depicting on your vision board?

- What does this image or vision board tell you about yourself that you otherwise would not have known?

Outsider Witnessing

Therapists and clients might also choose to create and process vision boards with other members of the client's system. When clients create their own vision boards simultaneously in session, or have others present during the creation of their own vision board, ask questions focused on the differing perspectives held by outsider witnesses or other members of the system. For example:

- What was it like to see _____ create their vision board?
- What is it like to hear _____ talk about the items in their vision board?
- How did it make you feel when _____ described the images and/or quotes on their vision board?
- How might your vision board differ from _____'s?
- What similarities do you see between _____'s vision board and your own?

The following vignette provides an example of using digital vision boards as a narrative therapy intervention when working with a couple.

Vignette

Brian (68) and Samantha (66) live in Nashville, Tennessee. Both have recently retired from their respective jobs as an engineer and middle school English teacher. Brian is a heterosexual, White male who does not practice religion. Samantha is a heterosexual, biracial female (Haitian and White) who recently returned to Catholicism. Both are college graduates. They have three children. Amy is a 37-year-old engineer. June is a 33-year-old school-based counselor. Josh is a 22-year-old recent graduate with a bachelor's degree in marketing. Brian and Samantha are saving up for a once-in-a-lifetime vacation that they have been looking forward to for years. However, Josh's move across the country to California to begin a job as a marketing intern for a start-up nonprofit has caused many issues between Brian and Samantha. Samantha supports Josh's new chapter, but Brian is disappointed and unsure of Josh's future.

The difference in emotions between the couple continues to cause arguments. During their fourth session, the therapist introduced the vision board activity to the couple. The therapist informed the clients of the purpose of the vision board, which was to help them reach their goal of communicating better and being able to go on their once-in-a-lifetime vacation. The therapist described the steps to create the vision board. Because Brian and Samantha had never before created a vision board, the therapist showed them an example of one so they could get a visual idea of what a digital vision board might look like.

Additionally, the therapist informed the clients that they were free to include anything they wanted on their vision board as long as it related to their decided goal. The therapist gave the couple 30 minutes to create their vision boards separately. At the end of the session, the therapist told the clients to finish their vision boards outside of therapy and to come prepared to share them in the next session.

In the couple's fifth session, the therapist asked Brian and Samantha to share their vision boards. Brian's vision board had pictures of him and Samantha before they had children, beach and ocean photos, activities the couple did together in the past, such as swimming with stingrays and skydiving, and an old picture of him teaching Josh how to throw a baseball (see Figure 19.2). Samantha's vision board included pictures of

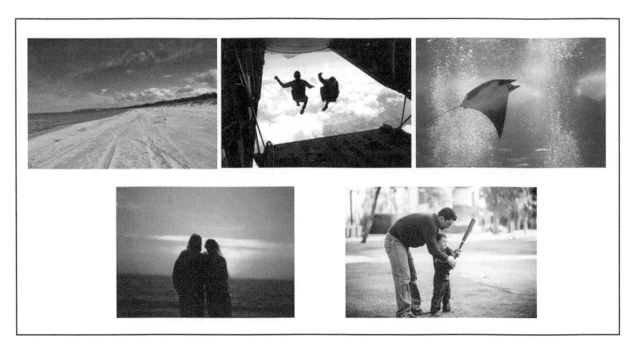

Figure 19.2 Brian's vision board. Credit for photos: Unsplash.

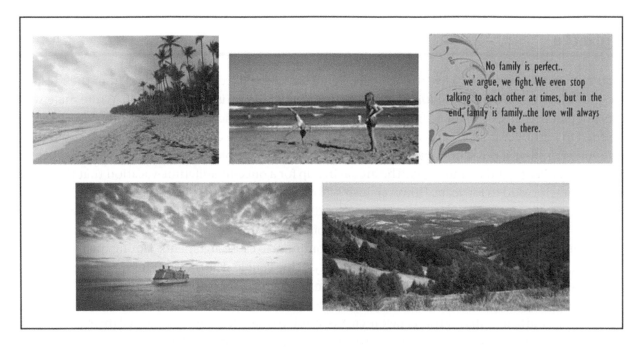

Figure 19.3 Samantha's vision board. Credit for photos: Unsplash.

family vacations to the beach and mountains, a photo of a cruise ship, and a quote from one of her favorite authors about the importance of family (see Figure 19.3).

While each individual shared their vision board, the therapist helped the clients process how they felt and how the photo or saying related to their goals for therapy. For example, when Brian pointed to the photo of him teaching Josh how to throw a baseball, the therapist asked, "How come you chose this specific photo of you and Josh when he was so young?" Brian responded that he saw great potential for his son, and watching his current journey worries him. Another example included when Samantha read the saying about the importance of family, and the therapist asked, "What does this specific quote mean to you?" Samantha responded emotionally, realizing she felt torn between Josh and Brian. Similarly, as the clients shared different portions of their vision boards, the therapist asked them what those pictures or sayings represented, why they chose those specific ones, what the image or saying meant to them, etc. The goal of the vision board is to process the reasons clients choose certain elements to put on their vision board and how it relates to their current therapeutic problems and future goals.

Suggestions for Follow-Up

You can ask clients to complete a joint vision board in future sessions. If clients create a shared vision board, work with them to collaboratively determine their vision for the board. For example, a family might decide that they want to create a vision board where everyone in the family gets along with one another. Clients must work collaboratively to determine what photos and quotes to include. If they have previously created their own vision boards in therapy, they may choose to combine relevant images and text that they included in their individual vision boards if they are relevant to their shared goal(s). When processing a jointly created vision board, ask questions about their experience of working together on this project, how the images and text included relate to preferred narratives, and how they might also work together to make parts of their jointly created vision manifest. For example:

- What was it like to work on this vision board with your [partner/spouse/etc.]?

- When choosing the specific images or text, was it difficult to come to a consensus? If so, how come, and what could have made it easier?

- How do your images or text represent your [goals/needs/desires]?

- When looking at your vision board, how do you plan on applying the images or text you have chosen to your real life?

- Thinking about how you worked together to create this vision board, what are other ways you can work together outside of this room?

  - What specific roles would you both need to take on to successfully work together, and how do you decide these roles?

Vision boards are an ever-evolving activity that can be implemented at any stage of therapy to help clients process identified problems and concretize therapy goals. Throughout the therapy process, return to identify which goals have been accomplished and which remain. Clients can create them annually to compare and contrast newly created boards with their old ones to evaluate how their stories and goals have shifted over time.

Contraindications

Depending on the client's level of independence, it might be helpful to adapt the intervention. For example, you might want to help clients gather materials for the vision board over several sessions. If clients cannot complete a vision board independently, consider how you will help them maintain autonomy within this activity. Another consideration is to make sure that clients use trusted sites like Unsplash, a website that provides access to free images to utilize for any project, if they use pictures from the internet or an online vision board–creation website. It may be helpful to have a list of safe websites that have a variety of images that are suitable for the activity.

The clients' access to vision board–creation programs might be an additional barrier to this intervention. If clients don't have access to a computer and use their phones for teletherapy sessions, it might be helpful for them to create traditional vision boards with paper and share photos of the boards in session.

References

Benedict, B. C. (2021). Using vision boards to reflect on relevant experiences and envision ideal futures. *College Teaching, 69*(4), 231–232. https://doi.org/10.1080/87567555.2020.1850411

Burton, L., & Lent, J. (2016). The use of vision boards as a therapeutic intervention. *Journal of Creativity in Mental Health, 11*(1), 52–65. https://doi.org/10.1080/15401383.2015.1092901

Conderman, G., & Young, N. (2021). Vision boards: Students look into their futures. *Kappa Delta Pi Record, 57*(2), 90–94. https://doi.org/10.1080/00228958.2021.1890446

Etchison, M., & Kleist, D. M. (2000). Review of narrative therapy: Research and utility. *The Family Journal, 8*(1), 61–66. https://doi.org/10.1177/1066480700081009

Gladding, S. T. (2008). The impact of creativity in counseling. *Journal of Creativity in Mental Health, 3*(2), 97–104. https://doi.org/10.1080/15401380802226679

Waalkes, P. L., Gonzalez, L. M., & Brunson, C. N. (2019). Vision boards and adolescent career counseling: A culturally responsive approach. *Journal of Creativity in Mental Health, 14*(2), 205–216. https://doi.org/10.1080/15401383.2019.1602092

White, M., & Epston, D. (1990). *Narrative means to therapeutic ends*. W. W. Norton & Company.

CHAPTER 20

GUIDED GROUNDING IN TELETHERAPY INTERVENTION

Kayla Sellers

Materials for Therapists and Clients: None.

Objective

The 5–4–3–2–1 grounding technique (Dolan, 1991) is used to help stop dissociation and guide clients away from past- and/or future-oriented thoughts and toward their present sensory experience. This chapter describes ways in which to implement this intervention via teletherapy.

Rationale for Use

Grounding is defined as guiding one's attention to the present moment, away from past, destabilizing events, leading one toward a present safety (Pitluk et al., 2021). By facilitating the reconnection of the brain's focus to present sensory experiencing, participants experience stabilization of the limbic system through intentional increased use of prefrontal cortex processes (Siddiqui et al., 2008). This is key in addressing dissociation with clients who have experienced trauma.

When clients demonstrate signs of dissociation in teletherapy, this can be particularly concerning to therapists due to the lack of control that therapists have in the client's physical environment. If it appears that a client is outside of their window of tolerance (Siegel, 2020) during a teletherapy session, therapists may use grounding techniques to safely address dissociation occurring in the current moment.

The following adaptation of the 5–4–3–2–1 grounding method (Dolan, 1991) instructs participants to name five things they see, four things they hear, three things they feel, two things they smell, and one thing they taste. Though this activity is focused on the individual, it can be applied to work with partners, families, or groups by having each person in session practice the activity simultaneously and then processing together after its completion. Unlike in-person services in which the therapist and client experience some of the same sensory input, implementation of this exercise via teletherapy requires clients to utilize a more detailed description of their senses to fully convey their experience to the therapist. As a result, the therapist gains a better understanding of the client's experience of their environment through the client's narrative. Clients are also afforded the opportunity to reorient to their present senses, experience a sense of stabilization within the present moment, and regain emotional stability. This exercise fits particularly well within

DOI: 10.4324/9781003289920-24

the framework of an experiential approach to therapy (Geller & Greenberg, 2012), though it can be applied to work with clients from any guiding theory or model.

Setup

When working with clients who have a history of trauma, preemptively assess for dissociation, continuously monitor for signs of dissociation during session, and collaboratively develop a plan for ways in which to address dissociation if signs should occur in session. This plan may include practicing the 5–4–3–2–1 grounding technique prior to any experience of dissociation so that clients are familiar with the exercise before it is ever needed.

Instructions

1. ***Familiarize clients with guided grounding.*** Introduce clients to guided grounding by providing a brief description of what it is. Ask clients if they are familiar with guided grounding, explain the difference between guided grounding and meditation, and describe potential benefits.

2. ***Invite clients to get into a comfortable position of their choice.*** This may look like remaining seated with both feet flat on the floor. It may also be sitting or lying on the ground. If clients choose to change their position for this activity, work with them to move their camera so that you can maintain visual contact during the activity. Visual contact allows for continued monitoring of signs of dissociation and of the client returning to the present moment (e.g., changes in pace of breathing).

3. ***Guide clients through taking three deep breaths.*** In a softened, relaxed tone, count for clients to breathe in for five seconds, hold their breath in their lungs for five seconds, and breathe out for seven seconds. Timing may be adjusted based on the needs of each client. For example, someone may desire to exhale for a slightly longer count in the sequence, or they may wish to continue deep breathing longer than three deep breaths. The first time that this activity is introduced, explain the sequencing prior to implementing the breathing exercise. Instruct clients to continue breathing at their own pace and count if the internet were to go out or if there is a lag in audio. This is critical because some clients may be inclined to continue holding their breath longer than they should if they are waiting on the therapist's prompt while technological glitches inhibit this process.

4. ***Instruct clients to name five things they can see.*** Encourage clients to explore items in their immediate environment rather than items on their screen. Invite clients to then verbally list the five visual items they identified. Clients may choose to show you their items on the screen if they are portable, but this is not necessary. Should they list one or more items in your background, this can be explored further during the processing stage.

5. ***Instruct clients to name four things they can feel.*** Explain that they can move as desired to complete this step but that you would like to ensure that they stay within range of the camera so you can continue to see them. Instruct them to describe the first tactile experience before moving on to the second, then the third, and finally the fourth.

6. ***Instruct clients to name three things they can hear.*** To help clients who struggle to focus, you may offer to count within your head a number determined by the client (e.g., five to ten seconds) and alert them when that time is up to share one thing that they heard during this time. Repeat the

process two more times, or until three sounds have been identified. It may be difficult for therapists to help guide clients to different noises in their environment because they may not be able to hear them through the computer. You may make suggestions to listen to sounds within the client's room, external to their room, or even within their own body. If clients struggle to identify three different sounds, they are welcome to repeat prior responses if necessary. It is more important that they engage in auditory exploration of their environment than to identify three unique sounds.

7. ***Instruct clients to name two things they can smell.*** Let them know that they may actively seek out olfactory input and are not limited to what they can smell within the air. Because of the different physical locations, you may not be able to help identify smells in the room as you might be able to do when working in an in-person setting. Rather, you may offer suggestions to smell things in the client's immediate physical environment, such as their clothing, hands, or other things in their environment. Ask clients to share the first scent description before moving on to the second.

8. ***Instruct clients to name one thing they can taste.*** Clarify that you are aware of the limitations of this portion of the exercise and can't offer a mint or chocolate like you might be able to do if the meeting was in person. If clients struggle to name something they taste, invite them to seek out another form of sensory input. Instruct them to describe the taste they are experiencing or the alternative sensory experience if chosen. If they choose to seek out a different form of sensory input, process this choice within the processing stage.

Processing

The 5–4–3–2–1 grounding method emphasizes the here-and-now sensory experience of clients. While the intervention does not require subsequent processing for effective implementation, making efforts toward processing the client's experience may help them to better identify internal sensations, emotional links to sensory experiences, and regulatory effects of the intervention. As clients are better able to understand the experience and identify possible benefits, they are more likely to independently integrate the intervention as a coping mechanism outside of sessions. Possible processing questions include but are not limited to the following:

- What was this experience like for you? Were there any parts that were harder to do than others? What supports might you need, if any, to successfully practice this exercise again in the future?

- What sensations do you notice within your body?

- What emotions are present for you? Do they differ from those you were experiencing before you engaged in the exercise?

- When you experience the emotions you had before (or after) participating in grounding, how do you typically notice or react to them?

- How might you [become aware of/explain/understand] the stressors you are facing differently after engaging in grounding?

- How would you assess your current environment in this moment?

- What did you notice about separating the different senses to focus on them one at a time? How did this change how you experienced them?

When working with more than one client in session, the following questions may be used to engage discussion:

- Take note of your feelings of connection to one another before and after engaging in this exercise. What changed? How did it change?

- How might you support one another in this exercise in the future? For example, is it helpful to hold hands while feeling things in the environment, or would you rather not be touched during the activity?

Vignette

Guided grounding presents as an excellent experiential intervention when working with individuals experiencing incarceration due to its emphasis on connecting with present sensory experiences. During incarceration, individuals are likely to experience sensory reduction and/or deprivation as a result of the generally confining and restrictive nature of the environment. Within this context, sensory deprivation can take place through lack of access to outdoors, removal of sunlight, mandatory lights out and silence, solitary confinement, and more. One of the most consistent reductions of the senses is the denial of human touch. Sensory reduction and deprivation can result in increased anxiety, depression, anger, emotional withdrawal, delusions, and hallucinations (Philippe-Beauchamp, 2021). To decrease overactivation of the limbic system's fight, flight, or freeze reactionary response process, clients intentionally engage the frontal lobe. Doing so enhances their capacity to use problem-solving skills, voluntary behavioral control, executive function, and emotional control capacities (Fuster, 1980). The following provides an example of the application of guided grounding with an incarcerated individual.

Jennie (28), a White, unmarried, self-identifying female incarcerated within the local county jail, was referred for teletherapy services through the jail's programs department. She was referred due to persistent increases in anxious symptoms as well as difficulty acclimating to the incarceration setting. This was Jennie's first reincarceration following an 18-month prison sentence that she was released from two years ago.

In session, Jennie reported lifelong difficulty coping with stressors, both in and out of incarceration settings. She shared fears for her future, stating that she had concerns that she would continue to be in and out of jail for the remainder of her life. Jennie discussed high levels of shame for her actions, especially when it came to her role as a mother. She also shared what she described as brief experiences of disconnect during times of high anxiety.

With Jennie frequently presenting in session in a state of heightened anxiety, the therapist noticed that moments of Jennie connecting with her immediate thoughts and feelings were often fleeting. Jennie frequently appeared to have trouble connecting with her present experiences and displayed minor signs of dissociation such as staring off into the distance and decreased ability to articulate her feelings when discussing topics of concern. The therapist thought she would be an appropriate candidate for the 5–4–3–2–1 guided grounding intervention.

Amid a session in which the therapist noticed Jennie appearing to dissociate she asked Jennie to pause to notice her present emotions. When Jennie struggled to do so, the therapist introduced the intervention as a coping mechanism, stating that she hoped it would help Jennie regulate her heightened threat response system both in and out of session by attuning to her immediate sensory inputs. Jennie expressed interest in trying the exercise. The therapist explained that Jennie would get herself comfortable, take three deep breaths, and then name five items she saw, four things she felt, three things she heard, two things she smelled, and one thing she tasted. The therapist stated that if Jennie desired to move around during the session to help become aware of different sensory inputs, she was free to do so as long as Jennie remained within view of the camera so she could continue to see her throughout the activity and only if Jennie's position and movement would not generate any alarms for engaging in behaviors against jail or prison policy.

As the intervention was underway, the therapist observed Jennie becoming teary-eyed as she named the items she saw and felt. Jennie began to cry as she continued to list the things that she was hearing. Jennie's crying came to an end as she listed the things she smelled and tasted.

Upon completion of naming her sensory experiences, the therapist asked process questions related to Jennie's engagement in the intervention. The therapist asked if she noticed any emotional changes or reactions as she was exploring her environment. Jennie told the therapist that she became overwhelmed with sadness and grief because she sees the same "stark white walls" and reinforced, clouded windows every day. She discussed the noises of the guards' keys, continuous locking and unlocking of the metal doors, and inmate fighting as incredibly distressing. Jennie shared that she didn't realize how upsetting the jail environment was without her conscious awareness of the sights, sounds, and sensations she regularly takes in. Jennie became emotional again as she shared that she wanted to feel a hug from a loved one, something she had not felt in several months. As the therapist inquired about Jennie's present emotions when exploring taste and smell, Jennie shared that she noticed herself shutting down and "feeling numb," something she often found herself doing when she felt unable to meet her own hygiene and hunger needs.

As the therapist validated Jennie's shared feelings, she probed for Jennie's awareness of how she normally experienced the feelings of sadness, grief, frustration, and loneliness that occurred during the activity. Jennie pointed out that whether she was incarcerated or not, she had always struggled to allow herself to feel emotions as they arose, frequently resulting in her emotional withdrawal, anxious state, and subsequent substance use. Jennie pointed out that she had never felt understood by loved ones. As the therapist and Jennie continued to process both Jennie's experience participating in guided grounding and the subsequent curiosities Jennie posed while processing, the therapist noticed Jennie's body language shift to a more relaxed state.

As the session closed, the therapist reframed Jennie's earlier description of shutting down and feeling numb as a form of dissociation that often occurs when people feel they are outside of their window of emotional tolerance. The therapist shared that struggling to connect to present feelings, as Jennie experienced prior to the exercise, is also a sign of dissociation. The therapist reminded Jennie that the exercise is a tool that she could use as a coping skill outside of sessions, especially when experiencing dissociation. The therapist informed Jennie that it was also a tool that could be utilized to connect with loved ones during phone calls and video visits when she felt herself struggling to be present in the conversation.

Suggestions for Follow-Up

The 5–4–3–2–1 grounding intervention can be used in subsequent sessions to aid in grounding clients in their present experiences. It can also be recommended for use outside of sessions. In cases in which clients are physically separated from their loved ones, such as incarceration, clients can introduce the intervention to others over phone calls or virtual visits to acquaint one another to their physical surroundings and help bridge the physical divide between them. When clients discuss their use of the intervention outside of sessions, further process their experience by exploring the emotional states that they were experiencing before and after use of the intervention.

Contraindications

Use best judgement in utilizing this exercise. This intervention should not be introduced with less than 25 minutes to complete. Though it may not take 25 minutes each time, ample time must be allowed for clients to be present within their environment, connect with their senses, and collaboratively process their experience.

References

Dolan, Y. M. (1991). *Resolving sexual abuse: Solution-focused therapy and Ericksonian hypnosis for adult survivors*. Norton.

Fuster, J. M. (1980). *The prefrontal cortex: Anatomy, physiology, and neuropsychology of the frontal lobe*. Raven Press.

Geller, S. M., & Greenberg, L. S. (2012). Experiential approaches: Somatic, emotion-focused, creative, and relational approaches to cultivating therapeutic presence. In S. M. Geller & L. S. Greenberg (Eds.), *Therapeutic presence: A mindful approach to effective therapy* (pp. 207–230). American Psychological Association. https://doi.org/10.1037/13485-011

Philippe-Beauchamp, X. (2021). A meagre world: Phenomenological corporeity in prison. *The Humanistic Psychologist, 49*(3), 423–434. https://doi.org/10.1037/hum0000163

Pitluk, M., Elboim-Gabyzon, M., & Shuper Engelhard, E. (2021). Validation of the grounding assessment tool for identifying emotional awareness and emotion regulation. *The Arts in Psychotherapy, 75*, Article 101821. https://doi.org/10.1016/j.aip.2021.101821

Siddiqui, S. V., Chatterjee, U., Kumar, D., Siddiqui, A., & Goyal, N. (2008). Neuropsychology of prefrontal cortex. *Indian Journal of Psychiatry, 50*(3), 202–208. https://doi.org/10.4103/0019-5545.43634

Siegel, D. J. (2020). *The developing mind: How relationships and the brain interact to shape who we are* (3rd ed.). The Guilford Press.

CHAPTER 21

SOLUTION-FOCUSED TELETHERAPY FOR SUICIDE INTERVENTION

Benjamin T. Finlayson, Jaclyn Cravens Pickens, and Ethan Jones

Materials for Therapists and Clients: None.

Objective

Solution-focused brief therapy (SFBT) is effectively used in face-to-face treatment modalities with clients experiencing thoughts of death by suicide (Kondrat & Teater, 2010; Quick, 1998; Yeager, 2002). This chapter describes ways in which to utilize SFBT for teletherapy suicide intervention.

Rationale for Use

SFBT is a goal-oriented, evidence-based approach that focuses on existing solutions that clients may have to presenting problems (De Shazer, 1994, 1997). A common misconception of SFBT is that it excludes discussion of problems. Though SFBT is goal focused and solution oriented, its effective application allows space for clients to discuss problems and for therapists to validate feelings and concerns.

SFBT is also not solution pushing. Through the process of *listen, select,* and *build*, therapists engage in the client's problem talk while looking for exceptions to existing problems and solutions to problems that have worked in the past. Listening for strengths and competencies assists in developing and achieving concrete, measurable, and realistic goals (de Jong & Berg, 2013; Georgiades, 2008). SFBT works effectively when therapists relinquish control of preconceived meanings of words (e.g., depression) and negotiate meaning with the client's experience (De Shazer & Berg, 1992). Therapists and clients thus co-construct practical and sustainable solutions to presenting problems.

SFBT is effective across presenting concerns (e.g., anxiety, domestic violence, substance use, postpartum depression; Georgiades, 2008; Kramer et al., 2014; Norman et al., 2018; Novella et al., 2020; Ondersma et al., 2007) and translates well across crisis-care treatment modalities (De Jong & Berg, 2013). In hospital emergency rooms and managed-care environments, SFBT can be integrated in existing care and discharge protocol to clarify presenting problems, expand solutions, and increase hope and agency for patients with suicidal ideation (SI; Kondrat & Teater, 2010; Quick, 1998; Yeager, 2002). Adapting solution-focused language across a teletherapy platform while actively intervening in suicide empowers both clients and therapists to make the most of the moment they have together.

DOI: 10.4324/9781003289920-25

Setup

At the onset of therapy, obtain the physical address of clients as a part of the paperwork process. Before any teletherapy session, confirm the physical location of clients, and have the local dispatch number for the client's address available in the event of an emergency. When clients are in a new location in subsequent sessions, ask for the address of the location and identify the local dispatch number for that area as well.

Instructions

Utilizing common techniques in SFBT demonstrates a significant effort to see beyond the problem and skillfully drops the client and therapist just on the other side of the crisis (Wells & McCaig, 2016). SFBT starts at the "end" of traditional suicidal interventions by building into client strengths and attributes first rather than investing in the many ways that problems feel inescapable in the present moment. When a client is experiencing thoughts of suicide or presents with a recent history of behaviors to end their life by suicide, capitalize on strengths-based resources more profoundly than you typically would with a traditional solution-focused approach and with deliberate safety in mind.

The following describes specific ways in which SFBT techniques can be applied via teletherapy when working with clients who are experiencing thoughts of death by suicide.

Miracle Question

The miracle question is an SBFT technique in which therapists ask clients to imagine that a miracle has occurred overnight and that the concerns that brought them to therapy have gone away. Only, no one knows that a miracle has occurred. Clients are asked to describe the things that they and others might notice when they wake up in the morning that might indicate that a miracle has occurred (De Shazer, 1999). The miracle question should address that change is immediate and unlikely to occur without a miracle. Yet, clients cannot know the miracle has happened. Ask clients to describe immediate, noticeable change after the miracle (Jordan, 2017). For more instructions on constructing a miracle question, see Strong and Pyle (2009).

For teletherapists, the miracle question is a powerful technique that meets clients where they are, with the resources they have access to, for tapping into hope (Fiske, 2008). Teletherapy is likely to occur in a place where clients spend much of their time, making the miracle question a unique intervention for clients to create an in-the-moment positive association, or shift, in a space that may be associated with the problem. The miracle question provides therapists with insight into what is meaningful and who might be meaningful in the attainment of that miracle.

The miracle question is a valuable resource to center clients in a solution-saturated story in conversations about suicide. To state a disclaimer, the miracle is not death by suicide. Through this collaborative model, therapists can affirm the difficulty of the client's present moment and not endorse death by suicide as a workable solution. The therapist then asks questions regarding the miracle that are aligned with the client's preferred future that doesn't involve death by suicide.

Exception Questions

Clients typically experience times when their presenting problem does not occur or does not occur fully, whether clients are aware of this or not (Fisk, 2008). For example, therapists might ask clients, "Can you think of a time when you didn't consider suicide as an option?" or "Can you think of a time when you were less likely to consider suicide?" Therapists may then ask about what was happening in those instances to help identify solutions. Exception questions allow therapists to strategically tap into what clients want and uncover reasons for living. As clients speak with you via teletherapy, they have already done so much (e.g., get out of bed, turn on their computer, log into session)! If clients feel that they have done nothing that day, gently remind them that they showed up to their appointment and the accomplishment of this task!

Scaling Questions

Scaling questions are a useful solution-focused tool that can be used to assess a client's safety. Scaling questions allow therapists to process the current state of clients and the state of difference between one number and the next by asking about noticeable, achievable, and realistic small steps (Greene et al., 1996). Scaling questions maximize the unknown through teletherapy by providing the clinician confidence in safety through the descriptions clients offer. For example, "On a scale of 0 to 10, where 10 demonstrates your confidence in achieving the first small step we identified toward your goal, and 0 is just the opposite of that, where would you place yourself?" Then, the therapist might follow up, "Wow, it sounds like you are at least a bit more confident to take that step. What would it take to go from there to just a little above that?" This continues the conversation around safety and resources and may even provide space to affirm that part of their confidence may be increased by self-admittance to a mental health clinic.

Scaling questions may also be used to identify client progress. For example, therapists may ask, "So let's say that I put this miracle on a scale, where 10 is [client's response to the miracle question, matching their language as much as possible] and 0 is when you scheduled your appointment with me. Where are you today?" The language in this scale is intentional and implies that change has already occurred. Indicating that 0 is the time that the client made the appointment shows that presession change or presession coping techniques have allowed them to make it from phone call to intake to appointment.

Scaling paired with circular questioning can bring awareness to interconnectedness with others and help in identifying small steps toward identified goals (Softas-Nall & Francis, 1998). For example, "What would your friends notice that would indicate to them that you have moved from a 3 to a 4?"

Scaling might also allow clients to recognize their own agency. For example, a therapist might ask, "And at what number would you say, 'I need additional help'?" This question normalizes the ebb and flow of progress and utilizes the client's agency to remind them they can ask for help when needed.

Listen, Select, and Build

The following process, *(1) listen, (2) select*, and *(3) build*, is a poststructuralist way to actively stay in the present experience of the client's language while engaging in SFBT. This process is not linear and presents a recursive pattern between the therapist and client as they continue to build collaborative working goals.

1. **Listen.** *Listen* to what is most meaningful to clients. To start the listening process, utilize a resource-loaded question such as, "What would [family member/friend] see you doing that would indicate that, as you look back on this meeting, our time was helpful to you?" This question implies: (1) a visible change in behavior (i.e., what they would see), (2) an accountability resource within (i.e., who would see them), and (3) that time will also pass (i.e., looking back), which erases that static nature of time clients in distress may experience. Responding with curiosity amplifies perceptions and guides you in *selecting* (step two) what is meaningful to clients (de Jong & Berg, 2013).

2. ***Select.*** Notice what is meaningful to clients or moments of difference that are exceptions to the "rule." It is through problem talk that the therapist is most likely to *select* what is meaningful to clients to *build* (step three) into preferred futures. As you select either resources, exceptions, or statements that indicate change, it is important to go further and discuss what makes this a solution. A therapist selecting a moment to build into might sound like, "Oh, so it is important for your kids to see you as a good dad?" In this example, the therapist has intentionally selected a resource to then start the building process. This example of a resource also implies an emotional connection that the therapist can build into.

3. ***Build.*** *Build* into the client's exceptions and solutions by discussing how they will achieve their preferred future or by asking what difference this preferred future might make. It is in the building process that the therapist diligently builds into what clients have done and would like to see more of that makes it solution focused. There is even an indication within "But I haven't even showered" that the client is aware that showering is important to them. They are aware they haven't done it, and they know that showering is something that they do when they are "doing better." As you build with the client, teletherapy can open the door to new positive connections in the client's physical space by inviting contextual "witness" of the preferred future. For example, a therapist might say, "Ah, and I see a bird just outside your window. Would they see a difference? What might they see?" or "What might your cat see when they wake you up in the morning?"

Safety Planning

The aforementioned SBFT techniques and interventions can be used in the application of safety planning with clients who are experiencing thoughts of death by suicide. The following outlines specific steps that can be followed to develop a safety plan using SBFT via teletherapy intervention.

- Teletherapy does not allow therapists to automatically know the physical location of clients. When working with clients experiencing SI, knowing physical addresses is critical so that police or emergency contacts can be sent to ensure client safety in the event of active SI. Obtain the address of the physical location from which clients will be attending teletherapy sessions at the onset of therapy. At the beginning of each session, obtain the physical address of the client if they appear to be attending from a different location.

- Have the phone number of the client on file so that you can call immediately if the internet drops and you need to immediately reconnect during active SI. Try calling them during your first session to ensure that the number you have on file is correct and to practice troubleshooting.

- Discuss the names of family/friends/others who could be contacted if you are concerned about active SI. An example of a solution-focused question might be: "You mentioned that later today, you'd be connecting with your best friend. Is this someone that you'd agree would be a good person for me to call in case of emergency?"

- Discuss confidentiality and when it could be broken.

- Identify emergency numbers, suicide hotlines, and other crisis services available in the client's physical location that can be accessed in the event of SI.

- Co-create a suicide prevention plan. A solution-focused approach to this might entail including preferred future resources and using scaling to identify when to utilize those resources. Scaling questions may help clients notice small changes that they might otherwise miss that would indicate the need to access support. For example, a therapist might say, "If you notice that you go from a 6 to a 5 on the scale, which of the resources that we've identified might help to get you back up a point?"

If you are concerned that a client may actively take steps towards completing suicide, take further steps in ensuring their safety. Discuss whether the client would like to make the call or if they would like the therapist to make the call to their emergency contact (and possibly the police). Remain on the teletherapy platform while the call is made, and keep attention and conversation on the client until emergency response arrives. For example, a therapist might state, "My goal is to keep you as safe as possible as you make changes that are meaningful to you. Right now, I think that it will be helpful to bring in additional resources that we previously identified. Let's bring up the safety plan that we created together. Who should we contact from this plan? Would you like to make the call, or would you prefer that I make the call? I'll stay on the teletherapy platform with you while the call is made. What else would be most helpful at this moment?" In this example, the therapist has recognized that a higher level of care may be in the client's best interest, yet, through language, has implied that the client may also hold agency in how they proceed in making the call. Additionally, the therapist is calling on resources formerly identified by the client and therapist, using solution-focused language to empower the client for change in the moment of crisis. If members of the client's family or intimate partners are present, they can help to make the call with the client present and should travel with the client to in-patient triage.

The following vignette (adapted from Finlayson et al., 2021) demonstrates the use of listening, selecting, and building using a SFBT approach in teletherapy when working with a family with a member who recently attempted to complete suicide.

Vignette

Julia (42) initiated therapy in a very distraught place, because in her words, she had just found out that her 15-year-old son had tried to "commit suicide." Being in a rural community, she was concerned about lack of access to resources, including local therapists. During the intake session, she and her husband Robert (45) shared that they had been married for 20 years and had three children, an 18-year-old daughter, a 15-year-old son, and an 8-year-old son. All children were still in the home but were not present during the session. Both Julia and Robert identified as European American, middle class, reported having steady careers, identified as Christian, and stated that they attended services at least monthly. Julia did the majority of the talking and explained how easy their life was until two years ago, when Wesley, their 15-year-old, came out to them as bisexual and gender nonbinary (he/they) and had since battled depression and thoughts of suicide. This battle culminated in the week prior, when he had a serious conversation with his father about no longer wanting to be alive. After the initial meeting, the therapist asked to meet with Julia, Robert, and Wesley together.

The following provides an example of the therapist's initial conversation with Julia, Robert, and Wesley, highlighting components of *listen, select*, and *build*.

(1) Listen

Therapist: Tell me, before we get started, how do you each spend your days?

Julia: I usually wake up first. I start my day by getting ready for work. I usually am at work by 8:30 a.m. I spend most of my day working and then come home around 5:00 p.m. and am usually greeted by the family. I cook dinner for everyone and then go for an evening walk. I guess the rest of the evening is spent in the living room, watching TV before bed.

The therapist highlights strengths in Julia's day.

> **Therapist:** Oh wow, you fit so much into a day! And Robert, how would you say you spend your days?

> **Robert:** I'm not an early riser, but I wake up shortly after Julia and then get the kids up and ready for school. I can get to work later in the morning, so I help get the kids going. I work in finance, so the job itself is not that fun, but it's something.

The therapist details strengths in Robert's day and switches to Wesley.

> **Therapist:** So you're not an early riser, but you figure out how to help everyone in the morning. And Wesley, how would you describe your days?

> **Wesley:** I think my days are all right mostly. I don't wake up easily mainly because I just don't want to go to school. It feels like a waste of my time and so it's hard for me, but I go. I like it more once I'm there and I see a few of my friends. After school, I go to marching band rehearsal for about an hour and a half. Then I go home, have dinner, go to my room, and work on school or play games online.

> **Therapist:** Wow! It too sounds like you put so much into the day. What would your teachers say is your strongest subject in school?

The therapist asks questions that presume strength in the response. The therapist listens for strengths and resources surrounding the client. The therapist does not direct a response. Through questions asked, the therapist begins assessment for safety resources and reasons for living.

> **Therapist:** So, online may be a new experience, but you all are here. Can I ask a funny question for our first day? Okay. You have all taken time to meet here today, and there will be a moment when we must end our time together. I am curious, what will have happened here today, together, that when you leave, you might say, "Oh that was worth our time?"

> **Julia:** I am so worried about Wesley. He came out to us, things haven't been the same, and he feels distant to me. I'm not sure what to do. So, we are here. I guess talking about that might be helpful for us today.

(2) Select

> **Therapist:** Wow! Julia, you are so worried for your son. I can tell you are a mom that cares about her kids, and being close to your kids is important for you.

> **Julia:** Yes, it is so important to be close. I never had a close family, and I want to be a mom that does better for her kids.

(3) Build

> **Therapist:** Oh, you don't have a close family and you want to be a mom that does something different. What would you say close families do?

> **Julia:** A close family is one in which we can share things together and support each other. Close families have intentional time together. I feel like close families deal with hard things together and I don't think we do that. I push and I push to keep us close, but it just doesn't work.

(1) Listen

Robert: I am also concerned. Wesley said that he has had serious thoughts about suicide and has acted on these behaviors. He came to me in confidence, and now I feel I've pushed him away by telling his mother and our coming here. I think I fractured our relationship and trust. I'm not sure if his identity is a cause, or if being bisexual and gender nonbinary just has its repercussions. I know LGBTQIA people really suffer with depression. I know this life is going to be hard for him. I just want him safe.

(2) Select

Therapist: So being here today, there would not be a fracture. You want to see Wesley flourish and be safe.

Robert: Yes, safe. I worry that whatever is causing this is keeping him unsafe and I'm being a bad dad somehow because I can't protect him. I can't shield him like I used to when he was young.

(1) Listen

Wesley: I guess I am just here because I know it will help somehow and my parents really want me here. I'm not sure what I want to get out of this except I do know that I'm not happy, and I want to be that again. It just all feels too much and too heavy.

Therapist: Thank you for being here. So, you want to be happy, and at times, there are moments it feels too heavy.

The therapist normalizes feelings and breaks the client's description of static time (i.e., "it all") by gently introducing "and at times." This offers the presumption that it is not all times.

(2) Select

Therapist: I think even a lot of adults would not have shown up today when feeling like you have. But something about this moment says it will help, that happiness will happen more.

Wesley: Yeah.

(3) Build

Therapist: What does happiness mean to you, Wesley? What do people see you doing when you are happy?

Wesley: I think I would be hopeful in the morning again and excited for school. I think Mom sees me less resistant to going to school. School has been so hard right now. I would be normal.

Therapist: Wow. You would be hopeful again and feel normal again. It is nice to feel like ourselves. What would you do if you woke up and felt hopeful? Have there been times since you talked to your parents that this day of feeling hopeful and normal has happened? Even if just for a moment? As you have described it, can you show me the items in your house that you said make you feel normal? Hopeful?

The therapist listens to Wesley describe what it is like to feel hopeful and normal. The therapist uses the client's response to highlight the items/resources that surround the client that may also encourage normalcy and hope. In this case, SFBT in teletherapy becomes a "resource discovery" to create newer positive associations with the client's immediate surroundings. As a family, it can be critical to understand what the client in crisis defines as "hopeful and normal" and do more of it. For example, the therapist may ask the family to move therapy to the dining room table after the client describes this as being a moment that felt normal.

Clients in crisis may be looking for a miracle that feels too far out of reach for this moment. By asking about moments or even glimpses of when this has happened, it helps clients expand resources within the conversation. In teletherapy, this can be immediately helpful because clients can associate memories and somatic responses to their environment.

Suggestions for Follow-Up

Scaling is a useful resource to measure change within and between sessions. Scaling questions offer clients agency to produce observable desired change. When working with clients expressing severe thoughts of death by suicide, demonstrate that small steps may be the most realistic and attainable.

In this vignette, the therapist might follow up with, "Wesley, on a scale of 0 to 10, where 10 is that place you mentioned where you are waking up more hopeful and you'd brush your teeth, and 0 is just the opposite of that, where are you today? At what number would you say, 'You know, I need to talk to someone about this'?" Scaling questions are relational and seek to tap into the hope within the family that each member can play a part in the difference.

Contraindications

Using SFBT and the miracle question for the first time may feel uncomfortable for some clients. You may need to shift from solution-focused conversations and proceed with other screening methods for clients who are active in thoughts of suicide and do not appear grounded using this technique (Gilmore & Ward-Ciesielski, 2019).

References

De Jong, P., & Berg, I. K. (2013). *Interviewing for solutions* (4th ed.). Brooks/Cole Cengage Learning.

De Shazer, S. (1994). *Words were originally magic*. W. W. Norton & Company Inc.

De Shazer, S. (1997). Some thoughts on language use in therapy. *Contemporary Family Therapy*, *19*(1), 133–141. https://doi.org/10.1023/A:1026170718933

De Shazer, S. (1999). *Beginnings* [From the BFTC-website]. https://www.sikt.nu/wp-content/uploads/2020/06/SdeS-Beginnings-.pdf

De Shazer, S., & Berg, I. K. (1992). Doing therapy: A post-structural re-vision. *Journal of Marital and Family Therapy*, *18*(1), 71–81. https://doi.org/10.1111/j.1752-0606.1992.tb00916.x

Finlayson, B. T., Jones, E., & Pickens, J. C. (2021). Solution focused brief therapy telemental health suicide intervention. *Contemporary Family Therapy*, *45*(1), 49–60. https://doi.org/10.1007/s10591-021-09599-1

Fiske, H. (2008). *Hope in action*. Routledge.

Georgiades, S. D. (2008). A solution-focused intervention with a youth in a domestic violence situation: Longitudinal evidence. *Contemporary Family Therapy*, *30*(3), 141–151. https://doi.org/10.1007/s10591-008-9067-1

Gilmore, A. K., & Ward-Ciesielski, E. F. (2019). Perceived risks and use of psychotherapy via telemedicine for patients at risk for suicide. *Journal of Telemedicine and Telecare*, *25*(1), 59–63. https://doi.org/10.1177/1357633X17735559

Greene, G. J., Lee, M., Trask, R., & Rheinscheld, J. (1996). Client strengths and crisis intervention: A solution-focused approach. *Crisis Intervention*, *3*(1), 43–63.

Jordan, S. (2017). Solution-focused brief therapy. In *The SAGE encyclopedia of marriage, family, and couples counseling* (Vol. 4, pp. 1576–1580). SAGE Publications, Inc. https://doi.org/10.4135/9781483369532

Kondrat, D. C., & Teater, B. (2010). Solution-focused therapy in an emergency room setting: Increasing hope in persons presenting with suicidal ideation. *Journal of Social Work*, *12*(1), 3–15. https://doi.org/10.1177/1468017310379756

Kramer, J., Conijn, B., Oijevaar, P., & Riper, H. (2014). Effectiveness of a web-based solution-focused brief chat treatment for depressed adolescents and young adults: Randomized controlled trial. *Journal of Medical Internet Research*, *16*(5), Article e141. https://doi.org/10.2196/jmir.3261

Norman, P., Cameron, D., Epton, T., Webb, T. L., Harris, P. R., Millings, A., & Sheeran, P. (2018). A randomized controlled trial of a brief online intervention to reduce alcohol consumption in new university students: Combining self-affirmation, theory of planned behavior messages, and implementation interventions. *British Journal of Health Psychology*, *23*(1), 108–127, https://doi.org/10.1111/bjhp.12277

Novella, J. K., Ng, K., & Samuolis, J. (2020). A comparison of online and in-person counseling outcomes using solution-focused brief therapy for college students with anxiety. *Journal of American College Health*, *70*(4), 1161–1168. https://doi.org/10.1080/07448481.2020.1786101

Ondersma, S. J., Svikis, D. S., & Schuster, C. R. (2007). Computer-based brief intervention: A randomized trial with postpartum women. *American Journal of Preventive Medicine*, *32*(3), 231–238. https://doi.org/10.1016/j.amepre.2006.11.003

Quick, E. K. (1998). *Doing what works in brief therapy: A strategic solution focused approach*. Academic Press.

Softas-Nall, B. C., & Francis, P. C. (1998). A solution-focused approach to suicide assessment and intervention with families. *The Family Journal: Counseling and Therapy for Couples and Families*, *6*(1), 64–66. https://doi.org/10.1177/1066480798061014

Strong, T., & Pyle, N. R. (2009). Constructing a conversational "miracle": Examining the "miracle question" as it is used in therapeutic dialogue. *Journal of Constructivist Psychology*, *22*(4), 328–353. https://doi.org/10.1080/10720530903114001

Wells, K., & McCaig, M. (2016). The magic wand question and recovery-focused practice in child and adolescent mental health services. *Journal of Child Adolescent Psychiatrist Nurses*, *29*(4), 164–170. https://doi.org/10.1111/jcap.12159

Yeager, K. R. (2002). Crisis intervention with mentally ill chemical abusers: Application of brief solution-focused therapy and strengths perspective. *Brief Treatment and Crisis Intervention*, *2*(3), 197–216. https://doi.org/10.1093/brief-treatment/2.3.197

CHAPTER 22

A PEEK INSIDE

VIRTUAL HOME VISITS FOR HOARDING DISORDER

Jennifer M. Sampson and Leslie Shapiro

Materials for Therapists: Hoarding disorder assessment(s).

Materials for Clients: Portable, cord-free device with working camera connected to cellular data or Wi-Fi.

Objective

Hoarding disorder (HD) is defined by (a) the acquisition of and failure to discard a large number of possessions, (b) clutter that precludes activities for which living spaces were designed, and (c) significant distress and impairment in functioning caused by these behaviors (APA DSM-5, 2013). Telehealth clinicians have a unique opportunity to conduct "in-home" assessments without the clinician being physically in the client's home. The following outlines the process for conducting a virtual home visit with clients for whom there are concerns related to potential hoarding behaviors.

Rationale for Use

Given that symptoms of HD are connected to the level of physical clutter that exists and the severity at which it prevents the use of living spaces in a client's home, in-office sessions, by nature, do not provide a direct avenue for clinical observation of this behavior. Telehealth sessions conducted from the client's home lend themselves well to the more accurate assessment of and treatment planning for HD than an in-office assessment would allow. Evidence-based therapeutic approaches to treating HD successfully focus on addressing the underlying cognitive-behavioral contributors to hoarding behaviors (Frost & Steketee, 2014). They fall short, however, as the physical nature of the disorder (i.e., the gross accumulation of possessions) is often not taken into consideration when therapists do not offer home visits or clients are unwilling to allow therapists into their home. A home visit is necessary to address these concerns, as the HD impairs functioning physically, not just emotionally and psychologically. Being able to see inside the home of people who hoard by doing telehealth therapy allows therapists to accurately address this.

DOI: 10.4324/9781003289920-26

Unlike most any other mental health disorder, HD directly involves the external "consequences" of the client's behaviors as a diagnostic consideration. For example, the accumulation of possessions in a home may pose significant health and safety hazards for individuals living in the home (Ayers et al., 2010; Frost & Gross, 1993; Kim et al., 2001). For a thorough assessment of the client and the state of the home to be done accurately, the utilization of assessment inventories along with an in-home safety assessment should be conducted. Yet due to a variety of factors including lack of funding, accessibility, and time, in-home therapy sessions can be difficult to conduct.

The use of telehealth during the screening and assessment process allows clinicians access to clients' homes with ease and without invasiveness. Clinicians can conduct visual home-visit safety assessments, in addition to typical verbal or written diagnostic inventories, to develop a comprehensive picture of living environment, potential safety risks, and overall scope of problem to determine appropriate intervention for clients who struggle with hoarding-related challenges.

Setup

Before conducting a visual inspection of the home, conduct initial screening, administer any necessary diagnostic instruments, and prepare clients for the visual inspection of their home.

Initial Screening

Throughout the initial intake and interview process, be mindful of the client's surroundings as sources of clinical information toward developing an accurate diagnostic picture of the client's situation. Some examples of observations that may indicate the need for additional assessment include:

- The client struggles to find a place to sit down to meet for sessions.

- Piles of seemingly disorganized items around the person's home are blocking or interfering with people's use of a given room for its intended purpose (e.g., blocked doors, windows, utilities, appliances).

- Stacks of items appear that they could cause a safety risk if they were to tip over.

- Unsanitary conditions exist, such as piles of garbage, rotting food, or dirty dishes that do not seem to get addressed between sessions.

In these situations, ask questions that directly address potential hoarding behaviors and the outcomes of their symptoms. Introduce questions during the interview process by saying something like, "I've noticed some areas of your home behind you that might be important for us to talk about as a part of our therapy work. Would you be willing to let me ask you a few additional questions about your living space?" These questions may include:

- Are any areas of your home difficult to walk through because of clutter?

- Are you unable to use any parts of your home for their intended purposes? For example, cooking, using furniture, washing dishes, sleeping in bed?

- Do you find the act of throwing away or donating things very upsetting?

- Do you have strong urges to buy or collect things for which you have no immediate use?

- Have you ever been in an argument with a loved one because of the clutter in your home?

If the client responds "yes" to any of these questions, there may be a need for more focused diagnostic assessment. Screening for HD must be conducted, as many other mental health diagnoses may underlie behaviors related to hoarding (e.g., anxiety, depression, limitations in physicality).

Even if a clinician does not directly observe disorganized or unsanitary conditions, it is wise to ask some questions related to the aforementioned challenges listed, as clients may only be presenting a small area of their home in their video screen, or they may use a virtual background, inhibiting the clinician's ability to gain a full visual assessment of the state of the home.

Administration of Diagnostic Instruments

Have the following assessment tools available for use in either paper or digital format:

- Structured Interview for Hoarding Disorder

- Hoarding Rating Scale

- Hoarding Assessment Tool

- Uniform Inspection Checklist

The Structured Interview for Hoarding Disorder (Nordsletten et al., 2013) is a reliable and valid diagnostic tool that utilizes an interview structure to guide diagnosis through the six criteria of HD and its two specifiers. This tool can be used to work through a full diagnosis of HD.

The Hoarding Rating Scale (Tolin et al., 2010) is a five-item, self-report measure that takes about two to three minutes to conduct. It assesses the severity of the main features of hoarding, which include: (1) clutter, (2) difficulty discarding, (3) acquisition, (4) distress, and (5) functional impairment.

Either of these diagnostic instruments can be delivered verbally via telehealth, with the clinician asking the client the questions for each item and recording their scores.

In the weeks leading up to the home tour, clinicians can utilize the Hoarding Assessment Tool (Frost & Steketee, 2007) as a resource for outlining relevant narrative information that will assist with developing a comprehensive and systemic treatment plan. The therapist should ask questions related to onset and duration of the hoarding problem, home environment and contents, thoughts and feelings about possessions, current acquiring, reasons for saving, strategies for organization, role of family, friends, and community members, immediate long-term threats to health and safety, problems resulting from hoarding, previous intervention attempts, personal goals and values with regard to current and future use of home, other contributing factors that might affect clinical intervention, and any impediments to change.

Preparation for Visual Inspection of the Home

Once it is determined through screening that the client needs a further clinical and functional assessment for HD, prepare clients for the visit by following these steps:

1. Explain that a home "tour" will need to be conducted during a future session to check for safety concerns and identify the severity of the hoarding. This gives clients time to prepare themselves psychologically for the "visit." Prior to the "visit," ask that clients not attempt to clean up so that you can see the home as it normally is. Explain to them that this is part of the therapeutic process to ascertain the level of hoarding and what type of hoarding behaviors they are having. In the absence of significant concern for the client's safety, do not rush into this process. Doing so may result in a breach of trust in the client–therapist alliance, which may be detrimental to the therapeutic process.

2. Prepare the client for the visit, as anxiety will likely be high. Present coping strategies that clients can use during the visit. Discuss with clients the need for them to have a portable, cord-free device with a working camera connected to cellular data or Wi-Fi for the tour.

Instructions

The home tour should be scheduled for two hours. Come to the session prepared with tools for assessing health and safety that might indicate higher priority of intervention. The Uniform Inspection Checklist (Matthews, 2014) helps pinpoint specific "targets" related to health, safety, and harm reduction that are important to note as clients show you around their living space. Utilizing formal assessments is ideal, as this allows for stating the facts about safety in the home rather than reliance on more subjective assessments made by the therapist. Formal assessments also allow clients to start to become aware of what needs to be prioritized (i.e., areas of highest risk of safety or health concerns).

1. Begin as you would normally begin your sessions, in the same location in the home, with an area that you have already seen before in previous meetings.

2. Let clients know that you will want to see as much of their home as you're able during your session, that it may take some time to do that, and that you are not in a rush.

3. Tell clients that you will be taking notes and that you will go over these with them during your next session.

4. Ask clients to use their device to show you the room they are in and to move slowly around each room, attempting to show you as much as they are able and willing. Some areas of a home may be inaccessible due to the amount of accumulation, but when it is possible, the main goals of the tour are to examine the standard rooms in a home (e.g., living room, kitchen, bedroom(s), bathroom(s)), plus any additional spaces (e.g., attic, basement, garage, laundry/utility room, yard, vehicles).

5. Ask clients to show you where all the means of exit are in each room (i.e., windows and doors), as well as the placement of electrical outlets and switches, appliances, or other fixtures.

6. Ask additional questions related to structure and safety (e.g., unstable floorboards).

7. Inquire about any additional storage spaces that the client may lease outside of their home property.

8. Once you have seen as much of the client's space as they will permit and as time will allow, ask them to return to the place that they usually occupy for their sessions and summarize your assessment with them.

Throughout the process, simply take notes, politely ask clients to move the camera to allow assessment of various areas of the home, thank them, and ask them to move on to the next space. Ensure ease of conversation during the tour so as not to seem punitive or judgmental. Use respectful language, utilizing the client's language when describing possessions and avoiding words like "trash," "junk," or even "hoarding."

Processing

When processing the home tour assessment with clients, focus on any emotional regulation that could be beneficial in the moment, and directly address any issues with the safety of their home.

Emotional Regulation

Once the client allows you to see their space, it can be difficult for them to not feel shame or stigmatized. Following a home tour, some client resistance can be expected. Rather than problem solving, use empathy with clients to decrease the likelihood of embarrassment, shame, anger, frustration, or feeling incapable.

Engaging clients in emotional regulation strategies, like grounding exercises, can be helpful following home visits. It can be extremely stressful to have someone observe their living conditions, and clients may experience high levels of stress and anxiety after the experience. Normalize this and help clients to develop a stress-management plan to utilize when they experience emotional overwhelm following the session.

Reviewing the Results of the Home Assessment

If safety concerns have presented themselves during the visit, it may be necessary to address these items immediately. If there are no imminent safety concerns, review any completed inventories and discuss your home assessment with clients at the time of your next session.

At the following session, do a check-in to gauge levels of distress since the previous visit. If clients seem dysregulated, attend to that before discussing the assessment summary. Once clients appear regulated and ready to discuss the assessment summary, use information gathered from the assessment instruments to structure the conversation. Highlight areas marked as concerns on the Uniform Inspection Checklist (Matthews, 2014), and discuss with clients if they would like assistance with coordinating a plan to address these issues.

Be clear and concrete about your concerns regarding the clients, their home, and relationships with others affected by the hoarding (e.g., neighbors, family members). Be direct and specific about the safety measures that need to be in place to alleviate these concerns. Use clear and quantifiable data to emphasize safety. This allows for the promotion of healthy changes and increases the likelihood to motivate change, empowerment, and self-efficacy.

If you are uncomfortable or anxious reviewing the assessments, identify your own feelings and values about cleanliness and organization of a home to ensure you are not letting your own personal values cloud clinical judgment.

Vignette

Barb is a 56-year-old, single White agnostic cisgender female. She came to therapy for treatment for depression. During her last teletherapy session, Barb complained of poor sleep and noted that she had been sleeping in her recliner. She stated that she was fearful of losing her job, as she had been consistently tardy due to struggling to stay organized (e.g., noted that she loses her keys and can never find things she needs). When the therapist inquired about medication management, she admitted that she consistently forgets to take medication, as she loses track of where she puts her prescriptions, and some are expired. While Barb appeared to have good intentions to complete weekly goals set during sessions, such as donating items that she had put aside, she reported never getting around to them.

During the telehealth session, the therapist was able to see into the client's home, as her camera captured the entire room. As she was searching for something that the therapist and client were discussing in session, the therapist noticed that there was an excessive amount of clutter in the living room (i.e., stacks of boxes and newspapers piled high above eye level that looked disorganized and likely to fall over). The therapist also noticed that the kitchen counter was completely covered, and the sink was full of dirty dishes. The therapist also saw narrow paths around the room, similar to a maze. The therapist recognized these signs as potential clinical indicators of HD and determined that further screening was needed. The therapist let the client know that during their next session, they wanted to do a more focused assessment to see if there were any clinical or mental health concerns connected to the reason they were coming to therapy.

At the next session, the therapist began with diagnostic assessments and determined that the client met criteria for HD. The therapist worked with the client over the next few weeks to prepare for a virtual home tour and focused on understanding the client's narrative about her history with hoarding behaviors. They worked with the client on developing self-soothing strategies so she would have tools for emotional regulation if things became too distressing for her during the home tour. A week prior to the virtual home visit, the therapist reviewed coping strategies with the client and discussed any questions she had about the upcoming tour.

On the day of the tour, the therapist began the telehealth session by checking in with the client about her emotional state heading into the visit. The client reported that she was experiencing some anxiety about the session, so the therapist engaged the client in some grounding exercises, including some deep breathing, and let the client know that it was fine to stop the session and do a breathing exercise at any point necessary. Once the client felt grounded enough to begin, the therapist asked the client to turn the camera around on her phone and asked her to walk through the home, slowly scanning each room. The therapist guided the client using gentle directions (e.g., "Can you please pan to the left a little bit?"; "I see there is a door behind that pile of boxes. Can we go over there and take a look? What's behind the door?"; "I see that the light doesn't work in this room. Can you tell me about that?").

Following the virtual visit, the therapist determined that the client's household required a coordinated collaborative response. This included a team of service providers such as a professional organizer who specialized in HD to help with the coordination of a harm-reduction plan to get the home to safety, while the therapist focused on treatment related to distress tolerance and emotional regulation during the process. This was an arduous task that was planned out with the client to minimize safety hazards and increase self-efficacy. Once the home reached levels of "safe enough," the therapist shifted treatment goals to focus more on the underlying factors contributing to hoarding behaviors.

Suggestions for Follow-Up

A harm-reduction approach is often the best option available to offer support around imminent health and safety risks related to HD. In a harm-reduction approach, the goal is not to eliminate the hoarding behavior itself but to minimize consequences that accompany the behavior (Tompkins, 2015). Harm reduction is ideal for working with individuals with cognitive impairments or people unwilling to seek treatment. Tompkins (2015) offers harm-reduction strategies for clinicians working with more severe hoarding situations. Steketee and Frost (2013) offer additional resources for designing treatment plans and interventions related to hoarding behavior.

Contraindications

Virtual home tours are not possible for all clients. For example, clients may have a physical disability, coupled with high falling hazards due to the hoarding conditions in their home. If clients are at high risk of danger with low cognitive capacity (e.g., severe mental health impairments, developmental disability), you may need to include legal guardianship or conservatorship in intervention (Saltz, 2010).

References

American Psychiatric Association. (2013). *Diagnostic and statistical manual of mental disorders* (5th ed.). American Psychiatric Association. https://doi.org/10.1176/appi.books.9780890425596

Ayers, C. R., Saxena, S., Golshan, S., & Wetherell, J. L. (2010). Age at onset and clinical features of late life compulsive hoarding. *International Journal of Geriatric Psychiatry*, *25*(2), 142–149. https://doi.org/10.1002/gps.2310

Frost, R. O., & Gross, R. C. (1993). The hoarding of possessions. *Behaviour Research and Therapy*, *31*(4), 367–381. https://doi:10.1016/0005-7967(93)90094-b

Frost, R. O., & Steketee, G. (2007). Compulsive hoarding. In *Obsessive-compulsive disorder* (pp. 76–93). Elsevier Science Ltd. https://doi.org/10.1016/j.cpr.2003.08.002. PMID: 14624821.

Frost, R. O., & Steketee, G. (Eds.). (2014). *The Oxford handbook of hoarding and acquiring*. Oxford University Press. https://doi.org/10.1093/oxfordhb/9780199937783.001.0001

Kim, H. J., Steketee, G., & Frost, R. O. (2001). Hoarding by elderly people. *Health & Social Work*, *26*(3), 176–184. https://doi.org/10.1093/hsw/26.3.176

Matthews, M. (2014). *Uniform inspection checklist-hoarding excessive clutter*. North Shore Center for Hoarding and Cluttering. https://thecluttermovement.com/wpcontent/uploads/2018/06/UIC-Quick-Reference-combined.pdf

Nordsletten, A. E., de la Cruz, L. F., Pertusa, A., Reichenberg, A., Hatch, S. L., & Mataix-Cols, D. (2013). The structured interview for hoarding disorder (SIHD): Development, usage and further validation. *Journal of Obsessive-Compulsive and Related Disorders*, *2*(3), 346–350. https://doi.org/10.1016/j.jocrd.2013.06.003

Saltz, E. (2010). Hoarding and elders: Current trends, dilemmas, and solutions. *Journal of Geriatric Care Management*, *20*, 4–10. https://doi.org/10.1017/S1041610216002465

Steketee, G., & Frost, R. O. (2013). *Treatment for hoarding disorder: Workbook*. Oxford University Press.

Tolin, D. F., Fitch, K. E., Frost, R. O., & Steketee, G. (2010). *Hoarding Rating Scale – Self-Report (HRS-SR)* [Database record]. APA PsycTests. https://doi.org/10.1037/t35976-000

Tompkins, M. (2015). *Clinician's guide to severe hoarding: A harm reduction approach*. Springer.

CHAPTER 23

VIRTUAL COGNITIVE STIMULATION THERAPY

A GROUP INTERVENTION FOR OLDER ADULTS WITH MEMORY LOSS

Matthew Amick, Max Zubatsky, and Marla Berg-Weger

Materials for Therapists: Some session interventions may require the use of sounds or digital images that may be easily acquired via the internet. For additional information on intervention implementation, therapists may review "Making a Difference" Version 1: The Manual for Group Facilitators. This manual can be found at: https://hawkerpublications.co.uk/product/making-a-difference.

Materials for Clients: Some session interventions may require the use of common objects found within the household (e.g., spices).

Objective

Cognitive stimulation therapy (CST) is an evidence-based nonpharmacological intervention for those with mild to moderate dementia (Spector et al., 2003). This chapter will present virtual cognitive stimulation therapy (vCST) for use with groups of older adults with memory loss via teletherapy platforms.

Rationale for Use

CST is based on reminiscence therapy, validation therapy, and reality orientation and incorporates key features of other holistic therapies within an evidence-based curriculum. Reminiscence therapy involves the recall of life events using visual and auditory aids (Huang et al., 2015). Validation therapy empathetically responds to the emotional content of an individual's words or expressions to alleviate negative feelings and enhance positive moods (Livingston et al., 2005). Reality orientation involves the presentation of personal and current information through various activities (Spector et al., 2000). Utilizing main components of each of these approaches, CST demonstrates improvement in quality of life (Orrell et al., 2005, 2014; Spector et al., 2003), processing and recall (Aguirre et al., 2013; Spector et al., 2003; Spector et al., 2010; Spector et al., 2011), and mood (Carbone et al., 2021; Stewart et al., 2017) in people with dementia.

DOI: 10.4324/9781003289920-27

Principles of CST are defined by Spector et al. (2006) as follows:

- Mental stimulation
- New ideas, thoughts, and associations
- Using orientation sensitively and implicitly
- Opinions rather than facts
- Using reminiscence as an aide to the here-and-now
- Physical movement
- Providing triggers and prompts to aid recall and concentration
- Implicit (rather than explicit) learning
- Stimulating language
- Stimulating executive functioning
- Person-centeredness
- Maximizing potential
- Involvement and inclusion
- Respect
- Choice
- Fun
- Building/strengthening relationships
- Continuity and consistency between sessions

A virtual adaptation of CST allows clients who might not otherwise be physically able to commute to an in-person office the ability to participate. Ideal candidates for vCST are aged 60 years and above. Participation is optimal when all members have identifiable memory loss (e.g., mild cognitive impairment or early-stage dementia) and are generally at the same level of functioning evident by a brief cognitive assessment. There is no designated number of participants needed to begin a group. However, having between five and eight participants may be favorable in providing avenues of connection without overstimulation. Recent literature (Perkins et al., 2022) highlights the implementation of vCST for group therapy with older adults. The following provides additional details on the specifics of vCST and certain considerations for those looking to facilitate these groups.

Setup

Setup for implementation of vCST involves having an appropriate teletherapy platform and group facilitators. Group norms must also be established prior to the start of the therapy.

Teletherapy Platform

Successful implementation of technology-based interventions for older adults is contingent on accessibility, affordability, and ease of use (Chung et al., 2016). For these reasons, Zoom videoconferencing software is an ideal platform for vCST. It is accessible on any smartphone, tablet, or laptop, is free to download, and is user-friendly. vCST facilitators may need to provide technology support, including training, and attend to participants' experience of technology during sessions.

Participants may also need to rely on caregivers for arranging in-home videoconferencing (Cheung & Peri, 2021). Therefore, caregivers should be present for the first session and potentially the first few minutes of subsequent sessions to assist with technology. The completion of appropriate paperwork (e.g., confidentiality agreement) for any support people must be considered prior to their participation in any sessions. It is up to the facilitator to explain expectations and decorum of caregivers "attending" a session. Caregiver involvement is limited to support with technology, but their presence often provides encouragement and comfort to participants during the beginning stages of vCST. They become an extension of the group process, as participants often look to caregivers for validation in the beginning of the process. The need for a caregiver's presence typically diminishes as participants get more comfortable with facilitators and other participants.

Group Facilitation

Two facilitators are preferred for the implementation of vCST. One facilitator manages the virtual presentation (i.e., screen-share content) while the other complements exchanges between participants and expands group engagement through conversation. Effective facilitators are high energy, directive, intentional, and explicit while remaining flexible and spontaneous.

Setting Group Norms

Facilitators must clearly create group norms and establish a culture that reverberates principles of CST among both participants and caregivers. Successful implementation of the social component of vCST is evident when the principles are systemically observable in group dynamics. Facilitators must offer gentle reminders for all participants and caregivers' adherence to the principles in all sessions. Because these principles often introduce new ways of communicating with loved ones, caregivers may innocently violate principles in their attempt to help. For instance:

> **Facilitator:** Oh wow, I think you are referring to that old Beatles song, but I can't remember which Beatle sings it. It could've been John, Paul, George, or . . . oh no I can't think of the last one.
>
> *Pauses to allow participants to respond to the social cue to help finish the sentence.*
>
> **Caregiver:** Come on, Dad, you know it is Ringo. You love the Beatles!

During this exchange, the caregiver not only cut her father's cognitive process short but also potentially robbed him or another group member of the sense of accomplishment from helping the facilitator name the fourth Beatle. If no one responds, the facilitator could spontaneously "remember" and continue, or even if another participant answered, "His name was also John," the facilitator could remark, "No wonder I forgot his name. I couldn't keep up with all the Johns!" Encouraging caregivers to focus on the process rather than the outcome helps them be a valuable member of the vCST practice, even though their role is limited in vCST. Facilitators model principles through their interactions with participants. Caregivers witness positive responses, teaching and motivating them to adopt principles of CST in their own interactions with the participant and their family system. Offering live demonstrations and implicit feedback to the caregivers makes vCST a more systemically focused intervention than traditional CST, from which caregivers are typically absent.

Instructions and Processing

Each session includes an introduction, main activity, and a close. Continuity between sessions provides comfort in routine.

Introduction

Facilitators welcome participants individually by responding to something they notice on screen. The facilitator welcomes the group, identifying them by their chosen group name. Facilitators encourage conversation by mentioning a calendar or current event to orient to the beginning and their own time and place. Facilitators can screen-share pictures to serve as prompts to the upcoming session themes or general pictures associated with calendar dates or upcoming holidays to aid in orientation (e.g., jack-o-lantern image if nearing October). Allow reality orientation, reminiscence, and validation therapy to shape comments, questions, and responses. Facilitators may begin each session with the following:

- *Reality orientation.* Help participants ground themselves in the "here and now." The following statements and questions are examples of things that may help to accomplish this task:

  - It is [day] and [time], and I am joining you from [location].

  - Are any of you joining us from outside [the facilitator's location]?

  - What season does it feel or look like there today? How can you tell?

- *Reminiscence.* Allow participants to recall information to improve long-term memory. For example:

  - What does the displayed image remind you of?

  - Is the displayed image something you and [caregiver's name] would do together?

- *Validation.* Help participants improve socialization and mood by tracking conversations and providing strength-based conversations. For example:

  - Does anybody have anything they want to share today about the displayed image?

  - Is the group in agreement about what this [word/picture/sound] represents?

  - What do you think is interesting about the perspective that [name of person] made?

Once the group and participants are oriented, the facilitator plays the group song. Each new vCST group establishes a group song and group name in the first session. Participants ideally choose their own group name and song, although some groups may need more prompting from facilitators such as gauging music genres and time periods generally liked by all members. Establishing a group song and name serves as a group icebreaker, aids in orientation at the start of each session, and establishes continuity in subsequent sessions. Attempting to compensate for the minimal physical activity associated with virtual attendance, incorporation of a physical component to the song is accomplished by facilitators instructing participants to mimic simple sitting arm stretches while the song plays.

Main Activity

The chosen song cues the transition from introduction and orientation to the main activity in each session. After the song ends, facilitators introduce the session's theme and activity (Spector et al., 2006).

Fourteen themed sessions are each structured to last 45 minutes (Perkins et al., 2022; Spector et al., 2006). vCST allows facilitators the flexibility to be creative in each theme's virtual adaptation. The following offers ideas for ways in which to implement each theme in a virtual format.

1. ***Physical games.*** Select games or other physical activities that participants can do in session. For example, challenge participants to pat their head while simultaneously rubbing their belly.

2. ***Sound.*** Play audio clips of different sounds (e.g., musical instrument). Have participants guess what makes the sound and/or discuss other things that make similar noises.

3. ***Childhood.*** Ask caregivers to have participants gather old photos or items that remind them of childhood memories to discuss with other group members during this session.

4. ***Food.*** Ask caregivers to make two spices (e.g., cinnamon, rosemary) available for session. Facilitators could make a game where each participant describes their spices without showing them and others process what spice is being described. With a higher-functioning group, participants may plan a meal or make a recipe with the spices.

5. ***Current affairs.*** Encourage group members to discuss relevant world or local issues to help engage in conversation and provide personal opinions about news topics. Facilitators can share news posts or other online articles with the group members.

6. ***Faces/scenes.*** Display a series of faces on the screen and ask prompting questions about participant reactions and preferences. This theme helps group members associate a face or scene with a personal emotion or feeling.

7. ***Word association.*** Present the group with a series of words, where the individuals associate a feeling or thought with that word.

8. ***Being creative.*** Encourage members to utilize their knowledge or skills to come up with ideas in the group. This is a chance to activate areas of the brain through expansion of new ideas. For example, facilitators may ask caregivers to provide the participant with a paper for drawing or for use in a facilitator-led origami tutorial.

9. ***Categorizing objects.*** Provide an opportunity for participants to come up with ways that objects could be similar or different. For example, show a picture of four animals and ask participants to explain which ones can be grouped together.

10. ***Orientation.*** Encourage group members to discuss topics that help orient them to places, events, past memories, and other remembrances in their lives. For example, discuss memorable moments in the country's history such as the moon landing or notable places often visited in a lifetime such as the Washington Monument.

11. ***Using money.*** Give members specific questions and exercises to help them recall how to use money and provide creative solutions to spend money.

12. ***Number games.*** Provide an opportunity for members to arrange numbers and find patterns to activate parts of the brain.

13. **Word games.** This is a fun, interactive activity in which participants can be creative in filling in words to well-known phrases or idioms. For example, have participants finish sayings like "It is raining cats and _____." Use these phrases to then prompt discussions regarding the idiom's origin or times when participants may have heard or used those phrases.

14. **Team quiz.** During the last session, split the group up into teams, and have them try to identify correct answers or ideas from the questions asked by the facilitators. For example, give the participants a list of well-known "old wives' tales" and ask them to determine which ones are true before reconvening to discuss answers.

Difficulty of each theme's main activity can be adjusted to the group's level of functioning. For example, the using-money theme can range from simply showing a picture of a common grocery item and asking participants to guess the cost to a more difficult task of asking participants to build a grocery list for supper using $10. vCST offers the opportunity to share an endless array of images, songs, and stimulating content to further expand conversation and engagement with session themes. Activities should be stimulating, socially engaging, inclusive, and adjustable according to the group's level of functioning. Creativity in tailoring the 14 main activities to each group keeps vCST exciting and stimulating. A good activity is measured by how engaging it is for participants in session rather than any postsession outcomes. Caregivers may be asked to equip participants with materials needed. Facilitators may choose to share screen images to provide context to the conversations as they arise.

Questions prompted by facilitators should be open-ended and elicit opinions rather than facts. Activities and interactions must avoid putting participants on the spot to answer "right or wrong." Two important guidelines every facilitator should instill are engaging new ideas from discussions and emphasizing opinions rather than facts. Removing "do you remember" from a facilitator's vocabulary takes practice but is necessary. As relationships are built, facilitators can gather more information to ask about that is unique to participants, making them feel especially included. Occasional pauses (e.g., stop screen share) may be necessary to improve interactions with this population.

Close

At the end of each session, facilitators should check in with each person about a goal or something that they are looking forward to during that week. Sometimes, participants will summarize what they enjoyed about the group or if there were additional things that they wanted to address with other members. Facilitators may also provide some tips for participants to think about from that day's theme or activity. If the facilitators are in contact with participants' caregivers, they may discuss topics and what group members might be able to work on outside of the group or in the home.

Vignette

The following provides an edited sample of fun and engaging vCST sessions with Mary, Betty, Margaret, and Gale, pseudonyms of real participants, where no confidentiality is revealed through this script.

Facilitator 1: Good morning, everyone! It is 10 o'clock on a Monday morning, and that means you are with us for the next hour to listen to music, play games, and whatever else we can get into. Betty, it looks like you were on the phone when you joined. Was that your daughter giving you your CST alarm?

Betty: Yes, that's my daughter, Victoria. She calls me to make sure I don't forget.

Facilitator 1: You must be lucky to have a daughter to keep you on task! Gale, it looks like you got your hair done in the last week. I see your partner behind you. You all must have made a trip to the salon recently.

Gale: Maybe we did. He always takes me to the beauty shop. I don't remember going this week.

Facilitator 1: Maybe you're just having a good hair day with no professional help!

Facilitator 1 continues greeting each member until everyone has been addressed.

Facilitator 2: It is so good to see all the Memory Keepers this morning. As you all may know, America celebrated July 4th on Saturday. It was 99° in St. Louis, meaning it is peak summertime. The heat almost kept me from going to a BBQ. That is what I think about when I celebrate the 4th of July. What do you think about when someone mentions the 4th of July?

Mary: Fireworks.

Facilitator 1: Of course you need fireworks, Mary! Margaret, did you see any of the fireworks Mary is talking about?

Margaret: I did not see any. I don't think I went outside.

Facilitator 1: I don't blame you, probably because of the heat! Margaret, if I recall correctly, you have lived in Missouri your whole life. Do you think 99° is the hottest it has ever gotten here?

Facilitator 1 continues until everyone is oriented and welcomed.

Facilitator 2: I am going to play our group song. Can everybody see Facilitator 1's screen? He is wearing a blue shirt today. I want you to watch his screen and try to do every movement he does while the song plays.

Facilitator 2 shares sound only while Facilitator 1 performs various arm stretches.

Facilitator 1: I emailed your caregivers before the meeting and asked them to set aside a few spices for you today. You may have guessed by now, but today, we are going to be talking about my favorite topic. Food! I see Betty is already holding her spice up to the camera, so we'll start with her. What I want you all to do is describe your spice to the group, how it smells, the color, whether it is made of little leaves or is a powder. What do you have, Betty?

Betty: I have cinnamon. It is red, it looks like a powder, and smells 'cinnamony' and sweet.

Facilitator 1: Mmmm . . . Betty has a good spice, great pick! Betty, do you think you would eat more cinnamon in the summertime or the wintertime?

Gale: You eat cinnamon during the holidays.

Facilitator 1: That's a good point, Gale. I know I eat tons of cinnamon around December. Do you agree, Betty?

Betty: Yes, it reminds me of apple pie.

Facilitator 1: Betty, was there a special apple pie recipe or tradition around the holidays with apple pie?

Betty: Yes, my mother would make one every year.

Facilitator 2 shares their screen with images of two apple pies.

Facilitator 2: So I have an important question for Betty and the group. Did your mother's apple pie look like the one on the right, with a lattice pie crust, or more like the one on the left, with the more traditional vents cut into the top?

Betty: Hmmm, it did not look like either. We used little cinnamon crumbles on top like a streusel. It made it so tasty!

Facilitator 1 follows up with Betty's memory and engages all members, asking about their own choice or versions of apple pie, before moving on to the next participant/spice.

When the activity concludes and time is up, the facilitators praise all participants for their involvement, highlighting specific instances of progress or positivity shown. Before ending the meeting for everyone, the facilitators remind participants that they will meet again on the same day and at the same time with a new and exciting activity.

Suggestions for Follow-Up

Avoid referencing previous sessions. This places participants in a situation where they are pressured to recall specific events. Participants often have difficulty remembering attendance and content from previous sessions. Therefore, continual tracking from participants is often limited. Participants' explicit feedback may not always be reliable, which may warrant asking a caregiver for their assessment of the participant's tracking and mood immediately after sessions. However, a participant's nonverbal feedback is generally reliable, evidenced by increased engagement and positive mood throughout the course of vCST. Discussions about entering maintenance CST (Aguirre et al., 2011) may be appropriate if a caregiver and participant are interested in participation beyond the original 14 sessions. This decision should be based on enjoyment and perceived benefits rather than identifiable improvements.

Contraindications

Medical, mental health, or paraprofessional facilitators require prior experience and training working with older adult health issues, including exposure to psychosocial groups. Prospective participants with advanced deficits of memory to the point of not tracking conversations and topics in the group may not be appropriate. vCST requires specific visuospatial, ordering, and cognitive processing abilities that demand participants' attention. Participants should have adequate hearing and vision to track the group conversations. Older adults with existing medical issues or disabilities that prohibit them from sitting and engaging in group dynamics for long periods of time are not appropriate. Deficits in these areas compromise group utility by potentially causing frustration in the participant and/or disruption of group process. Those that do not fit criteria are encouraged to begin individualized CST (Yates et al., 2014).

References

Aguirre, E., Hoare, Z., Streater, A., Spector, A., Woods, B., Hoe, J., & Orrell, M. (2013). Cognitive stimulation therapy (CST) for people with dementia – who benefits most? *International Journal of Geriatric Psychiatry, 28*(3), 284–290. https://doi.org/10.1002/gps.3823

Aguirre, E., Spector, A., Hoe, J., Streater, A., Woods, B., Russell, I., & Orrell, M. (2011). Development of an evidence-based extended programme of maintenance cognitive stimulation therapy (CST) for people with dementia. *Non-Pharmacological Therapies in Dementia, 1*(3), 197–216.

Carbone, E., Gardini, S., Pastore, M., Piras, F., Vincenzi, M., & Borella, E. (2021). Cognitive stimulation therapy for older adults with mild-to-moderate dementia in Italy: Effects on cognitive functioning, and on emotional and neuropsychiatric symptoms. *The Journals of Gerontology: Series B, 76*(9), 1700–1710. https://doi.org/10.1093/geronb/gbab007

Cheung, G., & Peri, K. (2021). Challenges to dementia care during COVID-19: Innovations in remote delivery of group cognitive stimulation therapy. *Aging & Mental Health, 25*(6), 977–979. https://doi.org/10.1080/13607863.2020.1789945

Chung, J., Demiris, G., & Thompson, H. J. (2016). Ethical considerations regarding the use of smart home technologies for older adults: An integrative review. *Annual Review of Nursing Research, 34*(1), 155–181. https://doi.org/10.1891/0739-6686.34.155

Huang, H. C., Chen, Y. T., Chen, P. Y., Hu, S. H. L., Liu, F., Kuo, Y. L., & Chiu, H. Y. (2015). Reminiscence therapy improves cognitive functions and reduces depressive symptoms in elderly people with dementia: A meta-analysis of randomized controlled trials. *Journal of the American Medical Directors Association, 16*(12), 1087–1094. https://doi.org/10.1016/j.jamda.2015.07.010

Livingston, G., Johnston, K., Katona, C., Paton, J., & Lyketsos, C. G. (2005). Systematic review of psychological approaches to the management of neuropsychiatric symptoms of dementia. *American Journal of Psychiatry, 162*(11), 1996–2021. https://doi.org/10.1176/appi.ajp.162.11.1996

Orrell, M., Aguirre, E., Spector, A., Hoare, Z., Woods, R. T., Streater, A., Donovan, H., Hoe, J., Knapp, M., Whitaker, C., & Russell, I. (2014). Maintenance cognitive stimulation therapy for dementia: Single-blind, multicentre, pragmatic randomised controlled trial. *The British Journal of Psychiatry, 204*(6), 454–461. https://doi.org/10.1192/bjp.bp.113.137414

Orrell, M., Spector, A., Thorgrimsen, L., & Woods, B. (2005). A pilot study examining the effectiveness of maintenance cognitive stimulation therapy (MCST) for people with dementia. *International Journal of Geriatric Psychiatry: A Journal of the Psychiatry of Late Life and Allied Sciences, 20*(5), 446–451. https://doi.org/10.1002/gps.1304

Perkins, L., Fisher, E., Felstead, C., Rooney, C., Wong, G. H., Dai, R., Vaitheswaran, S., Natarajan, N., Mograbi, D. C., & Ferri, C. P. (2022). Delivering cognitive stimulation therapy (CST) virtually: Developing and field-testing a new framework. *Clinical Interventions in Aging, 17*, 97–116. https://doi.org/10.2147/cia.s348906

Spector, A., Davies, S., Woods, B., & Orrell, M. (2000). Reality orientation for dementia: A systematic review of the evidence of effectiveness from randomized controlled trials. *The Gerontologist, 40*(2), 206–212. https://doi.org/10.1093/geront/40.2.206

Spector, A., Gardner, C., & Orrell, M. (2011). The impact of cognitive stimulation therapy groups on people with dementia: Views from participants, their careers and group facilitators. *Aging & Mental Health, 15*(8), 945–949. https://doi.org/10.1080/13607863.2011.586622

Spector, A., Orrell, M., & Woods, B. (2010). Cognitive stimulation therapy (CST): Effects on different areas of cognitive function for people with dementia. *International Journal of Geriatric Psychiatry, 25*(12), 1253–1258. https://doi.org/10.1002/gps.2464

Spector, A., Thorgrimsen, L., Woods, B., Royan, L., Davies, S., Butterworth, M., & Orrell, M. (2003). Efficacy of an evidence-based cognitive stimulation therapy programme for people with dementia: Randomised controlled trial. *The British Journal of Psychiatry, 183*(3), 248–254. https://doi.org/10.1192/bjp.183.3.248

Spector, A., Thorgrimsen, L., Woods, R. T., & Orrell, M. (2006). *Making a difference: An evidence-based group programme to offer Cognitive stimulation therapy (CST) to people with dementia.* Hawker Publications.

Stewart, D. B., Berg-Weger, M., Tebb, S., Sakamoto, M., Roselle, K., Downing, L., Lundy, J., & Hayden, D. (2017). Making a difference: A study of cognitive stimulation therapy for persons with dementia. *Journal of Gerontological Social Work, 60*(4), 300–312. https://doi.org/10.1080/01634372.2017.1318196

Yates, L., Orrell, M., Leung, P., Spector, A., Woods, B., & Orgeta, V. (2014). *Making a difference 3: Individualised CST–A manual for carers.* Hawker publications.

Part 5

Intimate Relationships

CHAPTER 24

STRUCTURAL INTERVENTIONS FOR INTIMATE RELATIONSHIP THERAPY

CAPITALIZING ON THE LIMITATIONS OF TELEHEALTH

Veronica P. Viesca and Parker Leukart

Materials for Therapists and Clients: None.

Objective

Structural therapy interventions can be used to capitalize on the limitations of telehealth. This chapter explains how to address common difficulties of teletherapy through structural therapy as an effective therapeutic intervention with intimate relationships.

Rationale for Use

Prominent difficulties of online therapy when working with intimate relationships include (Burgoyne & Cohn, 2020; Wrape & McGinn, 2019):

- Partners attending sessions from different devices and/or locations

- Environmental distractions

- Clients turning off their camera or walking out of view of the camera

- Overuse of the "mute" function

Applying a structural lens to teletherapy allows therapists to see commonly occurring limitations of teletherapy with intimate partnerships as part of the structure of the client system. The additional layer of technology overlaid onto therapy adds unique potential for innovation of intervention. The shortcomings of telehealth, therefore, can become its strengths. For example, partners attending teletherapy from different locations may find that physical distance supports opportunities for emotional regulation during difficult conversations to ultimately strengthen the partner subsystem. By applying this new perspective, therapists can identify new opportunities for therapeutic intervention that not only address the limitations of telehealth but help clarify boundaries, realign hierarchy, and restructure the client system.

DOI: 10.4324/9781003289920-29

The following tenets of structural therapy can be used to inform interventions and to overcome natural barriers of online therapy within intimate relationships (McDowell et al., 2017).

- *Reframing* occurs when the therapist challenges client assumptions, thoughts, or beliefs and offers a new way of viewing things.

- *Structure* maintains identified problems within the client system. Structural imbalance is often seen when there are overly rigid or diffuse boundaries around or within client systems.

- *Boundaries* are the psychological and emotional barriers or limits that exist within a family system. Boundaries determine the degree of separation and connection between family members.

- *Subsystem*s describe smaller, interconnected groups or relationships with the family unit. Examples of this are parents, siblings, or more specific pairings like father–daughter relationships.

- *Hierarchy* identifies who is in charge of what within a client system. In a family, a well-functioning executive subsystem manages its responsibilities to provide care, protection, socialization, and other important functions. This executive subsystem is at the top of the family hierarchy. Different hierarchies, however, may exist for different functions within the same system.

- *Restructuring* occurs when the structure of the family is reorganized. This can happen through the process of *unbalancing* or using *enactment*s, which help shape interactions through interruption, invitation for emotional expression, and coaching of communication.

Instructions

The following offers suggestions for online therapy with intimate partnerships based on the aforementioned tenets of structural therapy. Intervention ideas are organized by prominent difficulties of online therapy.

Location of Therapy

Each client may join online sessions from the same location, or they may join from separate locations. Reflecting on the structure of how clients show up can inform clinical hypotheses regarding the structure of the client system and illuminate areas for intervention. The following questions may guide evaluation that considers client perspectives:

- How does the environment that you're in during session impact your ability to focus on your relationship during our time together?

- What does your partner's chosen location for teletherapy indicate as it relates to your relationship with one another? For example, logging in from work could be a sign of disconnect, or it could evoke thoughts that "my partner cares so much about our relationship that they made time for us out of their workday."

- Would you feel closer or more distant if you met from [the same physical location/different physical locations]?

With answers to these questions and clear hypotheses of the client's presenting problems, therapists can develop structural interventions that will perturb the client's existing structure. Consider potential therapeutic outcomes of all available options for joining teletherapy sessions (i.e., meeting from the same location, meeting from different devices in different locations, or rejoining in the same physical location after meeting from separate locations). Then, provide clients with clear directives that align with structural theory to support therapeutic goals.

- ***Instruct clients to meet from the same location.*** This increases the potential for direct interaction and co-regulation. It also allows clients to be physically close, offering therapists the opportunity for additional assessments (e.g., how close do clients sit to one another, do they touch to comfort one another) and *enactment*. This also ultimately serves the purpose of strengthening the partner subsystem by delineating a clear boundary around the partnership as the singular client in therapy. Some clients who prefer to meet from separate locations for convenience may need a clear directive from the therapist that explains the importance of meeting from the same location.

- ***Instruct clients to meet from different devices in different locations.*** This creates physical distance between clients and may increase the ability to address complex topics when overly distressed. Clients with enmeshed boundaries may benefit from reorganizing therapy in this way to allow them to more clearly speak for themselves in therapy or to allow space for their partner(s) to speak in therapy.

- ***Instruct clients who have been meeting from separate locations to rejoin therapy from the same location.*** If this directive is provided mid-session, this may allow clients to come together in a moment of emotional vulnerability to heighten the experience and further strengthen the partner subsystem (Perel, 2020).

Environmental Distractions

When environmental distractions occur regularly in teletherapy, consider what this means with regards to the boundary surrounding the intimate relationship. Identify who or what is allowed into the intimate relationship. For example, children, animals, or even the use of technology may regularly be invited into the clients' intimate relationship, thus leading to a weakened partnership. A child interrupting regularly may indicate a diffuse boundary around the intimate partner subsystem. Likewise, if a child's care provider were to interrupt during session to indicate that there was an emergency and both partners were to avoid addressing the situation until the conclusion of session, this may indicate a more rigid boundary surrounding the intimate partner subsystem.

Use these patterns to inform structural interventions in teletherapy. Structural interventions related to environmental distractions might include:

- Requiring that clients have childcare available during sessions so that clients can focus on their relationship.

- Asking clients to turn on "do not disturb" mode and close all other windows on their devices.

- Inviting clients to leave the device they use for therapy out of arm's reach. This suggestion limits the temptation to click and scroll during the session.

- Inviting clients to leave their phones out of the room or place them face down so they do not see incoming notifications and are not tempted to pick up their phones.

Each of these directives serves the function of clarifying boundaries around the partner subsystem. This allows partners to focus on strengthening their relationship with one another in session and translates into setting up similar structures outside of therapy. Environmental distractions in teletherapy may also be used to inform strategic therapy interventions (see Chapter 25).

Use of the Mute Functions

"Mute yourself" is a common video meeting courtesy in professional settings to limit distractions. However, if partners mute themselves in therapy, the therapist may miss out on small reactionary sounds or comments. It is best practice to instruct clients to be unmuted for the entire session.

However, therapists may use the mute function to their advantage when working with partners who have a tendency to interrupt one another when meeting from separate locations. In this instance, inform clients in advance that you will interrupt them to help focus on goals of therapy or to allow space for their partner(s) to speak. If they do not follow this directive, you may use the mute function to allow this space. If and when this does occur, it is important to process this experience with clients afterward and to assess for any impact on the therapeutic relationship. This ultimately places the therapist at the top of the *hierarchy* in therapy and creates a clear structure for maintaining space for all partners involved in therapy.

Clients Who Turn Off the Camera or Walk Out When Distressed

Many clients feel distressed when seeing themselves tearful or in heightened states of arousal like anger or rage. Being on camera with their emotional state looking back at them in the "self-view" often results in clients turning off their camera or closing their computer when they become distressed. This ultimately serves to create a rigid boundary between themself and their partner(s). The following suggestions address how to navigate these situations in session to clarify boundaries and prevent disengagement:

- Give clients the directive at the start of therapy to turn off their self-view so they cannot see their reactions.

- Use the reflection of self as an intervention. If the client has the self-view on, this can be an opportunity to challenge assumptions, ask clients what they see when they look at themselves in the emotional state and what they think their partner(s) see(s), then check in with their partner(s) about what they actually see. This intervention is also an opportunity for the therapist to offer a reframe of what they see happening for the client.

- Name the behavior at the start of therapy. The therapist may say, "Sometimes, when clients become distressed, they move away from their device, for example by walking away, closing their computer, or hanging up. Unfortunately, this makes it hard for me as a therapist to assess you and support you."

- Once the behavior has occurred, bring it up in the next meeting and negotiate an agreed-upon plan. One might suggest, "Instead of turning off your camera, can you write in the chat box or say verbally that you really want to turn the camera off right now?"

- Invite partners to read each other's body language or energetic feeling by saying something like, "It's hard for me to get a clear picture of [client's name]'s body language from this camera angle. Can you tell me what they're doing? What do you think this is communicating? Based on their body language, how do you think they're feeling?" This can encourage partners to increase their observations of one another and to ultimately strengthen the partner subsystem.

Processing and Follow-Up

The following questions may be asked to assess the impact of the aforementioned interventions:

- What was it like for you to change physical locations for teletherapy?
- What has it been like for you to keep your microphone off mute?
- What has it been like for you to be muted?
- What has it been like for you to keep your camera on?

Following each of these questions, ask clients to reflect on the following:

- How have you clarified boundaries in your relationship as a result?
- How have you strengthened your relationship with one another as a result?

Vignette

George (37, male) and Armida (35, female) presented to therapy reporting frequent arguing and conflict. A month prior to initiating therapy, the couple decided that George should move out. George stayed with friends and family or at hotels. Their two school-age children and two dogs lived in their home with Armida. The couple scheduled their session during the day while the children were at school. They attended on different devices from different locations, often between work meetings. During therapy sessions, Armida often emotionally shut down or became distressed, turned off her camera, and became challenging to reengage. Similarly, George had a tendency to overexplain and defend himself when he felt attacked. It was difficult for the therapist to get his attention and/or stop him when he was hyper aroused. The therapist often ended the session after deescalating George, having not received a further response from Armida. Armida would reach out to the therapist after the session, apologizing for her reaction and expressing a desire to continue the therapeutic work "for the sake of her children."

In working with George and Armida, the therapist first considered how the meeting time and location were impacting how the couple showed up for the session. Scheduling time while the children were at school appeared to be helpful, but code switching between work and therapy poses challenges for some clients. Some alternative options included scheduling at the start of the day, following a lunch break, or at the end of the day. These times were aligned with shifts in the day and could help ease the transition. The clients' proximity to each other was also relevant in this case. The therapist preferred that the couple meet together using one device to provide more information to assess the couple's relationship dynamics. However, the therapist also recognized practical limitations of the clients' situation and took the route of openly discussing alternative options to scheduling and offered their preference for them to meet together if possible. The therapist explained that meeting together could provide opportunities for co-regulation and directive interventions of therapy. Before asking them to decide, the therapist asked the couple, "How would it feel to sit in the room with one another right now?" Each person explained that this might afford the opportunity for them to feel closer to one another and that they rarely spent time with each other without the children present. George was able to rearrange his schedule so therapy could occur at the end of his workday, while the children were still at daycare. Though they were unable to meet together on a weekly basis due to concerns regarding traffic and commute time, the couple prioritized meeting together for therapy for several sessions. On these occasions, the therapist focused on an integration of experiential and structural interventions that strengthened the couple relationship (e.g., sitting closer to one another, holding hands to support grounding one another in the present moment when emotionally distressed).

Contraindications

Some telehealth limitations are too substantial to navigate. For example, when violence and safety are a concern, teletherapy may not be appropriate for working with partners (Wrape & McGinn, 2019). In these instances, clarify the need for a different treatment structure such as individual or in-person therapy.

References

Burgoyne, N., & Cohn, A. S. (2020). Lessons from the transition to relational teletherapy during COVID-19. *Family process*, *59*(3), 974–988. https://doi.org/10.1111/famp.12589

McDowell, T., Knudson-Martin, C., & Bermúdez, J. M. (2017). *Socioculturally attuned family therapy: Guidelines for equitable theory and practice*. Routledge. https://doi.org/10.4324/9781315559094

Perel, E. (Executive Producer). (2020). On again/off again (Season 4, Episode 10) [Audio podcast episode]. In *Where should we begin?* Magnificent Noise. www.estherperel.com/podcasts/wswb-s4-episode10

Wrape, E. R., & McGinn, M. M. (2019). Clinical and ethical considerations for delivering couple and family therapy via telehealth. *Journal of Marital and Family Therapy*, *45*(2), 296–308. https://doi.org/10.1111/jmft.12319

CHAPTER 25

DOORBELLS, BABIES, AND DOGS, OH MY

DISTRACTIONS AS METAPHORS IN TELETHERAPY WITH INTIMATE RELATIONSHIPS

Racine R. Henry

Materials for Therapists and Clients: None.

Objective

The client's physical environment may be ripe with distractions from teletherapy, which may serve as metaphors within intimate relationships. This chapter provides strategic suggestions for preparing clients for potential distractions, addressing distractions once they occur, and using interruptions to make treatment more efficacious.

Rationale for Use

Teletherapy has the immense benefit of clients not having to travel to the therapist's office for sessions and reduces the need for childcare as a possible barrier to treatment (Hardy et al., 2020; Maier et al., 2020; McKee et al., 2022). Both clients and clinicians indicate that attending teletherapy from home creates a less sterile and more "human" feeling to the experience (Hardy et al., 2020; Maier et al., 2020). Despite these benefits, conducting teletherapy with clients in intimate relationships in their home environment rather than the therapist's physical office is correlated with clients being more distracted and less able to focus during sessions (Hardy et al., 2020; Maier et al., 2020). These distractions include but are not limited to the unexpected presence of other people or animals in the client's physical location, doorbells ringing with the arrival of packages, dogs barking to announce their arrival, phones ringing, televisions blaring, other noises coming from other parts of the client's physical location, people walking by windows, and the sudden ending of internet connectivity. These distractions only tend to worsen with time. Challenges related to distraction in teletherapy for intimate relationships continue to increase after a three-month period (Békés et al., 2021).

Although these distractions may interfere with the existing flow of treatment, there are benefits to their occurrence. Strategic therapy posits that it is impossible to not communicate and that every communication

DOI: 10.4324/9781003289920-30

offers valuable information that is useful in the treatment process (Weakland et al., 1974). The types of distractions that occur and how clients respond to these distractions can be seen as manners of communication for that client system. Subsequently, any communication can be a metaphor for how the client system functions and can provide insight into symptomology of the larger, overarching problem to be addressed in therapy. Since clients mostly participate in teletherapy from their homes, clinicians have the unique opportunity to not only see how these distractions develop but also see a client's instinctual response and plan of action for the distractions. This approach to problem solving can also be repeated in their interactional pattern regarding the treatment issue and reveal a portion of or the whole pattern to be interrupted. Clinicians performing teletherapy can then incorporate the client's style of addressing problems into their treatment plans and eventual approach of creating second-order change.

Setup

While it is impossible to safeguard teletherapy sessions from all distractions and possible negative occurrences, ensure partners are aware of the need for a quiet and confidential space and are given practical tools for getting back on track when distractions do occur. Preempt as many distractions as possible by collaborating with clients to create a plan for things like loss of internet connection or interruptions from children (Maier et al., 2020). To begin this process, it may help to take note of distractions that spontaneously occur versus those that occur regularly and the ultimate impact they have on clients. See Chapter 2 for more suggestions on managing multiple therapeutic environments in teletherapy and Chapter 24 for using structural therapy to address environmental distractions and other limitations of telehealth.

Instructions

According to strategic therapy, members of the client system often perpetuate problems with their own attempted solutions. For example, when the distraction is related to a household responsibility such as childcare routines or preparing a meal, a partner may leave the room or multitask during session in an attempt to fulfil an important task to support their partner(s) or family. This can also heighten tension and reinforce preexisting animosity for their partner(s). A distraction during session, for example, can elicit suspicion that the offending partner is less committed to the process and, therefore, the relationship. Alternatively, when distractions occur, they can provide opportunities for partners to self-regulate by momentarily shifting their attention from each other to the interruptions and then experiencing a moment of reconnection.

When environmental distractions occur in teletherapy, consider the function of the distraction and each client's response. For example, when dogs approach clients during session, squeaking a toy and wanting to play, this may provide partners with an outlet to turn their attention to at times of relationship conflict, ultimately allowing them to avoid addressing relationship concerns. Alternatively, it may provide an opportunity for partners to reconnect in a moment of shared laughter or affection for their pet.

Reflect on patterns of interaction as they relate to distractions. Consider the following:

- Is the distraction a one-off experience, or does it occur regularly?

- Does the distraction play a part in the clients' pattern of interaction with one another?

- If so, at what point in the clients' pattern of interaction is the distraction most likely to occur?

After reflecting on the function of the distraction and ways in which it shows up in patterns of interaction, identify ways in which to maximize the benefit of this exchange. Therapists may offer a reframe of the distraction or a client's response to the distraction, offer a paradoxical intervention, raise the intensity of existing patterns, or highlight the double bind that occurs with the occurrence of the distraction.

One approach can be to reframe their perception of the disruption or their response to it. For example, the therapist might reflect on the function of an external distraction by saying, "Your daughter must know how hard this is for you. She keeps trying to save you from having to be vulnerable with one another!" The therapist might reflect on a client's distracting behavior by saying, "Your partner must really care for you. It's so hard for them to see you hurting that they need to focus their attention on something else." These reflections serve as reframes that have the potential to perturb the client system and break existing patterns of interaction.

Another good place to start may be to create a paradoxical intervention. To do so, the therapist initiates a conversation about the potential pitfalls to teletherapy, such as distractions and unforeseen interruptions, to initiate solutions for what is possible to occur. By acknowledging that the therapist and clients are at home, juggling other responsibilities like kids, pets, and preparing meals, clients will have an awareness of the potential for distractions to occur. This may prompt them to take steps to mitigate those possibilities (e.g., aligning their child's nap time with the session time). This also lays the groundwork for any future discussions about eventual distractions. Similar to discussing limits of confidentiality in the first session, talking about the "what ifs" creates a reference point for future distractions. It can also align with the systemic belief that setbacks are an expected part of any new behavior or process. In emphasizing this, how the partners recover from the distraction can be used as a strength.

Alternatively, therapists may use the presence of a distraction to raise the intensity of existing patterns so that the system must change. For example, if in-laws continue to interrupt sessions, the therapist may invite them to join them in therapy. The treatment process can then incorporate and embrace what could have been a distraction by gaining new perspectives or soliciting support in interventions aimed at healing the relationship. An alternative response in this situation could be for clients to decline the invitation to invite the distraction into therapy, thereby shutting down the distraction and altering existing patterns of interaction.

Therapists may also highlight any double binds that present when a distraction is highlighted. For example, "you've scheduled therapy during the baby's nap time, but you go to check on the baby each time you're asked to express yourself more openly." Therapists must then be prepared to reconcile possible triangulation that presents with uncovered distractions.

Processing

The following questions may be asked to assess the impact of the aforementioned interventions:

- What has it been like for you to prevent _____ from distracting you in therapy?
- How have you experienced your feelings in new ways as a result?
- How have you experienced your partner(s) in new ways as a result?
- How have your interactions with one another changed as a result?

Vignette

Margaret and Liam presented for treatment to discuss their adjustment to being first-time parents and renegotiate their domestic duties while working from home. At least once a session, their infant would make an appearance, and they would wordlessly pass her back and forth to keep her calm. The therapist highlighted how well the couple worked together to address their baby's needs without becoming distracted by her presence. After a particularly heated exchange, Margaret got up to get the baby, and when she returned, both she and Liam had huge, bright smiles on their faces. The therapist pointed out that the couple had chosen to mask their emotions with smiles rather than expressing how they really felt in the presence of their child. With this acknowledgment, the couple began to reflect on other ways they tried to maintain a peaceful and quiet environment in which to raise their daughter rather than engaging in the argumentative, loud, and chaotic communication patterns they each grew up in. This led to another heated conversation about who put in more effort to break their family-of-origin cycles. The therapist encouraged the discourse while pointing out that the baby was not negatively impacted by her parents disagreeing. After some time, the therapist began a deescalation conversation, and they resumed their normal habit of intuitively communicating when to hand the baby off. At one point, the baby began to coo loudly, and everyone laughed. The therapist stated, "I wonder if you can both ground yourself in this present moment and acknowledge your strengths as a couple. Throughout our time together so far, I've admired the way that you both rely on each other to share the responsibility of child-care. Regardless of the topic or level of expressed animosity, you're both able to access a more patient part of yourselves. Not only is that a great environment to have your baby in, it also shows that even though we're talking about emotional injuries and a recurring disagreement, you can still be kind and loving to each other. This tells me that with some intention and time, you can respond to each other from that same loving place in times of distress." While the comments the clients shared were positive in order to create a contrast to the tension, a potential downfall could be that they had developed a habit of hiding or cutting off productive conversations in an effort to only show their baby harmony and positivity. The therapist eventually facilitated a conversation about how they could create more balance between harmless fighting and getting along around their child so that caring for her didn't create an excuse for either of them to neglect their partner's needs or feelings.

Suggestions for Follow-Up

After identifying the distractions as metaphors, therapists can refer to this again in subsequent sessions. For example, when things get heated and clients need emotional regulation, the therapist might ask, "Can someone call Fido over for a quick play break?" Alternatively, the therapist might ask how Fido is doing and if he's worn out from playing too much.

Contraindications

Clients may have an adverse reaction to clinicians pointing out distractions or may insist that there is no way of avoiding them. If this happens, you may need to discuss the implications for treatment and set clear boundaries if therapy is otherwise contraindicated in their presence.

References

Békés, V., Doorn, K., Luo, X., Prout, T. A., & Hoffman, L. (2021). Psychotherapists' challenges with online therapy during Covid-19: Concerns about connectedness predict therapists' negative view of online therapy and its perceived efficacy over time. *Frontiers in Psychology*, *12*, Article 705699. https://doi.org/10.3389/fpsyg.2021.705699

Hardy, N. R., Maier, C. A., & Gregson, T. J. (2020). Couple teletherapy in the era of Covid-19: Experiences and recommendations. *Journal of Marital and Family Therapy*, *47*(2), 225–243. https://doi.org/10.1111/jmft.12501

Maier, C. A., Riger, D., & Morgan-Sowada, H. (2020). "It's splendid once you grow into it:" Client experiences of relational teletherapy in the era of Covid-19. *Journal of Marital and Family Therapy*, *47*(2), 304–319. https://doi.org/10.1111/jmft.12508

McKee, G. B., Pierce, B. S., Tyler, C. M., Perrin, P. B., & Elliott, T. R. (2022). The Covid-19 pandemic's influence on family systems therapists' provision of teletherapy. *Family Process*, *61*(1), 155–166. https://doi.org/10.1111/famp.12665

Weakland, J. H., Fisch, R., Watzlawick, P., & Bodin, A. M. (1974). Brief therapy: Focused problem resolution. *Family Process*, *13*(2), 141–168. https://doi.org/10.1111/j.1545-5300.1974.00141.x

CHAPTER 26

INTIMATE RELATIONSHIP DEESCALATION FOR TELETHERAPY

THE STRUCTURED PAUSE

Charity Francis Laughlin

Materials for Therapists: Note-taking implements, time-keeping device, and list of ideas for self-soothing.

Materials for Clients: None.

Objective

Escalations between intimate partners can be particularly difficult to manage effectively in teletherapy due to limited control over participation, spatial positioning of clients, and limited visibility of body language or other subtle cues indicating a client has moved out of their window of tolerance (Hogan, 2022; Wrape & McGinn, 2019). This chapter explains the use of the structured pause, a choreographed version of triangulation that decisively disrupts an escalation. The reassurance and containment provided by this directive therapeutic stance is particularly apt for the unique challenges of intimate relationship escalations in a teletherapy setting.

Rationale for Use

The structured pause is based on biofeedback research in intimate relationships, which suggests taking a calming break for at least 20 minutes if partner(s) become emotionally flooded during an interaction (Gottman & Gottman, 2017; Gottman & Silver, 2012). The structured pause allows the therapist to choreograph time to meet individually with each partner during session to support deescalation, emotional regulation, and validation. During this time, the therapist provides reflective listening and validation to each partner without having to worry about causing further distress in the observing partner(s). The individual time can also be used to gently challenge unskillful behavior when it would be difficult for the partner to receive this feedback in the presence of their partner(s). While the therapist is meeting with the partner(s), each partner should identify and engage in self-soothing practices. Teletherapy may offer more options for self-soothing during each partner's pause time, as clients may be in their own home

DOI: 10.4324/9781003289920-31

with access to familiar comforts such as a favorite calming space in the home, a beloved pet, tea in a favorite mug, aromatherapy, or ready access to the outdoors.

Setup

At the start of therapy, obtain consent from partners for you to take an active role in stopping or redirecting damaging interactions. With this consent established, introduce the structured pause if partners become escalated to the point that they are unable to self-regulate in the presence of their partner(s), are unable to give/receive compassion and validation in the presence of their partner(s), or are ready to leave the session due to their emotionally flooded state (Wrape & McGinn, 2019). You can prepare by remaining internally regulated and self-/other-connected, thus modeling regulation during difficult moments.

Instructions

Following are suggested guidelines for directly intervening in an escalation to provide containment and build trust in the relationship's ability to navigate conflict, rupture, and repair. Of paramount importance is your own self-compassion, self-regulation, and ability to attune to the system while maintaining healthy boundaries.

1. ***Interrupt the escalation.*** Be direct, calm, and firm. Offer an observation such as, "From what I'm seeing, you're having some difficult feelings that your relationship isn't quite able to hold right this moment, and it is not going to be possible to continue productively without a short break. I'd like to spend some time one-on-one with each of you. Then, we will come back together." Reassure partners that this is a chance to practice pausing, soothing, and reconnecting in session and that they can use a version of this outside of therapy to pause and reconnect when emotionally flooded during conflict.

2. ***Choreograph.*** Determine how much time to spend meeting individually with each partner. For a dyad, 10 minutes of individual time with each partner fulfills the suggested 20-minute minimum. When three or more partners are present in therapy, spend a minimum of 7 minutes with each client to meet this 20-minute requirement, though more time may be needed to adequately address the needs of each client. Client needs must be balanced with the time remaining in session. Then, discuss with clients who will be seen individually first. Clients may have a preference, though you may make suggestions based on the needs of clients. For example, the most dysregulated partner may need to be seen first. Agree on a method to reach the other partner when it is their time to come back to the session (e.g., the therapist or partner sending a text message or calling them when ready).

3. ***Create a self-soothing plan.*** Ask each partner to identify one or two things they will do during their break away from therapy to self-soothe. The activity chosen should be an alternative to rumination on the escalation. Some ideas include a brief walk outdoors, mindful breathing, coloring, listening to an app-based meditation, cuddling a pet, or noticing and naming feelings without judgment. Screenshare or email a document with some ideas for self-soothing if there is difficulty identifying activities (see Kauppi, 2020).

4. ***Meet individually with the first partner.*** Once the other partner(s) leave(s) the session, provide reflective listening and validation for the partner being seen individually. This may be enough to reduce emotional flooding to the point that you can explore together how this partner could have

agency over changing what is in their control while also holding compassion for their partner's experience. Once emotional arousal has decreased, invite the next partner to join session using the previously agreed-upon method.

5. ***Meet individually with the second partner.*** When talking with the second partner, there may be less need to deescalate if they've been able to self-soothe during the break. Offer reflective listening and validation as needed. Then, explore together how this partner could have agency over changing what is in their control while also holding compassion for their partner's experience.

6. ***Meet individually with other partners.*** When working with relationships in which there are more than two partners present in session, the aforementioned steps should be repeated with each remaining partner. Ensure that partners not present with the therapist take space separately from each other.

7. ***Rejoin.*** After individual time with each partner has been completed, invite all partners to rejoin the session.

Processing

Once all partners have rejoined the session, explore thoughts and feelings toward the process. If time allows, move to the content that precipitated the escalation, allowing all partners a chance to share thoughts and feelings in the speaker role while their partner(s) reflect(s) what they've heard as a listener, express(es) compassion, and ask(s) what is needed to move forward. Processing questions may include:

- What thoughts and feelings do you have about this process?

- What did you learn about yourself and your partner(s)?

- What do you appreciate about how you and your partner(s) showed up in this session?

- What helped you to self-soothe?

- What do you wish your partner(s) understood about your experience of becoming emotionally flooded?

- What can you do to self-soothe in future instances, and how can your partner(s) team with you to support your efforts?

Vignette

Gina and Nate presented in therapy to work on their relationship. Gina was 40 years old and identified as a heterosexual cisgender Latinx female. Nate was 39 years old and identified as a heterosexual cisgender European American male. Gina was a project manager at a technology company and experienced clinically significant anxiety. Nate was a middle school teacher and had an established, medicated ADHD diagnosis. They had been in a long-term committed relationship with one another for 12 years. They lived together and had a 5-year-old biological child. Gina was experiencing emotional and sexual attraction toward a mutual friend and wanted to discuss opening the relationship to include a deeper connection with this friend. While the couple had experimented with ethical nonmonogamy previously, the possibility currently felt threatening to Nate due to a larger sense of failure in meeting Gina's connection needs. During discussions around this issue, blame and attack became mutual as they struggled to view each other with positive regard. Gina fiercely pursued connection and resolution while Nate withdrew until he felt backed into a corner and lashed out. In the therapist's assessment of the couple's conflict cycle in their initial session, the therapist briefly described this pattern to them, and both expressed a desire for the therapist to actively intervene if she saw their negative conflict cycle occur in session.

In their second joint couples therapy session, Gina began expressing to Nate the many ways he had fallen short as a partner. While her feelings and desires were valid, her approach was not skillful, and Nate became defensive and attacking. Both their voices were raised as they expressed pent-up resentment, and the therapist did not trust that either could witness the therapist validate the other's feelings or that a gentle confrontation of unskillful behavior could be tolerated in each other's presence. After about a minute, the therapist interrupted them, saying, "This is the damaging communication cycle we talked about last session, and I respect your time and money too much to let it keep going here. I want to help you find a different way forward like we discussed."

The therapist told Gina and Nate that she wanted to spend some individual time with each of them. The therapist asked Gina, as the connection-seeker, to stay first because the therapist hypothesized that the time apart would further distress Gina, whereas Nate, given time to himself, would be able to self-soothe. If this had occurred later in therapy, the therapist may have opted to meet with Nate first to support both of their growth. But for this session, the therapist chose to start with what felt more natural to provide them an opportunity to experience success. The therapist emailed them both a list of soothing activities, and Nate chose to walk around the block and listen to a favorite comedian's podcast. He took his cell phone with him with the agreement that Gina would text him when she and the therapist were finished.

After Gina confirmed that Nate had left the room, the therapist validated Gina's feelings and desires and reflected the sadness and overwhelm the therapist sensed underneath her blaming approach. Gina began to cry and expressed relief at being understood, and the therapist was then able to offer perspective that the way she was approaching Nate was not getting her desired outcome. The therapist then provided alternative ideas for an approach more likely to invite connection. Together, they reviewed the self-soothing list, and Gina decided that while the therapist met with Nate, she would sit in her favorite chair in the house far enough away that she could not overhear Nate's individual time with the therapist. She would listen to her favorite meditation music playlist with her eyes closed. She texted Nate that it was his turn, and they switched places.

The therapist asked Nate how he was doing after the walk. He responded that he was "fine." The therapist then asked what had happened inside of him when Gina started to express her disappointment in him. Slowly, he was able to identify fear of not being enough and that Gina would leave him for this other person. The therapist reflected and validated his feelings and the strengths the therapist had observed him bringing to the relationship. Nate was cautiously able to take in this support. Together, they explored strategies for responding to Gina in a more skillful way than defense and attack, such as curiosity or naming his fear and the story he told himself about failing her.

Nate then texted Gina to invite her back into the session. The therapist asked Gina and Nate to reflect on what they had learned about themselves and what they appreciated in how they and their partner had showed up in the exercise. Collaboratively, they designed a structured pause homework experiment and identified a safe word that could be used outside of session to signal the need for a structured pause.

Suggestions for Follow-Up

Encourage clients to practice a structured pause outside of therapy when experiencing emotional flooding. Instruct clients that the pause should be at least 20 minutes but no longer than 24 hours, with an agreed time to reconnect that is initiated by the partner who requested the pause (Rosen et al., 2007). Implement a safe word that partners can use, whether in session or outside of therapy, when clients realize they are becoming flooded to a point that a pause is needed. Obtain agreement that the pause is not be used to avoid difficult conversations. When used at home, each person should soothe themselves with self-directed compassion and validation, engage in calming activities, and identify what they have agency to change in the situation. Ask each partner to create their own self-soothing ideas list to use during the pause.

Contraindications

Because the teletherapy format could create conditions where partner(s) can overhear what is happening during the individual time with each partner, explicitly discuss ways to avoid overhearing other partners' individual therapy time (e.g., moving to a room far away within the household, putting on headphones) and help problem-solve as necessary (Wrape & McGinn, 2019).

The directive therapeutic stance required for the structured pause should be evaluated for appropriateness through the lens of intersecting identities of the clients and the therapist, particularly when client identities carry less privilege in relation to therapist identities (Dee Watts-Jones, 2010).

Due to time constraints, the teletherapy session may end with the conversation unfinished and/or partners still escalated. In this case, instruct clients to continue engaging in self-soothing activities that have been identified in session. You may also consider asking partners to hold off on talking about topics that lead to escalation until the next therapy session.

Partners may become escalated in session to the point that emotional or physical safety is a concern. This must be immediately addressed, with no time to implement a structured pause. If safety becomes a concern, focus on safety planning immediately to stabilize each partner.

References

Dee Watts-Jones, T. (2010). Location of self: Opening the door to dialogue on intersectionality in the therapy process. *Family Process*, *49*(3), 405–420. https://doi.org/10.1111/j.1545-5300.2010.01330.x

Gottman, J., & Gottman, J. (2017). The natural principles of love. *Journal of Family Theory & Review*, *9*(1), 7–26. https://doi.org/10.1111/jftr.12182

Gottman, J., & Silver, N. (2012). *What makes love last? How to rebuild trust and avoid betrayal.* Simon & Schuster.

Hogan, J. N. (2022). Conducting couple therapy via telehealth: Special considerations for virtual success. *Journal of Health Service Psychology*, *48*(2), 89–96. https://doi.org/10.1007/s42843-022-00060-x

Kauppi, M. (2020). *Polyamory: A clinical toolkit for therapists (and their clients).* Rowman & Littlefield.

Rosen, K. H., Matheson, J. L., Stith, S. M., McCollum, E. E., & Locke, L. D. (2007). Negotiated time-out: A de-escalation tool for couples. *Journal of Marital and Family Therapy*, *29*(3), 291–298. https://doi.org/10.1111/j.1752-0606.2003.tb01207.x

Wrape, E. R., & McGinn, M. M. (2019). Clinical and ethical considerations for delivering couple and family therapy via telehealth. *Journal of Marital and Family Therapy*, *45*(2), 296–308. https://doi.org/10.1111/jmft.12319

CHAPTER 27

MAPPING THE CYCLE

A VIRTUAL EMOTION-FOCUSED INTERVENTION FOR CLIENTS PRACTICING CONSENSUAL NONMONOGAMY

Kk O. Lightsmith

Materials for Therapists: PDFs of blank diagrams (included as supplemental materials to this book) and PowerPoint or another computer program that allows text to be added to images.

Materials for Clients: None.

Objective

Consensual nonmonogamy (CMN) is an umbrella term for many types of conscious relationship structures beyond monogamous arrangements, such as multiple romantic, sexual, or domestic partners. CMN systems often have multiple schedules to coordinate, and members of the system may live in different houses or cities (Yuen, 2018). Teletherapy is a practical way to accommodate the scheduling needs of CMN clients. The following provides a procedural description of an online intervention based on emotionally focused therapy (EFT; Johnson, 2019) that uses interactive techniques to map negative cycles of interaction. Through this intervention, understanding and openness within relationships are encouraged by reframing conflict in terms of attachment needs and emotions.

Rationale for Use

EFT uses an empirically validated theory of adult bonding as the basis for conceptualizing and improving relationship problems (International Centre for Excellence in EFT, n.d.). EFT posits that powerful and positive relational change is possible through the conduit of a secure attachment connection (Johnson, 2019). EFT inventions reframe problems in terms of attachment needs and emotions and encourage understanding and openness to other system members' experiences (Furrow et al., 2022). Focusing on emotional experiences and attachment needs of system members is essential to reconnecting and strengthening secure attachment bonds (Johnson, 2019). EFT is an evidenced-based practice for a diverse range of partnerships and is effective in working with clients facing comorbidities such as depression and PTSD (International Centre for Excellence in EFT, n.d.).

DOI: 10.4324/9781003289920-32

In its original form, the "negative cycle" was created by Scott Wooley for clinicians to use as an assessment and note-taking tool with monogamous couples in in-person therapy (Furrow et al., 2022). In this assessment, the therapist diagrams each partner's actions in the cycle and their emotional process that drives these behaviors. The therapist then helps partners see how each person's emotions and actions work together with those of their partner to maintain an established pattern of interaction (Furrow et al., 2022).

This intervention has been adapted to working with CMN systems by creating space to interactively identify and track thoughts, feelings, and attachment needs that maintain negative interactional patterns between multiple people.

To accomplish this task via teletherapy, tools for mapping attachment bond cycles with CMN systems have been digitized and are included with the supplemental materials that accompany this book.

Setup

The following specifies steps required for setting up the intervention.

1. ***Describe the intervention and its purpose.*** Let clients know this intervention will take the entire session and will be utilized in future sessions. Describe how mapping conflictual interactions can be a step toward increased awareness and acceptance with each other, leading to more secure attachment bonds and better ability to problem-solve together. For example, "This activity will help us discover more about the feelings and needs that are under conflicts you experience. We will take this session to complete the diagram together. In later sessions, we will use this information to practice new ways of relating to each other that will help you feel loved, supported, and important. You may learn information about each other that surprises you, even in topics you've covered many times before."

2. ***Decide who to include in the activity.*** When deciding who to include, consider how the CNM system is structured and how decisions are made within the system (Kauppi, 2020). Because only some members of the CNM system may be active participants in therapy (i.e., clients), discuss with clients the potential of inviting other members of the CNM system to participate in the intervention. If a participant is not a client, such as a member of the CNM system who is attending only for support of other clients during this activity, consider what documentation is legally required for the participant to attend.

3. ***Predetermine the digital arrangement of all participants.*** Do not assume that all participants will be joining the session from the same physical location. Consider limitations of physical space and technical equipment (e.g., who owns headphones or has a private space available to them). Work with clients in advance to decide if participants will attend the session from the same or different devices and what physical space each participant will be in during the session. Arrangements requested by the therapist, such as which participants join from which screen, communicate clinician assumptions and knowledge about the CNM system (e.g., how it will impact relational dynamics or therapeutic rapport for a client to join from a location with one partner versus with a different partner).

4. ***Ensure each participant has access to the link and/or information necessary to log into the session.*** Even if participants plan on joining the session from the same device, sending all participants the necessary login information allows for flexibility of last-minute device or schedule changes.

5. ***Prepare the diagram.*** Open the template diagram image in PowerPoint or any program that allows you to easily and quickly add text to an image. Select the image that corresponds with the number of partners present in the CNM system (see Figures 27.1 and 27.2). It can also be helpful to have diagrams

available to map cycles between subsets of the CNM system (see Figure 27.3). Maximize or enlarge the program so that it takes up most of your screen while still allowing visual contact with client video. If possible, it may be helpful to have two computer screens for this activity (i.e., one for the diagram and one for client video). Alternatively, use a whiteboard function of a teletherapy platform to draw the diagram and add text to the image in real time.

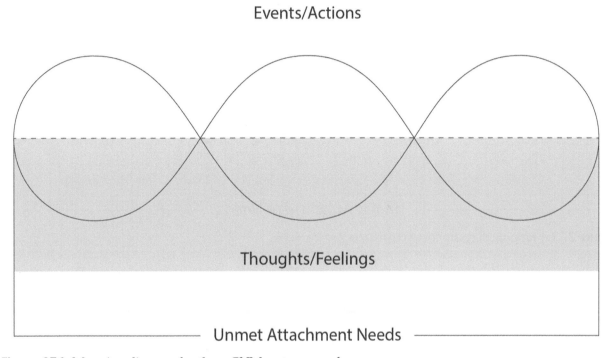

Figure 27.1 Mapping diagram for three CNM system members.

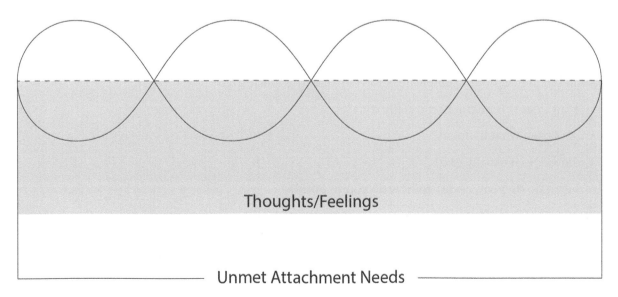

Figure 27.2 Mapping diagram for four CNM system members.

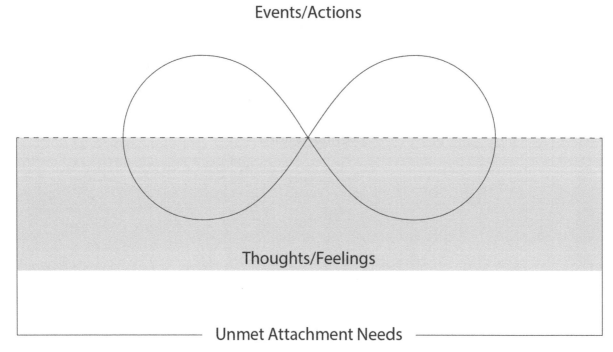

Events/Actions

Thoughts/Feelings

Unmet Attachment Needs

Figure 27.3 Mapping diagram for two partners.

Instructions

1. ***Start screen sharing or using the whiteboard.*** Use the screen-sharing or whiteboard option to share your screen with all participants. Ensure all participants can see the diagram or whiteboard.

2. ***Describe the diagram.*** Explain that all participants will help you to document on the diagram what usually happens during challenging interactions. Explain that each participant is represented by a loop, and all loops impact each other. Explain that part of the interactions are seen and heard (e.g., behaviors), and part of the interactions are not seen or heard (e.g., emotions, thoughts).

3. ***Gather and record information regarding visible and audible actions or behaviors.*** Prompt participants to describe the visible and audible actions involved in their challenging interactions. As participants speak, enter their responses into the diagram via text boxes or drawing with the whiteboard function. Example questions include the following:

   • How does this interaction usually start?

   • And then what happens?

   • How does it usually end?

   • What do they say, and then how do you respond?

   Participants may provide information about each other. When this happens, check in with the participant being discussed to clarify information shared about them by others. For example, one partner may volunteer, "They usually leave when I yell." The clinician may then ask that client directly, "Is there anything you would add or change about that description?"

4. ***Elicit and record information regarding thoughts and feelings.*** Prompt participants to describe their thoughts and feelings that are present during this interaction. As participants speak,

enter their responses into the diagram via text boxes or drawing with the whiteboard function. Example questions include the following:

- When [she/he/they] say(s) [statement made by another participant], what do you tell yourself? And what do you feel?

- When [she/he/they] do(es) [action of another participant], what do you think? And how do you feel?

- When you say [statement made by participant], what are you thinking? And what are you feeling?

5. ***Help each participant identify an unmet attachment need and record it.*** Based on the thoughts, feelings, and actions participants report in session, help each participant identify at least one attachment need that is unmet during the interaction, and write it in the diagram.

    Attachment needs include (Fern et al., 2020):

    - Mattering or making a difference to others

    - Expecting and receiving comfort, reassurance, and acceptance from others

    - Being able to rely and lean on others

    - Others responding when you call them

    The following are example client statements that may indicate unmet attachment needs:

    - "I can't count on them to be there for me."

    - "I expect them to criticize or attack me."

    - "I can't get their attention or time."

    - "I'm on my own in this relationship."

    - "I'm not seen or heard."

    - "I'm not enough."

    - "I'm unlovable."

    Record unmet attachment needs in positive language. For example, if someone states, "He never listens to me," work with the participant to identify the attachment need behind the complaint (e.g., a need to be heard).

Processing

After the completion of the intervention, utilize questions regarding clients' inner worlds, attachment needs, and emotional experience to promote emotional awareness, understanding, and openness in the relationship. These questions can be utilized immediately after the intervention and in future sessions while referencing the diagram.

Ask questions about clients' inner worlds. Use the client's language in framing questions (Johnson, 2015). Example processing questions include the following:

- Did you know before this process that [she/he/they] were feeling [afraid/sad/lonely/hopeless/ despair/helpless/confused/hurt] when in conflict?

- Had you heard before now that [she/he/they] want(s) to connect with you?

- Did you understand in a different way what [she/he/they] mean(s) when [she/he/they] say, "I miss you"?

Ask questions that validate and empathize with identified attachment needs. You might also ask questions that expose that unmet attachment needs drive insecurity and negative interactions. Explain that attachment needs are healthy and adaptive, yet when attachment needs are unmet and the emotional experience of system members is unknown, problematic patterns of communication arise (Johnson, 2004). Example questions may include:

- Did you know that [she/he/they] long(s) to be lovable?

- Have you ever wanted to be understood by someone who mattered to you?

- When [she/he/they] leave(s) the room after you argue, did you know they were longing to be comforted?

Encourage clients to share their emotional experiences. Change ultimately occurs through new emotional experiences and interactional events (Johnson, 2004). In processing, attend to client affect and interactions. Attend to nonverbal cues by noticing facial expressions, changes in posture, and other physical cues. To process verbally, ask questions that encourage clients to identify emotions within relational experiences. Example questions may include:

- When [she/he/they] said they believe they're not lovable, how did you feel?

- When you heard [she/he/they] reveal their need to be important, what happened inside of you?

- I noticed you turned away from your screen when they were talking to me. What was going on for you when that happened?

Vignette

Jon (35, he/him) and Melissa (32, she/her) had been together for three years and married for one. Melissa identified as bisexual and Latinx; Jon identified as heterosexual and White. They both identified as cisgendered and were U.S. born, able-bodied, upper middle class, and lived in an urban center. Lily (35, they/them) identified as queer and White. Lily and Melissa had been dating for five months. Lily identified as genderqueer, U.S. born, middle class, had chronic mental health concerns, and lived in the same area as Melissa and Jon. Melissa had come out as bisexual two years ago but had never dated anyone who was not cisgendered, heterosexual, and male-identified. Melissa and Jon had been discussing the possibility of Melissa dating someone else so she could "fully express her sexuality." Though neither Jon nor Melissa had practiced CNM before, they were hopeful that they could have a healthy marriage and Melissa could express herself.

The clients reported that Lily and Jon had met several times and that Jon initially got along with Lily. Five months into Lily and Melissa dating, Jon felt threatened by how important Lily seemed to Melissa and how much time she spent at their house. Melissa felt hurt and angry that Jon initially encouraged their relationship and then "took back" his support. Jon and Melissa reached out to the clinician, reporting that they "wanted couples therapy for communication problems." The clinician began therapy with Melissa and Jon as the clients.

Through assessment in the first two sessions, the clinician learned that there was no interpersonal violence in the client system. Melissa and Jon considered themselves to be "monogomish," which they defined as sharing finances and a house together, being sexual and romantic partners mostly with each other, and thinking of each other first when it came to making life decisions. Their agreements were that Jon would not have other partners and that Melissa was "allowed" to have other partners only if they were "not men." The clinician determined that Jon and Melissa were the "decision-making body" holding the most power to make agreements and decisions in the CNM system (Kauppi, 2020).

The clinician briefly described the mapping and reframing conflictual cycles intervention and explained that it would help to build understanding and empathy between all members of a CMN system, leading to the possibility of more secure attachment bonds between partners in the system. Melissa requested that Lily come to session as a guest for the intervention, and Jon agreed it would be good to have them present.

Before the session, the clinician sent a guest informed-consent document to Lily. They filled this out and returned it online. The document described the role of a guest versus a client and the clinician's privacy policies and legal requirements. The clinician suggested that all three members join the next session from separate screens and sent a link to each participant before the session. The rationale behind this request was that the clinician wanted to convey to Melissa, as a hinge partner (i.e., a sexual and romantic partner to both Lily and Jon, with no partnership bond between Jon and Lily) a respect for both of her partnerships by not putting her in a position to have to choose which partner to appear with onscreen.

At the start of the session, the clinician described the flow of the session and began the intervention. First, they asked Jon and Melissa to describe how their recent conflicts played out. Jon reported that Melissa spent more time than ever with Lily, and he often accused Melissa of caring for Lily more. The clinician gathered more information from Melissa about how she usually responded to this. Melissa reported she usually denied that there was any difference in her time spent away but admitted she probably did spend more time over at Lily's house now. The clinician supported Jon in identifying how he felt when Melissa left. He reported feeling lonely and afraid. The clinician asked Lily and Melissa what happened when Melissa came over to their house. Lily reported Melissa came over more often but that they felt suspicious and afraid. Lily often accused Melissa of "not being serious" about wanting to date them. The clinician invited Melissa to disclose how she felt when Jon accused her of caring for Lily more, and she reported that she was angry and hurt. The clinician asked Melissa how she felt when Lily accused her of "not being serious," and she reported she felt anxious.

Using the diagram as a guide (see Figure 27.4), the clinician narrated all members' influence of each other in their "dance" of interactions. The clinician noticed how Jon accused Melissa of caring for Lily more when he felt afraid, and Melissa, feeling angry and hurt, responded to the accusations by denying that any changes had happened. The clinician noticed that when Lily felt afraid and suspicious, they questioned Melissa's seriousness. Melissa, feeling anxious, responded to Lily by spending more time with them.

The clinician worked with each participant to identify one unmet attachment need, based on the emotions and behaviors they reported. Lily reported they had an unmet need for security. Melissa reported an unmet need for acceptance. And Jon reported an unmet need to be important.

The therapist left 15 minutes to process the intervention. The clinician asked questions to elicit each participant's inner world and emotional experience. Through these questions and the discussion of client answers, the clinician invited everyone to see the connection between unmet attachment needs and negative interactions.

- **Clinician to Jon:** When you hear Melissa say she longs to be accepted as a bisexual person, what happens for you?

- **Clinician to Lily:** As you hear about Melissa responding to Jon and you in this pattern, does anything change about your understanding of Melissa's commitment to your partnership?

- **Clinician to Melissa:** When you hear Jon wanting to be important to you and afraid that he is no longer important to you, what comes up for you?

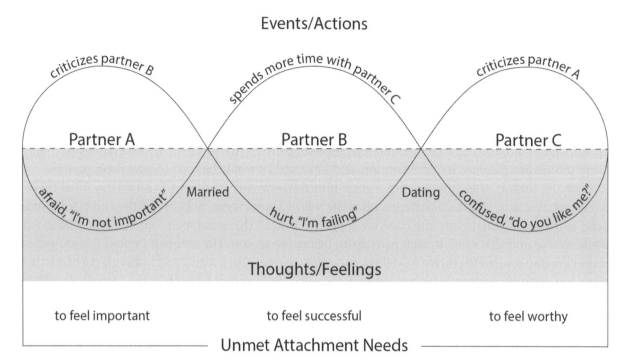

Figure 27.4 Mapping example with three CNM system members.

After the conclusion of the intervention, the clients reported an increased understanding of their interactional patterns and an increased openness to each other. Jon thanked Lily for coming to the session and shared that he now realized that his need to be important does matter to Melissa. Melissa reported her overall anxiety decreasing as her spouse and her lover witnessed her distress and efforts to be a good partner. Lily reported an increased sense of trust in Melissa.

Suggestions for Follow-Up

By conducting this intervention via telehealth, clinicians can easily save the completed diagram to add to the client file and reference in future sessions. Refer to the completed diagram in future sessions to support clients in healing attachment injuries and correcting harmful communication patterns. This intervention could also be repeated or modified throughout therapy to highlight or assess changes in the client system over time.

Contraindications

Before working with clients interested in or actively pursuing CNM, examine your own beliefs about CNM and relationship health indicators. Many clinicians "equate being CMN with attachment insecurity" (Fern et al., 2020, p. 118). A working assumption of this intervention is that a healthy, multiple partnership system is possible and achievable. Examine and reexamine internalized biases that may keep you from believing this assumption, and seek consultation, supervision, and continuing education as needed.

References

Fern, J., Rickert, E., & Samaran, N. (2020). *Polysecure: Attachment, trauma and consensual nonmonogamy*. Thornapple Press.

Furrow, J. L., Johnson, S. M., Bradley, B., Brubacher, L., Campbell, T. L., Kallos-Lilly, V., Palmer, G., Rheem, K., & Woolley, S. (2022). *Becoming an emotionally focused therapist: The workbook* (2nd ed.). Routledge.

International Centre for Excellence in Emotionally Focused Therapy. (n.d.). *EFT research*. ICEEFT.

Kauppi, M. (2020). *Polyamory: A clinical toolkit for therapists (and their clients)*. Rowman and Littlefield Publishers.

Johnson, S. M. (2004). *The practice of emotionally focused couple therapy: Creating Connection*. Brunner-Routledge.

Johnson, S. (2015). *The practice of emotionally focused couple therapy: Creating connection*. Routledge.

Johnson, S. M. (2019). *Attachment theory in practice: Emotionally focused therapy (EFT) with individuals, couples, and families*. The Guilford Press.

Yuen, J. (2018). *Polyamorous: Living and loving more*. Dundurn.

CHAPTER 28

MINDFULNESS-BASED SEX THERAPY

SETTING THE STAGE FOR SENSATE FOCUS VIA TELEHEALTH

Tina M. Timm

Materials for Therapists: None.

Materials for Clients: Common objects found in the home.

Objective

This chapter describes how to integrate an introductory mindfulness exercise into sex therapy via telehealth. The goal of the exercise is to help partners understand and practice mindfulness principles before engaging in prescribed sensate focus exercises in the privacy of their homes.

Rationale for Use

Sensate focus is a behavioral intervention commonly used in sex therapy. It is designed to shift the focus away from sexual performance and help intimate partners connect physically and emotionally using a series of at-home touching exercises (Masters & Johnson, 1966, 1970). The goal is to help partners to be in touch with their own experience, sensations, and pleasure rather than trying to please their partner(s). Sensate focus homework exercises themselves are done privately between sessions.

Mindfulness-based sex therapy is an effective treatment for sexual dysfunction (Brotto et al., 2016; Rashedi et al., 2022). Therapists may practice mindfulness exercises in session to help ground clients in their senses and to prepare them for mindfully experiencing their partner(s) during sensate focus homework assignments. The exercise described in this chapter is first done in session to teach basic concepts of mindfulness. The exercise itself includes elements of many standard mindfulness practices, prompting partners to focus on the five senses.

Though any theoretical orientation may be used in processing this activity, internal family systems (IFS) is applied here for processing the exercise in session (Anderson et al., 2017).

DOI: 10.4324/9781003289920-33

Setup

This exercise should be conducted when working with two or more partners in the same therapy session. For the most successful implementation, partners should be in the same physical location during session. Clients should ideally be at home and surrounded by things that help them to feel safe in their natural environment (e.g., a comfortable couch, a warm blanket, a cup of tea, comfortable clothing). Encourage clients to take 10 minutes before session to create a safe and comfortable space for therapy together. If clients have a laptop available, this may allow them to be more creative in choosing their location for therapy (e.g., cuddled up on a comfy couch rather than at a desk, seated in separate chairs). This helps clients to come to sessions already grounded so they can move more quickly into therapeutic intervention. Adjustments may be made to meet the needs of each client if all of the aforementioned conditions are not possible.

Instructions

This in-session exercise should be done the day the first sensate focus homework is assigned. The following offers step-by-step instructions on engaging partners in a mindfulness-based exercise in preparation for sensate focus homework:

1. ***Introduce the concept of mindfulness and the ways in which it relates to sex therapy.*** For example, "Mindfulness is about noticing and paying attention. It is about quieting the mind and being in the moment. It is about being aware of what we are thinking and feeling while practicing the skill of staying grounded in our bodies. Good connecting sexual experiences include many of those same elements."

2. ***Have each partner choose an item sitting near them.*** It can be anything (e.g., mug, phone, pillow). A benefit of doing this activity via telehealth is that this object may have already been seen and touched many times and is quite familiar to them. This offers an opportunity to experience a familiar object in new ways, similar to the goal of sensate focus.

3. ***Ask each partner to hold the object in their hands and silently notice everything they can about it.*** Encourage them to touch and notice the object as if it were the first time they had encountered it. Tell clients that the goal is to pay attention to what they are noticing, and if they are doing that, they are succeeding. Ask clients to focus on their own chosen object rather than the one(s) selected by their partner(s). Give them a few minutes to do this.

4. ***Encourage clients to use all five senses in exploring their objects.*** Propose the following questions to encourage further exploration of the object(s):

   - What details can you see about your object?

   - What textures, temperatures, or other things can you feel on your object?

   - Does your object have any discernible smells?

   - Does your object make a sound?

   - And as appropriate, how does it taste?

5. ***Have each partner take turns describing the things they noticed about their objects.*** Encourage partners to offer their descriptions in detail, out loud.

6. ***If clients struggle to go into detail, ask additional questions to further the exploration.*** For example, you might ask:

   - What do you notice about the item that is new to you?

   - Tap or shake the item. What sound does it make?

   - Can you feel where the item makes contact with your hand? Does it feel any different if you touch it to your arm or your leg?

   - Try putting it up to your nose. Can you discern any smell?

7. ***Once each partner has had a chance to fully describe their item, make the explicit connection between the mindfulness skills they used in this exercise and how you want them to approach the sensate focus activity.*** For example, "When you touch each other, I want you to move away from touching to please the other person. I want you to explore your partner's body using all five senses like you did with the item in session. Even though you have touched each other many times, I want you to do so with new eyes, taking in all the tiny details and noticing how that feels for you."

Processing

After doing the exercise, additional processing questions may include:

- What was the experience like for you?

- Did you notice anything happening in your body?

- What thoughts were you aware of?

- Were there any emotions or feelings that came up? If so, which ones? How intense were they?

- When you noticed [thought/feeling], what did you do?

- Were you concerned in any way about what your partner(s) was/were experiencing?

- What else would you like me or your partner(s) to know?

Being able to answer and openly discuss these types of questions is essential in processing sensate focus homework as it moves forward.

As with any mindfulness practice, it is not uncommon for people to experience a wide variety of thoughts, feelings, and reactions. Normalize this for clients. For example, if a partner feels anxious, this is a great opportunity to explore that part using IFS (Anderson et al., 2017). Sample IFS-oriented questions include:

- Where/how do you experience "the anxiety"?

- Are you compassionate toward the part that gets worried?

- What is that part afraid of?

- What would you like that part to know about why you are doing this work?

After the in-session activity, introduce clients to the sensate focus homework assignment. The following steps will prepare clients to relate their mindfulness-based experiences to the activity:

1. ***Give an overview of the sensate focus homework assignment.*** To learn more about the specifics of sensate focus and how to effectively integrate this into clinical practice, see Weiner and Avery-Clark (2017).

2. ***Encourage partners to set up a comfortable space to conduct the sensate focus activity.*** By encouraging clients to set up comfortable spaces from which to attend therapy, clients should already have some practice doing this. Ask clients to consider the temperature, lighting, and anything else that might create an enjoyable ambiance. It is standard practice to have clients do two sensate focus exercises between weekly sessions. Have partners alternate being the one who sets up the room, so this responsibility is shared equally.

3. ***Explain that you want them to explore each other during the sensate focus activity similarly to the way that they explored their objects in session.*** Partners have likely seen each other naked and have touched each other many times. However, over time, many partners go on autopilot or become "goal-focused," and quickly skip to sexual touch for the sole purpose of arousal and orgasm. Encourage them to notice the small details about each other just like they did in the exercise (e.g., the temperature and texture of their skin and how it is different in different places on the body, subtle sounds of touching crevices and indentations, different scents, taste of the body). This skill set keeps them grounded in their bodies and in a space of "noticing" rather than "performing."

Vignette

Connie (25) and Jared (26) are a heterosexual couple who presented for therapy due to chronic sexual pain when trying to engage in intercourse. Both grew up in the Mormon church but moved away from its teachings and were no longer affiliated with organized religion. Connie tried to "push through" the pain during the early years of their marriage, which led to intense physical and psychological distress. This culminated in them eventually stopping all sexual contact.

Connie grew up in a family with emotionally unavailable parents where she learned that she was all alone with her physical and emotional pain. Jared grew up internalizing negative messages about sex and sexual thoughts before marriage. He was overwhelmed and deeply ashamed of his sexual desires. While he did not overtly pressure Connie to continue to be sexual, it was only within the relationship that he felt he could express his sexuality. The combination of their upbringing, combined with not knowing how to communicate openly about sexuality and having little to no support system, left them feeling very isolated. Fortunately, they were deeply committed to each other, had a strong friendship, and were highly motivated to heal both individually and relationally.

In treatment, when it was time to start sensate focus, the therapist started the session with the mindfulness exercise described. Connie picked up a journal that she had been writing in. Jared used his phone for the exercise. Both did well in reporting what they saw with their eyes, for instance, describing the color and places that were worn, but needed more prompting with the other senses. The therapist asked them to close their eyes and explain what they noticed without being able to see it, using touch and smell. Connie seemed physically uncomfortable when asked to do this and started fidgeting in her seat. The therapist asked her to pay attention to what was happening in her body. She reported having fluttering in her chest. The therapist asked if she was willing to explore this more, and she agreed.

Connie reported not liking this anxiety, as she blamed it for keeping their relationship stuck and not being able to move toward reclaiming their sexual relationship. The therapist asked her what she was afraid would happen if the anxious part stopped shutting her down. She said it would lead to physical pain again. The therapist validated that fear and asked her to thank the anxious part for keeping her safe. The part was able to hear that, and when the therapist asked her again how she felt toward it, she reported feeling grateful and appreciative. Once it was clear Connie was operating more from a place of self, the therapist asked her to let the anxious part know what is different now (e.g., she is older, they are in therapy, her partner is safe), and if the part worries again that something feels scary, to let her know and that she would listen and keep her safe. The job the anxious part had been doing was very important, and while Connie wanted it to be less vigilant, it should always have permission to watch and protect as needed.

The first time the couple tried to do a sensate focus exercise at home, they started by doing a mindfulness exercise. Connie was acutely aware of how "activated" she was. She noticed there was a lot of internal "noise," or parts of her were worried about doing the touching. She had some flashbacks of times when touching led to painful sexual experiences and could feel her heart racing. Connie was able to communicate what was happening to her with Jared, and instead of doing the touching exercise just because they were "supposed to," they took time to process the fears that were coming up. This allowed them to stay close emotionally and make a decision together to not proceed with the sensate focus activity on that day as planned. Connie was able to ask for what she needed, which was simply to be held. As Jared held her, she noted the warmth of his embrace, the vibrant colors of his old shirt that she had seen a million times, the gentle scratchiness of his facial hair, the slight scent of toothpaste lingering on his breath, and the taste of his lips when she kissed him.

Jared was able to reassure Connie's parts that she was in control, and he would never make her do anything she did not want to do again. This was very reassuring to her parts and helped to establish more trust internally and relationally. When they came to session that week, even though they had not done the sensate focus homework as planned, the therapist celebrated all the wins of their interactions that were important.

In the following weeks, Connie and Jared were able to complete the sensate focus homework consistently. In each session, the therapist helped them process what they noticed in themselves when touching or being touched. The therapist then used those observations to intervene as needed.

Mindfulness activities and sensate focus homework did not provide an immediate cure for Connie and Jared's struggles. Yet through these activities, they built safety, connection, and more effective communication within their relationship. They learned to "listen" to their own bodies, to previously unacknowledged parts of themselves, and to each other.

Suggestions for Follow-Up

Subsequent sessions can be used to process sensate focus activities that clients have conducted between sessions. When discussing homework assignments, use processing questions like the ones used to discuss in-session activities. Continually assess whether clients should continue doing more of the same activities or if they are ready to move on to the next stage of treatment.

Contraindications

The activities described in this chapter are not recommended for partners with a history of interpersonal violence. When emotional and/or physical safety has been compromised, doing mindfulness with a partner and focusing on the senses can be deeply triggering. Even simple requests like closing eyes with an unsafe partner can feel unsafe and make the goals of the exercise unattainable.

References

Anderson, F. G., Schwartz, R. C., & Sweezy, M. (2017). *Internal family systems skills training manual: Trauma-informed treatment for anxiety, depression, PTSD & substance abuse*. PESI Publishing & Media.

Brotto, L. A., Chivers, M. L., Millman, R. D., & Albert, A. (2016). Mindfulness-based sex therapy improves genital-subjective arousal concordance in women with sexual desire/arousal difficulties. *Archives of Sexual Behavior, 45*(8), 1907–1921. https://doi.org/10.1007/s10508-015-0689-8

Masters, W. H., & Johnson, V. E. (1966). *Human sexual response*. Little, Brown, and Company.

Masters, W. H., & Johnson, V. E. (1970). *Human sexual inadequacy*. Little, Brown, and Company.

Rashedi, S., Maasoumi, R., Vosoughi, N., & Haghani, S. (2022). The effect of mindfulness-based cognitive-behavioral sex therapy on improving sexual desire disorder, sexual distress, sexual self-disclosure and sexual function in women: A randomized controlled clinical trial, *Journal of Sex & Marital Therapy, 48*(5), 475–488. https://doi.org/10.1080/0092623x.2021.2008075

Weiner, L., & Avery-Clark, C. (2017). *Sensate focus in sex therapy: The illustrated manual*. Routledge.

CHAPTER 29

ASSESSING APPROPRIATENESS OF TELETHERAPY FOR INTIMATE PARTNER VIOLENCE

Jaclyn Cravens Pickens and Aaron Norton

Materials for Therapists and Clients: Recommended items for supporting privacy include headphones and a noise machine.

Objective

Therapists must be familiar with forms of technology-facilitated intimate partner violence (t-IPV; Hertlein, 2021) and have a protocol to assess for intimate partner violence (IPV) in teletherapy (Springer et al., 2020). This chapter provides recommendations for assessing IPV with teletherapy clients, including an overview of ways technology is used to perpetrate violence, how t-IPV may connect with typologies of perpetration, and how therapists can assess appropriateness of teletherapy for clients experiencing IPV.

Rationale for Use

Because therapists have limited control of the end-user site environment (e.g., clients' home) during teletherapy sessions, special attention must be given to safety issues such as intimate partner violence (Wrape & McGinn, 2019). There are unique aspects of teletherapy, however, that complicate the assessment of violence (i.e., electronic surveillance).

Intimate Partner Violence

IPV is the experience of abuse or aggression by a current or former intimate partner (CDC, 2021). This may include physical, sexual, emotional, and psychological violence as well as economic and financial control, threats, and stalking. IPV can also range in frequency and severity. Johnson (1995) identified different types of partner violence, including situational couples violence, intimate terrorism, and violent resistance. Situational couples violence is a less severe form of violence that is typically related to partner conflict that escalates out of hand. It is not characterized by attempts to control another person and is generally bidirectional in nature (Johnson, 1995). Intimate terrorism is characterized by a coercive and

DOI: 10.4324/9781003289920-34

controlling partner that results in emotional and physical harm. It is typically male perpetrated and is severe in nature. Violent resistance occurs when a victim of intimate terrorism uses violence to defend themselves from abuse.

Technology-Facilitated Abuse

t-IPV includes forms of coercive control that are most likely to occur in instances of intimate terrorism. Cyberbullying and cyberpsychological abuse are categories of t-IPV. Cyberbullying is the intentional bullying of an individual via an electronic medium, including sending repeated harassing, threatening, or slandering messages online. Cyberpsychological abuse is the use of technology to engage in psychological abuse. This includes emotional abuse such as ghosting or blocking partners, denigration, posting compromising pictures, intimidation tactics, demanding passwords to accounts, using smart-home technology (e.g., controlling the thermostat), making private information public (e.g., revenge porn, outing a person), and cyberstalking, where technology is used to track or monitor a partner (Hertlein, 2021).

Cyberstalking is a coercive control tactic commonly used by intimate terrorists and is a risk factor for serious violence. Cyberstalking can occur by installing spyware on someone's computer, phone, or other device or through the use of phishing attacks that trick someone into clicking a link that will trigger the download of malware containing malicious files that hack the individual's device, giving the cyberstalker access to sensitive files or data. Spyware is tools (e.g., app, software program, device) that allow an unauthorized person to secretly monitor or record information on a device. These practices enable perpetrators to stalk, track, and harass victims. They can be difficult to detect and to remove once detected. Anything that a victim does on their device could be revealed to the perpetrator monitoring it (e.g., searching "detecting device monitoring" or "leaving an abusive relationship"). Beyond spyware, perpetrators may access their partner's information by accessing their browser history, reading text messages, or accessing their accounts (e.g., bank, email, social media). It is also possible a survivor of IPV or someone participating in violent resistance may use technology, such as cyberstalking, to know where the perpetrator is physically located as a means of protection.

Assessment and Treatment Considerations

A client's device potentially being monitored creates concerns about confidentiality and safety. Best-practice guidelines recommend that therapists assess for IPV as a routine practice, using multimodal assessments and conducting individual interviews with each partner (Stith et al., 2005). Teletherapy services at unsupervised sites (e.g., clients' homes) presents concern regarding lack of control over the clients' environment, including who else may be listening to the session or be present off-camera (Wrape & McGinn, 2019). While room scans, headphones, and a noise machine may reduce the likelihood of sessions being overheard or observed by others, cyberstalking remains a concern. If all recommended logistical considerations are addressed, therapists must consider whether teletherapy is safe due to the potential risk of an abusive partner monitoring a client's device. A perpetrator may become angry that their partner sought therapy, for discussing their relationship, or for talking about their experience of IPV. If cyberstalking occurs without the partner's awareness, therapists must know that retribution is a risk to client safety. Therefore, therapists providing teletherapy services must consider a routine assessment concerning technology privacy, especially when IPV is of concern.

Setup

Teletherapists must have adequate technological competence (AAMFT, 2015) and seek training as needed. Resources provided by the Safety Net project (NNEDV, 2018) are available to learn more about t-IPV.

Instructions

The following provides instructions for assessing t-IPV and the appropriateness of teletherapy services. Safety is always the primary concern, even with intake assessments (Stith et al., 2005). Therefore, assessment questions are designed to be intentionally vague to avoid alerting potential perpetrators of discussions about violence and cyberstalking.

1. ***Determine whether initial assessment will occur in person or via technology.*** When a potential client requests teletherapy services, one option is to request an in-person intake appointment, regardless of whether services will continue in person or online. For clients within a reasonable geographic distance and those able to travel safely to attend therapy in person, this option is recommended for direct assessment of IPV and cyberstalking. For those unable to meet in person for their intake, ask that potential clients speak by phone to assess the appropriateness of teletherapy services before scheduling the first appointment. When scheduling the call, explain potential ways in which privacy can be compromised, including having people in nearby rooms in which they can overhear conversations or smart-home devices (e.g., Alexa, Google Home).

2. ***Assess for t-IPV.*** Whether conducting the assessment in person or over technology, assess for technology monitoring. While privacy is a concern for all clients receiving teletherapy, the added risk of retribution related to IPV increases the significance of the impact of cyberstalking. For technology-facilitated assessments, ask the following questions to determine whether technology monitoring may be a risk (NNEDV, 2018):

   • From where are you calling?

   • Who is in the location with you?

   • What device are you using to call?

   • What device will you use to access teletherapy?

   • Is this device shared with other people? If so, who?

   • Is this device accessible by other people? If so, who?

   • Do you have concerns about the technology not working properly?

3. ***Use prepared responses to clarify the reason for asking these questions.*** This assessment may raise questions from the potential client, or if the perpetrator is monitoring the client's technology, inquiring about the client's devices may raise alarms with the perpetrator about technology monitoring being discovered. Take overt or covert approaches to answer questions, depending on whether the assessment revealed safety concerns (NNEDV, 2018).

   If there is any concern about a device being monitored, reduce risk of retribution by answering covertly. For example:

   • "I ask because it is necessary for teletherapy clients to have consistent access to properly working devices, and if a device is shared or not working properly, this will potentially disrupt therapy."

If there is no worry about monitoring, an overt answer may include:

- "I ask to ensure teletherapy can be conducted on a confidential and private device that does not risk your safety in a situation in which a current or former partner might be monitoring your device(s)."

This can also include a more focused IPV assessment by asking:

- "Are you concerned about your abuser or partner knowing where you are all the time?"

- "Are you concerned that your abuser or partner might be able to access your communication with others?"

- "Are you concerned about information that's posted about you online?"

4. ***Take steps to prevent t-IPV from interfering with safety planning.*** If an abuser is monitoring the device that the client is using to attend teletherapy, attempts to create a safety plan may be thwarted (e.g., abuser could learn about client's plan to leave and use this information to prevent it from happening). If t-IPV is a concern, take the following steps immediately prior to creating a safety plan.

- Encourage clients to call you back using a secure device.

- Provide clients with information about how cyberstalking occurs with different devices (e.g., cell phones, social media, email, tracking devices).

- Provide education about how technology can be used to monitor and track people and how to identify if a device is being monitored.

5. ***Create a safety plan.*** Follow established guidelines if safety concerns are revealed. This should include general safety planning (e.g., Stith et al., 2005) as well as t-IPV specific safety planning. Throughout safety planning, avoid victim-blaming (i.e., any response that covertly or overtly assigns blame for the violence to the victim).

To create a general safety plan:

- Provide psychoeducation on abuse, risk to safety (e.g., leaving an abuser is the most dangerous time in an abusive relationship), and safety planning.

- Identify signs of escalation (e.g., behavioral, cognitive, physical/somatic, sensory changes).

- Evaluate on a continuum the level of escalation (e.g., early warning signs, when client should use their safety plan).

- Develop strategies for leaving (e.g., where to go, what to take, who to call).

- Help clients develop a safety plan, a set of actions to help lower risk of harm from a perpetrator across different domains of the client's life (e.g., safety during escalation, safety at home/work/school, safety when preparing to leave).

- Provide clients with resources near their physical location (e.g., domestic violence shelters) as well as online resources for victims/survivors of abuse.

- Tell the client to keep any documentation of their safety plan or other IPV-related resources in a location the perpetrator does not have access to.

To support clients in t-IPV-specific safety planning:

- Warn clients about potential retribution from perpetrators should they stop using monitored devices or close accounts that their partner has gained access to (NNEDV, 2018).

- Discuss how to safely use devices in ways that will not alert perpetrators that the client is aware of the technology monitoring (i.e., keep using devices in ways that would not compromise safety).

- Support clients in opening accounts on unmonitored devices to have safe technology.

- Discuss how to collect evidence should they wish to take legal action.

6. **Create a plan to access therapy.** This should include how the client can identify a device that the perpetrator has not had physical or remote access to (e.g., library, friend, or work computer).

7. **Discuss how to safely communicate about therapy and send teletherapy links.** This may entail creating a new email account on a safe device not linked to existing accounts (NNEDV, 2018).

Suggestions for Follow-Up

Assessment for IPV and concerns about monitored technology or lack of privacy for teletherapy services should be ongoing. Over the course of therapy, watch for irregularities that might be evidence of a monitored device (i.e., odd sounds during the call, device shutting down without known reason, device running slow despite strong internet connectivity, unusual browser pop-ups, webcam recording without authorization). Discuss the need for synchronous communication with clients, and avoid responding to asynchronous electronic communication (e.g., email, text messages) about service-related information (e.g., scheduling teletherapy sessions) in case this communication is not actually from the client.

Contraindications

If assessment for teletherapy appropriateness reveals t-IPV, it's possible such behaviors represent forms of violence enacted by an intimate terrorist, and conjoint couples therapy would be contraindicated (Stith et al., 2005). Individual teletherapy services can proceed as long as the client has access to a safe device.

If assessment reveals concerns about compromised devices and clients cannot locate a secure device, teletherapy would be contraindicated. If in-person therapy is an option, therapy services should be shifted to this format. If in-person therapy is not an option (e.g., clients do not have access to transportation or are not allowed to leave their house), consider the risk of conducting therapy that is being monitored and the risk of clients not receiving services. If therapy cannot be continued safely, identify alternative methods to help clients safely access resources (e.g., work with a community partner to access unmonitored technology).

References

American Association for Marriage and Family Therapy. (2015). *AAMFT code of ethics*. www.aamft.org/Legal_Ethics/ Code_of_Ethics.aspx

Centers for Disease Control and Prevention (CDC). (2021, October 9). *Intimate partner violence*. www.cdc.gov/ violenceprevention/intimatepartnerviolence/index.html

Hertlein, K. M. (2021). The weaponized web: How internet technologies fuel intimate partner violence. *International Journal of Systemic Therapy, 32*(3), 171–193. https://doi.org/10.1080/2692398X.2021.1906619

Johnson, M. P. (1995). Patriarchal terrorism and common couple violence: Two forms of violence against women. *Journal of Marriage and the Family, 57*(2), 283–294. https://doi.org/10.2307/353683

National Network to End Domestic Violence (NNEDV). (2018). *Safety net project: Exploring technology safety in the context of intimate partner violence, sexual assault, and violence against women*. www.techsafety.org/resources/

Springer, P., Bischoff, R. J., Kohel, K., Taylor, N. C., & Farero, A. (2020). Collaborative care at a distance: Student therapists' experiences of learning and delivering relationally focused telemental health. *Journal of Marital and Family Therapy, 46*(2), 201–217. https://doi.org/10.1111/jmft.12431

Stith, S. M., McCollum, E. E., & Rosen, K. H. (2005). *Couples therapy for domestic violence: Finding safe solutions.* American Psychological Association.

Wrape, E. R., & McGinn, M. M. (2019). Clinical and ethical considerations for delivering couple and family therapy via telehealth. *Journal of Marital and Family Therapy, 45*(2), 296–308. https://doi.org/10.1111/jmft.12319

Part 6
Families

CHAPTER 30

DIGITAL PLAY GENOGRAMS

Rebecca A. Cobb

Materials for Therapists: PowerPoint or another computer program that can be used to create a genogram and compile images; clip art or other digital images. An initial set of images are included as supplemental materials to this book.

Materials for Clients: None.

Objective

Individual and family play genograms have been successfully used for in-person therapy assessment and intervention where therapists have toys available for use in the therapy room (e.g., Gil, 2015; McGoldrick et al., 2020). This chapter explains how to conduct genogram assessment and intervention via teletherapy using clip art or other digital images.

Rationale for Use

Genograms are used in individual and family therapy to assess family constellations, family history, and intergenerational patterns. Play genograms provide a medium through which children, adolescents, and adults can engage in these discussions in a playful way that captures and maintains attention. Additionally, play genograms allow clients to participate through nonverbal communication and to discuss through metaphors, reducing client resistance (Gil, 1994, 2011; Schaefer, 1993) and making the activity more engaging for younger and less verbal clients.

Setup

Place basic shapes necessary for the creation of a genogram in a digital file that can be used in session with clients. A variety of images that symbolize important constructs (e.g., anger, joy, nurturance, strength) should be selected and compiled in a digital file that can be shown to clients during session (e.g., a Power-Point slide). Include images that represent the clients' culture and faith traditions. An initial set of images are included as supplemental materials to this book. You may begin with this and add other images to it.

DOI: 10.4324/9781003289920-36

While clients could be asked to find their own images for the activity, this may feel overwhelming and require more left-brain cognitive processing than right-brain metaphorical/creative processing. For a variation of this activity, therapists with a robust play therapy room may take photographs of their miniatures and use these images instead. Clients who attend both in-person and teletherapy sessions may enjoy having the same toys available for use.

If you already know the composition of the family, you can also prepare the genogram prior to session.

Instructions

Begin by explaining what a genogram is and then share your screen to show the image of the genogram that you created prior to the session. If there isn't enough information to create the genogram prior to the session, you can create the genogram during the session with the assistance of the family. Then ask if the genogram needs any changes made to it. Once the genogram has all necessary components, explain that "each person is to pick one image or object to represent each person in their family, including yourself." You might consider starting with the youngest member present or the person who typically speaks less.

Ask the first participant to guide you on what images you should put on the genogram for each member of the family. As each image is selected, place the images on or adjacent to the shape representing the person that the image was selected for.

Once the first person has finished selecting all their images, go through the same process with the next person and continue until all members in the family have selected images. Upon completion, verify with the family that everyone had a chance to share everything that they wanted. During this stage, do not ask processing questions. Rather, reflect what you hear clients say if they choose to share information about what they selected and why.

Processing

After the completion of the genogram, ask processing questions that are in the metaphor of the images. For this activity, clients don't need to explain why they chose each object. Rather, by focusing on metaphors, the activity remains playful and engaging and allows right-brain creative processing.

Though genograms are traditionally used with transgenerational theories (e.g., Bowen's family systems theory; Platt & Skowron, 2013), this assessment/intervention can be processed with many different guiding theories (e.g., solution-focused; Kuehl, 1995; Weiss et al., 2010; narrative therapy; Chrzastowski, 2011; Kuehl, 1996). Keeping a guiding theory in mind may help to focus the types of questions that are asked. In addition, processing questions may be asked to facilitate discussion of both intrapersonal and interpersonal relationships (i.e., discussion of relationships between objects selected for the same family member and discussion of relationships between objects selected for different family members).

Narrative therapy allows client-generated metaphors to become a central part of the therapeutic process (Legowski & Brownlee, 2001). These metaphors can be identified as "problems" that are externalized and combatted by the family through the therapeutic process or as part of the clients' preferred story that is achieved through collaborative dialogue about said metaphors, restorying, and "thickening" (Geertz, 1978) the story of the preferred metaphor. Given the central focus of processing digital play genograms while staying in metaphor, this intervention may be particularly fitting with a narrative therapy approach.

Vignette

Sondra (38), Dylan (38), Chase (13), and Abby (6) presented in teletherapy reporting increased family conflict following the birth of the youngest family member, Sofia (5 months). At the start of the second session, the therapist introduced the digital play genogram as a way of conducting continued assessment and to facilitate discussion among family members.

Prior to the session, the therapist created a basic genogram on a PowerPoint slide depicting the members of the household. The therapist also compiled about 50 clip art images and placed them around the edges of the PowerPoint slide. Knowing a bit about the family, the therapist strategically selected a few images that might be of significance for this family's current circumstance (e.g., baby, bottle, cow nursing, mother holding baby). The therapist also selected a wide variety of other images.

During the session, the therapist introduced the family to the activity by first explaining what a genogram is. They then shared their screen to show the image of the genogram that they created prior to session. The therapist asked the family if the genogram looked right and if they needed to make any changes to it. They then explained that they would show them images on the screen and that "each person is to pick one image to represent each person in their family, including yourself." The therapist started with Abby, the youngest member present in session, and proceeded in ascending order by age. Because Sondra and Dylan were both the same age, the therapist asked Dylan to participate before Sondra, because Sondra appeared to be more engaged in the therapy process.

As each image was selected, the therapist placed the images on or adjacent to the circle or square representing the person that the image was selected for (see Figure 30.1). Without prompting, each member of the family explained why they selected each image for each person.

Abby selected an image of a witch for her mom, a robot for her dad, a couch for her brother, a baby for her little sister, and Lady Liberty for herself. She stated, "Mom is mean. Dad acts like a robot. Chase never does anything and just sits on the couch all day on his phone or playing video games. And my baby sister is just

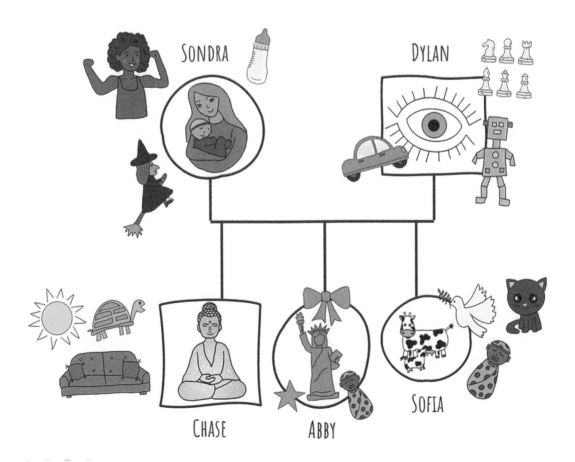

Figure 30.1 Example of digital play genogram.

a baby. I'm the only one in the family who sees that none of this is fair!" The therapist reflected what they heard Abby saying without asking additional questions.

Chase selected a strong woman for his mom, a car for his dad, a bow for Abby, a smiling cat for his baby sister, and the Buddha for himself. He stated, "Mom's pretty cool. Dad's gone a lot. Abby always seems to want everything to be perfect. Sofia is pretty cute. And I think I'm pretty chill." Again, the therapist reflected what they heard Chase saying without asking additional questions.

Dylan selected a woman nursing a baby for his wife, a turtle for Chase, a star for Abby, a dove with an olive branch for Sofia, and chess pieces for himself. Dylan explained, "Sondra spends so much time with the baby. It seems like she never gets a break. Chase's picture for Sondra is perfect. She really is Superwoman. Little Sofia is such a gift to our family, but she's a lot of work! Chase is slow with most things, but he's insightful. Abby is right; he spends a lot of time on the couch! Abby is my little star. She's smart, does great at school, and usually shines so bright! At first, she was excited about having a little sister, but something changed. She changed. She isn't as happy anymore. As for me, I picked the picture of the chess pieces. I like chess. I don't have much time to play it anymore." Sondra started quietly crying while Dylan spoke. The therapist allowed silence to fill the space.

Sondra selected the evil eye symbol for her husband, a sun for Chase, a baby for Abby, a nursing cow for Sofia, and a bottle for herself. She shared, "Dylan is our protector. He works so hard for our family. He keeps us safe. Though he's gone a lot. I try to keep up with everything while he's away. I don't think I'm doing a very good job. Chase is my sun. It's true; he's a little on the slow side, and he is on that couch a lot, but he's always in good spirits and knows how to make me laugh. I chose this baby cow nursing on its mom for Sofia. Sometimes, it feels like that's all I do. Nurse, change diapers, and repeat. I love that Chase and Dylan see me as a superwoman, but it doesn't always feel like that. I hate that Abby sees me as a witch. She's my little baby. I know she's six, but I still see her as my little baby. I guess we don't get to spend as much time together as we used to. I'm sorry, baby." Abby immediately appeared to soften. "It's okay, Mommy. Daddy's right. Sofia is a lot of work. But she *is* pretty cute. Sometimes."

The therapist reflected, "It sounds like everyone here has quite a fondness for baby Sofia, and also that she's thrown you for quite a loop!" "Thrown for a loop?" asked Abby. Dylan clarified, "We've gotten a bit mixed up, honey. And we need to figure out how to be a family again with our newest member."

The therapist thanked the family for sharing about the objects that they selected and asked if it would be okay to ask them a few questions about their genogram. All members of the family agreed, and the therapist proceeded to ask questions in the metaphor of the images:

- What does the mother think of the strong woman? What does the strong woman think of the mother? What might the strong woman say to the momma cow? And to the baby cow?

- When does the witch show up? Who does it cast spells on?

- How do the two babies get along? Who takes care of them?

- What happens when the kitten is playful? What happens when the kitten is upset?

- How does Lady Liberty get along with the cat? How does Lady Liberty get along with the baby cow? What does she think about the robot? What injustices does Lady Liberty see? Does anyone else stand up with her against injustice?

- When does the star shine its brightest?

- What does the eye see that others might not notice?

- Where does the car go? How do the others feel when it's away? How does the car feel when it's away? Where would these characters take the car if they could go anywhere? Who would go?

- Do any of these characters ever spend time on the couch?

- How do the robot and the turtle get along? What do they do together?

- When does the turtle go into his shell? When does he come out of it?

- How did the Buddha get so wise? How does he remain so calm? Who does he share his wisdom with? What does the Buddha do when the babies are crying?

- Who does the sun shine light on? What happens when the sun goes down?

Through discussion of these images, the therapist and family learned the following:

- The sun shines on everyone.

- The couch is lonely.

- The turtle usually stays out of his shell, but others rarely visit him.

- The Buddha gained his wisdom from the eye.

- The car is often gone and would like to be home more often. Most everyone would like to go somewhere together with the car.

- The babies get along and like each other quite a lot. One of the babies often gets jealous of the other and would like to be held by the mom more to help scare away the witch.

- The strong woman has been working out and thinks she might be able to hold both babies at the same time.

- The Buddha has been sitting by himself on a couch and thinks he might be able to spend more time with the babies if the strong woman would let him. He's also interested in learning how to play chess.

- The eye sees an amazing and loving family that wants to care for one another. The eye is confident that they'll figure it out.

Hypothesizing but not assuming that the images on the genogram were metaphors for this family's current dynamics, the therapist deducted that Chase brought joy to everyone in the family but was lonely and wanted to spend more time with his dad. He might also be willing to help with his sisters if his mom was okay with it. Sondra appeared to want to spend more time with Abby, and if she were to allow Chase to help with Sofia, this might free up more time for her to do that. Dylan appeared to miss his family, too, and wanted to spend more time with them. Chase, specifically, might benefit from more time with Dylan. If they were to play chess together, this might also allow Dylan to reengage with one of his favorite hobbies.

The therapist used this information to engage in further discussion with the family, both in and out of the metaphor of the images. Following this activity, Dylan began taking fewer work trips so he could spend more time with his family. He made a point of teaching Chase how to play chess. Chase began watching Sofia a couple times a week, allowing Sondra to have more time to spend with Abby. The whole family sat on the couch more with Chase, and Abby seemed to shine a little brighter. In a subsequent session, the therapist engaged the family in a follow-up intervention, having the images on the genogram plan a trip, decide where they would go, and what they would do. The family ended up taking a road trip similar to the one that the images suggested. The trip was difficult at times with a baby, and they reported that it was good.

In this example, family members were all high in verbal skills and appeared to gravitate toward cognitive processing. Because each member of the family, starting with the youngest, chose to explain their selection, the therapist allowed the clients to lead. The therapist, however, stayed in the metaphor of the images when asking their own processing questions. In this instance, the clients were responsive to this more playful approach as well.

Suggestions for Follow-Up

Hypothesizing but not assuming that the images on the genogram are metaphors for the family's dynamics, the therapist can use information gathered from this activity to engage in further discussion with the family, both in and out of the metaphor of the images. One of the benefits of doing genograms via teletherapy is the ability to save the actual genogram for future use, rather than simply making note of what objects were selected by whom. Keep a copy of the genogram in the client's file to use in future discussion. Gil (2015) suggests making note of which clients select which objects for each family member to facilitate further processing.

Contraindications

If clients struggle to remain actively engaged in session, you may offer the opportunity for the family to create the play genogram themselves and guide them throughout the process while they share their screen. Each participant may take turns selecting and moving images. Younger children may receive assistance from other family members as needed.

References

Chrzastowski, S. K. (2011). A narrative perspective on genograms: Revisiting classical family therapy models. *Clinical Child Psychology and Psychiatry*, *16*(4), 635–644. https://doi.org/10.1177/1359104511400966

Geertz, C. (1978). *The interpretation of cultures*. W. W. Norton.

Gil, E. (1994). *Play in family therapy*. Guilford Press.

Gil, E. (2011). Family play therapy igniting creative energy, valuing metaphors, and making changes from the inside. In C. E. Schaefer (Ed.), *Foundations of play therapy* (pp. 207–225). John Wiley & Sons.

Gil, E. (2015). Individual and family play genograms. In C. S. Sori, L. L. Hecker, & M. E. Bachenberg (Eds.), *The therapist's notebook for children and adolescents* (2nd ed., pp. 13–20). Routledge.

Kuehl, B. P. (1995). The solution-oriented genogram: A collaborative approach. *Journal of Marital and Family Therapy*, *21*(3), 239–250. https://doi.org/10.1111/j.1752-0606.1995.tb00159.x

Kuehl, B. P. (1996). The use of genograms with solution-based and narrative therapies. *The Family Journal*, *4*(1), 5–11. https://doi.org/10.1177/1066480796041002

Legowski, T., & Brownlee, K. (2001). Working with metaphor in narrative therapy. *Journal of Family Psychotherapy*, *12*(1), 19–28. https://doi.org/10.1300/J085v12n01_02

McGoldrick, M., Gerson, R., Petry, S., & Gil, E. (2020). Family play genograms. In *Genograms: Assessment and treatment* (4th ed.). Norton.

Platt, L. F., & Skowron, E. A. (2013). The family genogram interview: Reliability and validity of a new interview protocol. *The Family Journal*, *21*(1), 35–45. https://doi.org/10.1177/1066480712456817

Schaefer, C. E. (Ed.). (1993). *The therapeutic power of play*. Jason Aronson.

Weiss, E. L., Coll, J. E., Gerbauer, J., Smiley, K., & Carillo, E. (2010). The military genogram: A solution-focused approach for building resiliency in service members and their families. *The Family Journal*, *18*(4), 395–406. https://doi.org/10.1177/1066480710378479

CHAPTER 31

TELEHEALTH FAMILY SCULPT

SO MANY PEOPLE, SO LITTLE SPACE

Nathan C. Taylor, Paul R. Springer, and Richard J. Bischoff

Materials for Therapists: Picture or video of what a family sculpt looks like (included in supplemental materials to this book).

Materials for Clients: Moveable camera (e.g., tablet or laptop) or flexible tripod. Stuffed animals, dolls, figurines, modeling clay, paper, and drawing utensils are optional, depending on the chosen method for the sculpt.

Objective

Sculpts are experiential interventions used when working with intimate relationships and families (Satir, 1983). Sculpts can be administered via telehealth with some alterations to their traditional in-person format (Taylor et al., 2021). The purpose of this chapter is to explain the adaptation of this intervention for use in telehealth.

Rationale for Use

Experiential approaches, such as sculpts, increase awareness, insight, and understanding of systemic relations (Satir, 1988). Key to experiential interventions are spontaneity and emotional presence, both of which can be impaired in telemental health sessions (Taylor et al., 2021). While barriers do exist, telemental health doesn't have to be without emotion or experiential activities.

Family sculpts consist of clients arranging family members or items that represent family members in positions to portray each person's perception of the family using space symbolically and metaphorically (Duhl et al., 1973). Sculpts can be used to explore family systems as a whole or to explore subsystems such as parent, parent and child, and sibling dyads. Because sculpts are not dependent on verbal communication, they are particularly useful for clients with limited or impaired communication abilities and patterns.

Sculpts are process oriented, meaning they focus on how problems are discussed and maintained and are therefore beneficial to transition away from session content or the extraneous details around specific problems. By focusing on the process or the internal experience of clients, clinicians can identify overarching

DOI: 10.4324/9781003289920-37

patterns within client systems rather than spending session after session discussing each new problem experienced by clients. For example, sculpts help to access emotion, heighten client awareness of their experiences with one another, and explore boundaries, roles, and hierarchies (Bell, 1986; Constantine, 1978). Sculpts are useful throughout the stages of treatment and can be used for initial assessment and intervention and to evaluate treatment progress.

One benefit of teletherapy is the ability to see families in their own homes. In some telehealth cases, clients may choose to place family members in the actual location where they are normally found within the household. For example, a family may be sculpted all in the same room, except for one person, who is placed in another room to represent disengagement.

Unique to telemental health is also the limited amount of space to conduct a sculpt, a problem that is compounded when working with larger families. The following describes the unique setup and instructions that therapists should follow to conduct a successful family sculpt via teletherapy.

Setup

1. ***Introduce clients to the activity.*** Explain that a sculpt is a visual representation of family dynamics and that each person will have an opportunity to shape other members of the family based on their experiences. Initial instructions for a family sculpt can be abstract and difficult to comprehend. For in-person sessions, guide clients in physically positioning family members to demonstrate the sculpting process. Over telehealth, trying to verbalize how family members could be positioned as a sculpt example can be more confusing. To ease setup, have a picture or short video of a nonclient family sculpt that clients can see to provide clarity of the intervention. A picture of a family sculpt is included with the supplemental materials that accompany this book to use as an example.

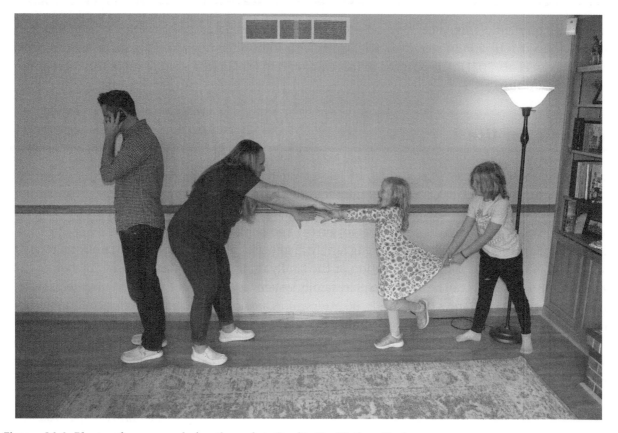

Figure 31.1 Photo of an example family sculpt. Credit: Dr. Nathan Taylor.

2. ***Evaluate the space available to clients to conduct the activity.*** Is there sufficient room to fit the entire family and move around, or does the family fit like "sardines in a can"? If limited space is available, ask clients if they have a larger room that they can move to for the activity. If a larger room is not available, discuss alternative options:

    a. Clients may conduct smaller sculpts of different subsystems within the family.

    b. Clients may use resources available to them in their current location to conduct a variation of a family sculpt. For example, clients may use items such as stuffed animals, dolls, or figurines to represent each member of their family. Alternatively, clients may use clay (Banker, 2008) or paper (Bell, 1986) to sculpt each member of their family. Discuss resources available to clients and their preferences in deciding on the method of family sculpt.

3. ***Assess the type of camera at the client's physical location.*** For example, are clients using a camera attached to a tablet or laptop that can be moved, or is the camera fixed?

4. ***Provide guidance on setting up successful visuals during the activity.*** Sculpts work best with a moveable camera to capture the differing perspectives of each participant. Encourage family members to use their cell phones that session if cell phones are available to them. This allows clients more flexibility in showing different angles of the sculpt as well as their own unique perspective in the family system. If clients will be using a phone, tablet, or laptop for the activity, provide instructions to have the device sufficiently charged prior to the sculpt to prevent technological problems that may disrupt the sculpting process. If clients will be using a desktop computer with a fixed camera, encourage the acquisition of a small, flexible tripod. This can ease challenges related to camera positioning and maximize the field of view. If a tripod is not available, clients can be creative in camera positioning. For example, positioning a stack of large books under the camera can help to obtain an angle that allows for a wider range of vision.

5. ***Prepare clients with emotion regulation skills prior to the intervention.*** Sculpts can be distressing for some clients and result in heightened emotions. Provide a list of resources if clients should need additional help deescalating (Springer et al., 2020).

Instructions

To conduct a sculpt via teletherapy: (1) describe the connection between physical and metaphorical space, (2) establish boundaries of the sculpt, (3) determine who will begin the sculpt, (4) construct the sculpt, (5) guide clients in repositioning the camera as needed, (6) document the sculpt, and (7) repeat the sculpt with each subsequent member of the family. The following describes each of these stages.

1. ***Describe the connection between physical and metaphorical space.*** While clients are in whatever position they have shown up to therapy in, ask them to describe the physical space between each of them. Is that space close together? Is it far away? Once the physical space is explored, connect this to the metaphorical space by asking what the physical space represents. For example, does the closeness or distance between members represent emotional, physical, or spiritual connection or disconnection? This is a vital precursor to conducting a sculpt via teletherapy due to the limited space available for the therapist to be able to see all family members at once in the screen. To remain in view, two family members may only be able to stand a foot apart. However, metaphorically, a foot may represent substantial disconnect in comparison with six inches between other family members. Have clients move closer and further away from each other to help illustrate the connection further. Discuss whether this elicits any emotions, and process these as they come up.

2. ***Establish boundaries of the sculpt.*** Determine the space that clients can use during the sculpt. If the client's camera is moveable, as is the case with a tablet, laptop, or phone, it is easier to extend the sculpt outside of any one particular field of view because you can instruct clients to move the camera as the sculpt evolves. If a tripod is available to hold the camera or if there is another way of placing the camera in the room in a way that allows for the entire sculpt to be seen, guide clients on positioning it in a way that maximizes the space included in view of the camera. Then, describe the boundaries of the sculpt within their physical space according to what can be seen on screen. If the camera cannot be moved throughout the room, it can be helpful for clients to mark the edges of the field of view with tape if tape is available to them. If clients decide to extend the sculpt outside the field of view, instruct them to increase the verbal description of what is occurring. While a family member positioned outside the field of view is not ideal, it may be a powerful and more accurate representation that a family member is not even in the picture.

3. ***Determine who will begin the sculpt.*** Different theoretical orientations may determine who you will ask to construct the sculpt. For example, a structural family therapist would choose to do a sculpt as a means to restructure family dynamics. In this case, the therapist is more likely to begin the sculpt with one of the parents as a means to support the parental hierarchy. If the purpose is to identify coalitions in the family, they may start with a sibling. If the goal is to enhance communication, it would be useful to start with the quietest family member whose voice is least often heard. With that said, the intended purpose of the sculpt and the therapist's theoretical orientation should be taken into consideration when determining the order in which family members lead the sculpt.

4. ***Construct the sculpt.*** The sculpt begins with a prompt, which is aligned with what the therapist hopes to achieve. This can include exploratory sculpts such as "how do you see others in your family?" or more focused sculpts such as "what would your family look like if they were all connected?" Inform the person beginning the first sculpt that they will be asked to provide interpretation of the sculpt from their own perspective. This minimizes pressure to construct a sculpt that captures everyone's experience and emotions. During all parts of the sculpt, constantly monitor the client environment for any signs of distress, and intervene when necessary.

5. ***Guide clients in repositioning the camera as needed.*** For example, if a parent is asked to describe the relationship among siblings and parents, the other parent should be asked to hold the camera while the children are placed in their positions. This allows the sculptor to move in between family members and to describe the physical space and how family members are positioned. The camera holder should be the last person to be included in the sculpt. When it is time for the camera holder to be positioned, instruct them to give the camera to the sculptor. The sculptor can then provide a panoramic view of the sculpt before ultimately positioning themself within the sculpt. At this point, ask the sculptor to give the camera to the person positioned the farthest away to provide the best visual of the final sculpt. When clients are responsible for holding and moving the camera, provide time at the end of the sculpt for all members of the family to be in the sculpt without holding the camera. Instruct clients to place the camera in a location in the room that allows the best view, acknowledging that it may not be perfect. Explain to the family that you really want them to experience what it feels like to be in these positions without having to worry about the camera. This will allow more opportunities for felt emotions and potential insights on the part of the clients.

6. ***Document the sculpt.*** With consent, have each client take a picture or video of the sculpt. When taking a photo, each member of the family should take a picture of the sculpt from their perspective. If a tripod is available, pictures can be taken with a timer from multiple angles to capture all family members' positions. The sculpt can then be explored, processed, or restructured in subsequent sessions.

7. ***Repeat the sculpt with each subsequent member of the family.*** Typically, it is helpful to construct the sculpt multiple times by different family members to gain a more holistic view of how family

members view the problem. For example, having different family members construct a sculpt based on the same prompt, such as, "How would you like to see your family?" provides information about the views of each family member. With each repetition, guide clients in documenting the sculpt.

Processing

Processing occurs both during the construction of the sculpt and following its completion. The processing of a family sculpt typically takes longer when delivered via telemental health than when conducted in person (Springer et al., 2020; Taylor et al., 2021), so allow adequate time to discuss before the conclusion of the therapy session.

Unique to telehealth, when the camera is moveable, pictures can be captured and shared to more fully explore all the perspectives from the sculpt. It can be incredibly powerful for clients to see their view of the family from the context of how they were positioned. It can also be powerful for clients to see themselves in the sculpt from the perspective of other members of their family.

Even when the camera is moveable, there are inevitably parts that cannot be seen. To aid in fully connecting the physical and metaphorical space, processing the telemental health sculpt requires more verbal descriptors to capture missed visual and auditory cues. For example, if you were to conduct a sculpt in person, you would be able to walk around and see that someone was sculpted with eyes looking slightly to the side of a family member. Over telehealth, it may incorrectly appear that the person is looking directly at their family member. When processing the sculpt, ask more questions to make up for missed visual and auditory cues.

Processing prompts and questions may include:

- Describe where everyone is looking. What meaning does that have for you?

- What was it like to position everyone in certain ways?

- What does it feel like to be positioned in this way?

- What does it feel like to see your family in this way?

- How do you think it feels for [family member's name] to be positioned in this way?

- What might it feel like to move closer together?

- What might it feel like to move farther apart?

- What would it feel like if you switched roles?

- What do you see or not see in the sculpt?

- What would I see differently if I was in the room with you?

Processing highlights the inner experience of each family member. This creates a more powerful experience for clients as they describe and listen to one another's perspectives.

Vignette

A family therapist worked with a mother (Kara), stepfather (John), 15-year-old girl (Jentry), and 12-year-old boy (Dave). The family came in shortly after Kara and John were married because the two children were beginning to act out in school and in the home. The therapist wanted each member of the family to experience how they were seen by other members of the family as well as the overall structure of the family system. The therapist decided that a family sculpt would be an excellent way to portray each family member's perceptions of what was happening in the family, what alliances had been formed, and the overall sense of belonging.

The therapist asked the family to bring in a fully charged tablet to session. With a moveable camera, it was not necessary for the therapist to help the family identify the field-of-view parameters. Jentry was invited first to sculpt the family in a way that represented her current experiences and her place in the family system. Jentry was chosen to go first because the therapist wanted to gather the children's perspectives prior to being influenced by the parental subsystem. In addition to being one of the children, Jentry was the oldest child and had some power in the family. The therapist hypothesized that if Jentry willingly participated in the activity, the other members of the family might as well.

Jentry was asked to sculpt all members present and her father with the prompt of "position your family to represent how they are connected." During the intervention, Dave was initially asked to hold the camera because he was old enough to be able to hold the camera steady for the therapist but young enough that standing in the same place for the entire time was difficult. At times, Dave was asked to move the camera around the room to capture the different perspectives of each family member. This allowed the therapist to maintain a presence throughout the process.

To include her father in the sculpt, Jentry was asked to go and pick a stuffed animal to represent him. Jentry started by placing "her father" (i.e., the stuffed animal) at the other end of the room. Without prompting, she described him as "sitting on the floor with his elbows on his knees and his face in his hands, in utter despair." Jentry put her mother and stepfather on one side of the room, holding hands and facing the center of the room. Her mother was also positioned with one arm reaching outward. Once her mom and stepfather were positioned, the therapist asked John to hold the camera to allow Jentry to position herself and her brother in the remaining part of the sculpt. Jentry then positioned her brother facing herself, with Jentry looking towards the opposite corner of the room.

The therapist inquired about what was happening in the sculpt and discovered that Jentry felt intense loyalty conflict. She was stuck between her reaching mother and her biological father, who was alone and hurt by the lack of time he could spend with his children. The therapist also explored why Jentry chose that specific stuffed animal to represent her father. This provided additional depth and understanding of how Jentry viewed her father and his role in the family system.

To connect the metaphorical space with the space in the room, the therapist asked Jentry to take one step toward Kara and to describe the emotions that were elicited. Jentry quickly began crying and said that as she took a step toward her mother, she could hear her father weep. Similarly, as Jentry took a step toward her father, she described feeling sick in her stomach because she would be hurting her mother. The therapist then included the rest of the family in processing their own experience of the sculpt. Because the therapist was not in the room, it became even more important to ask frequent questions about how each family member was "feeling" based on how they were being positioned in the room and responses to each other's experiences. This sculpt became the metaphor of treatment as the therapist worked to restructure the family so the children could be connected to both their father and mother without experiencing guilt or loyalty conflicts.

Suggestions for Follow-Up

It is helpful to ask families to construct sculpts at various times throughout the therapy process. This is a way to document change in families and provide a creative avenue for all family members to discuss their lived experiences. Prompts for conducting follow-up sculpts may include:

- Show me how your family has grown since coming to therapy.
- How would you like to see your family?

- How might your family look different if family therapy was a success?

- If everyone in the family could be their true self, what would that look like?

- What would healthy communication in your family look like?

One of the strengths of telehealth is the ease in taking pictures for use in future discussions about the sculpt. If the camera is movable, pictures can be taken from different angles to access the different perspectives of the participants. With permission of the family, the therapist can screenshot pictures and share them in future sessions, allowing experiences to be further explored long after the original sculpt. The sculpt is a useful resource to track or demonstrate progress. At the end of treatment, a sculpt can highlight therapeutic change and elicit explanations for changes in individual and family functioning. This can be particularly impactful when clients compare images of initial sculpts with subsequent ones that illustrate changes in the family over time.

Contraindications

Due to the intense emotions that a family sculpt may elicit, be cautious when using this intervention with clients that struggle with emotion regulation. Skills to navigate high emotion should be demonstrated prior to implementation.

Avoid making assumptions about availability of space or other resources that may limit the ability to conduct a family sculpt. Adapt to the needs of each client and provide alternative options as necessary.

References

Bell, L. G. (1986). Using the family paper sculpture for education, therapy, and research. *Contemporary Family Therapy*, *8*(4), 291–300. https://doi.org/10.1007/bf00902930

Banker, J. E. (2008). Family clay sculpting. *Journal of Family Psychotherapy*, *19*(3), 291–297. https://doi.org/10.1080/08975350802269533

Constantine, L. L. (1978). Family sculpture and relationship mapping techniques. *Journal of Marital and Family Therapy*, *4*(2), 13–23. https://doi.org/10.1111/j.1752-0606.1978.tb00508.x

Duhl, F., Kantor, D., & Duhl, B. (1973). Learning space and action in family therapy: A primer in family sculpture. In D. Block (Ed.), *Techniques of family psychotherapy* (pp. 47–63). Grune & Stratton.

Satir, V. (1983). *Conjoint family therapy*. Science & Behavior Books.

Satir, V. (1988). *The new people making*. Science & Behavior Books.

Springer, P., Bischoff, R. J., Kohel, K., Taylor, N. C., & Farero, A. (2020). Collaborative care at a distance: Student therapists' experiences of learning and delivering relationally focused telemental health. *Journal of Marital and Family Therapy*, *46*(2), 201–217. https://doi.org/10.1111/jmft.12431

Taylor, N. C., Springer, P. R., Bischoff, R. J., & Smith, J. P. (2021). Experiential family therapy interventions delivered via telemental health: A qualitative implementation study. *Journal of Marital and Family Therapy*, *47*(2), 455–472. https://doi.org/10.1111/jmft.12520

CHAPTER 32

STACKING THE DECK

A STRATEGIC APPROACH TO THE UNGAME

Rebecca A. Cobb

Materials for Therapists: The Ungame and PowerPoint slides with additional questions tailored to clients and their presenting problems. Some are included as supplemental materials to this book.

Materials for Clients: None.

Objective

The Ungame is a commonly used game in therapeutic practice that can enhance self-reflection, communication, and intimacy among family members (Swank, 2008). Each player takes turns selecting question cards from a deck and answering whatever question is asked on the card. Special cards allow players to ask a question to another player or make a comment on something that someone else has said. Players only talk when it's their turn or when the person whose turn it is asks them a question. There are no winners or losers in this game. This chapter presents a strategic approach to using the Ungame in teletherapy in which therapists intentionally select question cards for clients aimed at discussing presenting problems in a playful way.

Rationale for Use

Many families, and especially children, love playing the Ungame because it allows them to interact with one another in new and unique ways. As a result, families talk about things that they don't normally talk about and learn new things about one another that they might not otherwise learn.

From a strategic therapy perspective, new communication rules provided by the game (e.g., only listening when someone else speaks, discussing topics that might not otherwise be discussed within the family) perturb the family system and break existing patterns of interaction, allowing for the possibility of second-order change as it relates to family communication patterns (Fisch et al., 1982). Use of the Ungame may also assist in forms of assessment that are important from a strategic approach – assessing patterns within the family, identifying problems within the family, and identifying things that people have done to try to resolve problems (Watzlawick et al., 1967). Unique to teletherapy, clients may not have access to a physical

DOI: 10.4324/9781003289920-38

version of the game, thereby relying on the therapist to pick question cards from the deck. The therapist can use this limitation to the advantage of a strategic approach by adding questions to the deck that are aimed at addressing presenting problems.

Setup

The following outlines steps for setting up the game prior to session.

1. ***Acquire the Ungame.*** There are multiple variations of the Ungame, including full-size board versions (i.e., original, Christian, Catholic) and pocket versions (i.e., all ages, kids, teens, 20-somethings, seniors, couples, families, Christian). Although using a full-size board version for in-person therapy practice can be appealing to many families, pocket versions or simply using the cards available from the full-size board versions are ideal for teletherapy practice. The card deck from the original full-size board version of the game or card decks for all ages or families are ideal for working with families.

2. ***Transfer questions to digital format.*** After acquiring the Ungame, transfer questions from the cards to a PowerPoint file so clients can see the questions during therapy. Another computer program may also be used if preferred. Type each question on a separate slide within the file. You may type questions in random order to allow a variety of questions that are both fun and serious to show up during gameplay. Choose a fun and colorful slide background that allows the words to be easily seen.

3. ***Add new questions.*** Although the Ungame provides a good starting place for questions during gameplay, consider adding questions to the existing deck. The following is a list of questions that could be added for families experiencing death, divorce, or gender identity exploration. PowerPoint slides with these questions are included as supplemental materials to this book. Consider adding other questions to this list, paying special attention to questions that might represent each client's culture, religion, sexuality, gender identity, and presenting problems.

Death

-   Say something about death.
-   Why do you think people die?
-   What do you think happens to people after they die?
-   Do you believe in ghosts?
-   Would you rather be buried, cremated, or composted when you die?
-   Do you believe in heaven? If so, what do you think it smells like?
-   If you could be reincarnated as anything you want, what would you come back as?

Divorce

-   Say something about divorce.
-   Why do people fight?
-   How do you feel when your parents don't get along?
-   Why do you think divorce happens?
-   How do you think kids feel when their parents get divorced?

- Is there anything good that ever happens from divorce?

- What do you think it's like to have two homes?

Gender Identity and Expression

- Make a statement about gender expression.

- Alex identifies as nonbinary. People at school tease them and ask, "Are you a boy or a girl? What are you?" How do you think Alex feels?

- How would you feel if someone called you a boy?

- How would you feel if someone called you a girl?

- Tell us about a time that you may have crossed a gender-related boundary and someone disapproved. How did you feel?

- What's your favorite item of clothing to wear? Why?

- If you could change your name to anything you wanted, what would it be?

When adding questions, provide a balance of serious questions and fun questions that will bring levity to the game (e.g., "What's the silliest face you can make?"). Though there are multiple questions listed about each of the aforementioned topics, the therapist might only insert one or two questions about the family's presenting problem(s) in order to not draw too much attention to that topic.

Instructions

The following specifies instructions for this activity in eight steps.

1. ***Introduce the activity.*** Tell the family that you have a game that you'd like to play to get to know them better. Explain that the game is usually played using a deck of cards with questions on them but that you've transferred the questions to the computer so they can see them. You might consider showing the family the original deck of Ungame cards if you have them available.

2. ***Explain the rules.*** Begin by sharing the rules of the game. Explain that "To play this game, each player takes turns selecting question cards from a deck and answering whatever question is asked on the card. Special cards allow players to ask a question to another player or make a comment on something that someone else said earlier in the game. Players only talk when it's their turn or when the person whose turn it is asks them a question. If you have a question or comment that you'd like to make when it's not your turn, you can write it down so you don't forget. There are no winners or losers in this game."

3. ***Determine order of game play.*** You can determine the order in which family members play or allow the family to decide. If you decide, consider starting with the youngest member of the family and taking turns in order by age.

4. ***Show the slide deck.*** Share your screen so the family can see the PowerPoint.

5. ***Begin game play.*** Ask the first player to select a number between 1 and 10. Then select the corresponding slide. The person whose turn it is should read the slide out loud for everyone to hear. If someone can't read, you can read it for them. The person whose turn it is then answers the question while all other members of the family remain silent.

If the person selects a slide that says, "You may ask a player one question OR comment on any subject you choose" and chooses to ask a question of another person, that person may respond with an answer. Game play then moves to the next person.

6. **Move used slides.** Once a question on a slide has been answered, move the slide to the end of the slide deck to ensure that it doesn't get asked again and to allow other questions to move to the position of 1–10. If you continue moving used slides to the end of the deck, slides 1–10 should remain unused until all but 10 slides are left.

7. **Maintain structure.** Throughout the game, help to maintain structure of the session and ensure that the rules of the game are followed. Sometimes, people may decide that they don't like a question that is being asked and want to select another question or pass on their turn. It can be up to the family and/or the therapist to determine what is and isn't allowed. It's recommended that clients aren't forced to share things that they don't want to share. One rule that therapists should enforce, however, is the no-talking rule when others are sharing. Families may need several reminders for this throughout the game, but they typically get better about it as time goes on.

8. **End the game.** The game ends when the family decides that they're done playing or when the therapy session is almost over. It's recommended that gameplay end 10 or 15 minutes before the session is over to allow time for processing.

Processing

After the game is over, ask processing questions about the family's experience. The following is a list of questions that can be asked:

- What was it like for you to hear your [mom/dad/sister/brother/etc.] say _____?
- What was it like for you to share _____?
- What was it like to only be allowed to listen while others spoke?
- What was it like to be able to speak without anyone interrupting you or asking questions until their turn?
- What questions do you have that weren't answered?
- What questions did you hear that you wanted to answer?

As is the case with gameplay itself, it's important to provide a balance of serious and fun processing questions that bring levity to the conversation (e.g., "What was it like for you to hear your mom say that she was sad?" and "What was it like for you to see your mom make a face like a monkey?"). Although therapy doesn't always need to be fun, the balance of lightheartedness with seriousness in this game allows members of all ages to remain engaged, even while discussing difficult topics.

Vignette

Darnell (37), Daria (35), Dre (10), and Danielle (7), a middle-class Black family, presented in teletherapy reporting increased anxiety within the family after Darnell was pulled over and harassed by the police without having done anything wrong. In the initial intake, Darnell and Daria met alone with the therapist to explain their concerns. They stated that Dre was in the car with his dad at the time of the incident and appeared to be having an extra-hard time. Dre demonstrated high anxiety about going to school and appeared to worry any time his dad left the house. The family seemed generally embarrassed about the situation and hadn't spoken about it with many people. They indicated that Darnell and Daria spoke with the children about the event and had conversations about racial injustice and empowerment with them since they were very young. The children, however, didn't seem to want to talk about what happened.

For the second session, the entire family was present. After initial introductions, the therapist introduced the idea of the Ungame as a way of getting to know one another better. The family agreed to give it a try. During the game, the family appeared to have fun thinking about their responses and hearing what one another had to share. The family initially wanted to discuss responses to each question after each person went, but toward the end of the session, the therapist didn't need to remind them of the rules anymore, and they seemed to adjust to this new method of communication. For this initial time playing the game, the therapist didn't add any questions to the deck that directly tied to the family's presenting problem. Rather, the therapist wanted the children to gain comfort with the therapist and the process of therapy before moving onto more sensitive topics.

The therapist had the family stop playing 15 minutes before the end of session and asked them how they liked the game. The children spoke first, saying how much fun they had. Danielle said that she especially liked hearing that Mommy wanted to be a cat. Danielle said that she would want to be a cat too and wondered what Daddy wanted to be. Darnell shared that he would be a dog so he could chase Mommy and Danielle around the house! Dre said that he would be a dog, too, so he could chase the cats with Daddy. The family shared a big belly laugh with one another.

The therapist then asked what it was like to only be allowed to listen while others spoke. Everyone indicated that it was hard but noticed that they got better at it by the end of the game. The therapist asked what it was like to speak without anyone interrupting them. Dre said that it was kind of nice to talk without being asked any questions. The others agreed.

Danielle asked if they could play the game again, and the therapist said that they could if the rest of the family was okay with it. The others agreed.

The third session, game play began shortly after the session started. This time, the therapist added a couple of questions to the deck that could be instrumental in discussing the incident with the police. "Say something about the police" was added to slide #22. "Say something about justice" was added to slide #23. This positioning allowed each person to answer at least three questions, 12 questions in all, before the questions about police and justice appeared in slides 1–10. This allowed the family to warm up to the game again before discussing more sensitive topics. The therapist also made sure that there were enough lighthearted questions surrounding these slides and that a couple of question or comment cards appeared soon after the questions about police and justice.

Initially selected cards raised questions that appeared to naturally help discuss topics related to the family's concerns:

- "Share something you fear."

- "What do you do when you get angry?"

- "Complete this statement: I wish I felt free to . . ."

The questions prompted conversation about topics loosely related to what appeared to be at the forefront of everyone's mind. Daria shared that she is afraid of her kids living in fear. Darnell said that when he is angry he tries to not let it get the best of him. Dre said that he wishes he felt free to go anywhere he wants.

Other questions allowed the family to reflect on things that made them smile and laugh:

- "Give three reasons why you like yourself."

- "Tell about a funny experience."

- "Share one of the happiest days of your life."

Danielle shared that she likes herself because she's smart, funny, and pretty. Darnell told a funny story that made the whole family laugh so hard that Danielle snorted. Daria shared two of the happiest days of her life – the days that each of her children were born.

By the time that "Say something about the police" and "Say something about justice" showed up in the deck, the family developed a rhythm of discussing serious and happy topics in an open way. Danielle selected the question about the police. The family grew quiet before Danielle blurted out, "They're poopy heads!" Dre went next and selected the question about justice. He simply stated, "unfair." A few turns later, several question or comment cards appeared, allowing the family to continue the conversation about police and justice. With about 20 minutes left before the end of session, the therapist ended gameplay to process. By asking "What questions do you have that weren't answered?" and "What questions did you hear that you wanted to answer?" the family continued discussion beyond the game. Though they no longer had to talk according to game rules, the family continued to allow space to share without interruption and without asking many questions of one another. This new pattern of interaction appeared to allow the children to discuss their concerns more openly.

Suggestions for Follow-Up

Many children and adolescents who play the Ungame in therapy request to play the game in future sessions. Some make it a practice of playing every session. In-person use of the game does not easily allow therapists or clients to keep track of which questions have previously been asked. Online gameplay using PowerPoint, however, allows therapists to save a copy of the PowerPoint at the end of each session to keep track of which questions a family has answered. This allows new questions to be discussed in subsequent sessions. Alternatively, therapists might review questions that were discussed in a prior session and ask if anyone else wants to answer a question that has been asked of someone else or if anyone wants to ask the same question to a different member of the family.

Contraindications

There might be certain questions in the Ungame that aren't appropriate for all families in their original form. With alterations, the game can be made more inclusive for clients from all backgrounds. You might also consider changing the rules of the game to be more culturally attuned or letting the family come up with their own rules. Additionally, if questions prompt strong emotional reactions or trigger trauma responses, you may need to pause the game to attend to the needs of the client.

References

Fisch, R., Weakland, J. H., & Segal, L. (1982). *The tactics of change: Doing therapy briefly*. Jossey-Bass.

Swank, J. M. (2008). The use of games: A therapeutic tool with children and families. *International Journal of Play Therapy*, *17*(2), 154–167. https://doi.org/10.1037/1555-6824.17.2.154

Watzlawick, P., Bavelas, J. B., & Jackson, D. J. (1967). *Pragmatics of human communication*. W. W. Norton.

CHAPTER 33

VIRTUAL ALTAR-MAKING FOR GRIEF AND LOSS

Christie Eppler, J. Maria Bermúdez, and Rebecca A. Cobb

Materials for Therapists: None.

Materials for Clients: A computer program or application that compiles images (e.g., PowerPoint) and digitized photographs of people or animals who have died, photographs of things that belonged to the deceased, images of things that represent the deceased, images of flowers, the text of poems or prayers, or anything else that clients would like to include in their altar that represents loss, transition, or grief.

Objective

An altar is traditionally a decorated table, shrine, or shadow box that can be used as an intervention across a range of therapeutic modalities (Bermúdez & Bermúdez, 2002). Altars or shrines have been used for in-person therapy interventions to help individuals, partnerships, families, and groups experiencing grief and loss. This chapter explains how to support clients in creating a virtual altar for processing grief and loss in teletherapy sessions.

Rationale for Use

Grief and loss occur when people die, jobs are lost, communities lose resources, or anything else is experienced that has a profound, negative impact. Mourning can last months or years. Grief experiences can be ambiguous (e.g., life changes related to a global pandemic) or anticipatory (e.g., when death is forthcoming; Boss, 2016). Identifying multiple and complex feelings, reconstructing meaning and identity within a new reality, and the creation and reliance on social support promote resilience throughout the grief process (Boss, 2016; Eppler, 2008; Neimeyer, 2022).

According to constructivists, the grieving process includes meaning making, finding purpose after loss, and revising one's identity (Neimeyer, 2022; McCoyd et al., 2016). In general, art can be very beneficial in therapy, especially as a way to help couples and families to work together to externalize and face problems together (Bermúdez et al., 2009). A creative, virtual activity such as building an altar with grieving clients may support this process by helping them to express themselves through images and symbols and then reflect on this process (Bermúdez & Bermúdez, 2002).

Building an altar is a creative process, but it does not require artistic talent, and clients of all ages and developmental abilities can take part. The process of curating an altar may help therapists and clients invite

DOI: 10.4324/9781003289920-39

remembrance and honoring of the deceased, identify themes which contribute to stuckness in grief patterns (e.g., isolation, sadness, regret), embody emotions that may be difficult to express during mourning, and invoke new ways of coping. When working with partners, families, or groups, this activity may be used to promote communication and identify commonalities and differences among grief experiences. Building a virtual altar may be particularly helpful for clients who have difficulty verbalizing their grief experiences. Additionally, it can facilitate spiritually-integrated therapy for clients who wish to integrate faith practices or folk healing into treatment.

Setup

1. ***Introduce the idea of this activity to clients.*** Share that this activity offers an opportunity to remember, honor, and grieve the deceased in community with one another. It is important to explain that the word "altar," as it is used in this context, comes from Spanish, and an altar, as used in Mexico and other Hispanic cultures, is not meant to be a place to worship or idolize. An altar in this context is a space to honor and remember. For this activity, an altar would be a digital means to memorialize, remember, and honor a loved one. This should be explained prior to the session in which you intend to conduct the activity. This gives clients time to prepare for the activity outside of session.

2. ***Invite clients to collect photographs or other digital images that they would like to use for the activity between sessions.*** Digital objects may include photographs of people or animals who have died, photographs of things that belonged to the deceased, images of things that represent the deceased or other losses, images of flowers, poems, sayings, prayers, or anything else that they would like to include. Clients may transfer physical photographs to digital form and photograph other objects as a part of this process. Encourage clients to save files of all digital objects that they would like to include in their alter in one folder that they can easily access during the next session and share with others.

3. ***Ask if clients have a computer program or digital app that allows for the compilation of images.*** Explain that this would look like something similar to a collage. PowerPoint is also a readily available program that works for this activity.

Instructions

The following steps outline the process for creating virtual altars in teletherapy:

1. ***Confirm that all necessary digital objects and images have been collected.*** If clients have not gathered the things that they want to include in their altar, ask if they would like to do this during the session or if they prefer to wait to do the activity in the following session. Some clients may need additional support in the collection process and may prefer to do this while the therapist is present with them. They can also keep adding images over time, making this an ongoing process.

2. ***Share the client's screen.*** Once clients are ready with the digital objects that they have collected, request that they share their screen with you.

3. ***Make the altar/memorial/shrine.*** Invite clients to talk to one another (if there is more than one person in the session) to discuss how they would like to assemble their altar using the digital objects that they collected. Explain that they may use any computer program that they would like to compile the images. Once a new file has been created for this activity in their computer program of choice, ask

clients to take turns copying and pasting the digital objects that they collected onto this page. These objects may be resized and arranged any way that they would like. The process is as important as, if not more important than, the final product.

4. ***Collaborate with others.*** When working with partners, families, or groups, check in with clients on their process to ensure that everyone has the space that they feel that they need to include the digital objects that they would like to include. Support them in making any accommodations necessary to make space and honor the needs of others while simultaneously having their own needs met. For example, family members may need to resize their objects after placing them to make space for someone else to place their objects. This may be likened to creating space for others to grieve in ways that work for them when others might experience grief in different ways.

5. ***Save the altar.*** Instruct clients to save the completed altar to their device and to share this file with each other (if there is more than one person in therapy). Discuss the possibility of sending the file to you to save for use in future sessions.

Processing

Use observations and prompts to promote dialogue as clients co-create the altar and after its completion. Bermúdez and Bermúdez (2002) identify eight steps in the process of altar-making from a narrative therapy perspective. These steps include externalization, identifying unique outcomes, reconstruction, thickening the plot, and spreading the news, all of which may be used in processing this activity. You may use a narrative approach or your own theory of change to generate questions and reflections (e.g., focusing on defining boundaries or rules regarding grief from one's family of origin or assessing grief from hierarchal or structural perspectives of grief). Following is a list of transtheoretical questions that may be asked before, during, or after the altar-making process:

- Can you tell me something you learned about grief from your culture or from other family members?

- How does your grief differ from the experiences of others? How is it the same?

- Before you constructed the altar, what was your image or metaphor of grief? How has it changed?

- What would you like others to know about your grief and how it has transformed?

- In what ways have you seen family members cope with grief?

- How would you like to remember the deceased after this process?

- What thoughts or feelings might need to be transformed? How might your family system be affected by this transformation?

- Whenever you see or think about the altar, what is the first thing that comes to mind?

- Through the process of creating an altar, how has your family grown or changed?

- Would you like to create a physical alter/shrine/shadow box after seeing your digital altar? If so, who and what would you include?

Allow time and space for all clients to speak and respond. Throughout the conversation, reflect on clients' emotions and content that might facilitate healing.

Vignette

The Dominquez family sought therapy after the loss of their 20-year-old son/brother who died suddenly in a fatal car accident. He was the oldest of three children. The parents were experiencing enormous grief. However, they became increasingly distraught when the youngest son (14) began to show severe symptoms of depression. He did not want to attend school, be with friends, or do the activities and sports he once enjoyed and began to lose weight and have insomnia and night terrors. Their son's school was putting pressure on them to seek counseling for their son, and their church offered to pay for the sessions. As therapy unfolded, the parents, son, and their 17-year-old daughter began to discuss the ways in which the grief was taking over their lives. They were all deeply saddened and, two years later, still unable to regain the sense of strength they once felt. It became apparent to the therapist that this family could benefit from doing an activity together in session that helped them process their grief.

After the therapeutic alliance was established, the therapist asked the family if they would be willing to create an altar/shrine to share their memories and grieve their loss together in a focused and creative manner. After they agreed, the therapist began the process. The therapist asked who would be willing to take the lead, and the sister volunteered. Each family member thought of the things that were special to their son/brother and added them to the list. The therapist served in a supportive and facilitative role as the family mostly talked amongst themselves. At this point, they simply talked and made a list of what they would include in the altar. To help move them along, the therapist encouraged them to think of this shrine as if it were three-dimensional and not digital. The therapist asked them to think about what they would put in it if it were a shadow box. They mentioned things like his driver's license, a picture of his soccer trophies, high school graduation picture and ring, baby shoes, pictures together, pictures of his favorite foods, music, and video games. At the end of the session, the therapist encouraged the family to continue to add to the list if they wanted, but that when they were ready, they could start to take pictures of these things and save them to a file on their computer.

The next session, the family was ready to co-create their digital altar. The sister took the lead for the third session, and the son took the lead on the fourth session. By taking the lead, they were able to ask the rest of the family about the images they wanted to include, why they wanted to include them, and where they wanted them placed on the collage. In addition to using the pictures of the items they wanted to include, they also added images that were used for the slide show of their son's/brother's funeral. They placed all of the images into a collage that could be printed into poster-size print. They focused on the altar for five sessions in total. Throughout this time, therapy focused on working through their grief and offering strong emotional support for their son/brother and each other. The son continued to work with the therapist individually, and his parents and sister joined in his sessions a few more times. The son did well in sessions, and the altar-making sessions with his family therapy helped serve as a bridge for him to get more intensive individual therapy. Family therapy continued as needed.

Suggestions for Follow-Up

One of the benefits of a virtual altar is the ability to save it for future use. Clients may keep a copy of the altar and revisit it at any time, inside or outside of therapy. They may also choose to add to their altar at any point. You may also save a copy of an altar in the client's file to use in future discussion if clients are comfortable with this option. Virtual altars can be revisited in subsequent sessions during times of particular significance. For example, clients may wish to return to this activity and add to their virtual altar around the time of birthdays of the deceased, anniversaries of the death of loved ones, when clients experience another loss, holidays that may serve as reminders of the deceased, or *Día de los Muertos*

(Day of the Dead) for clients who choose to honor the dead by making *"ofrendas"* (offerings) around this time of year.

Contraindications

The availability of family photographs can be associated with wealth and privilege, especially for generations who had less accessibility to cameras in their youth. Some individuals and families have lost photographs in natural disasters, migration, and by other means. Also consider culture and spirituality as they relate to clients' comfort with this activity. The idea of creating an altar/shrine may be associated with religious beliefs that may not be compatible with clients' belief systems. It can be helpful to reframe this as a creative process and piece of art to help them grieve, honor, and remember their loved one(s). However, any hesitance in participating in this activity for these reasons should be met with understanding, and alternative interventions should be introduced.

References

Bermúdez, J. M., & Bermúdez, S. (2002). Altar-making with Latino families: A narrative therapy perspective. *Journal of Family Psychotherapy, 13*(3–4), 329–347. https://doi.org/10.1300/J085v13n03_06

Bermúdez, J. M., Keeling, M., & Carlson, T. S. (2009). Using art to co-create preferred problem-solving narratives with Latino couples. In M. Rastogi & V. Thomas (Eds.), *Multicultural couple therapy* (pp. 319–343). Sage Publications.

Boss, P. (2016). The context and process of theory development: The story of ambiguous loss. *Journal of Family Theory & Review, 8*(3), 269–286. https://doi.org/10.1111/jftr.12152

Eppler, C. (2008). Exploring themes of resiliency in children after the death of a parent. *Professional School Counseling, 11*(3), 189–196. https://doi.org/10.1177/2156759X0801100305

McCoyd, J. L. M., Walter, C. A., Sussman, S. W., & O'Connor, M. (Eds.). (2016). *Grief and loss across the lifespan: A biopsychosocial perspective*. Springer.

Neimeyer, R. A. (2022). *New techniques of grief therapy: Bereavement and beyond*. Routledge.

CHAPTER 34

MIGRATION JOURNEYS

INCREASING BONDS WITH SHARED STORIES AND GEOGRAPHICAL MAPS

Jacqueline Florian and Rebecca A. Cobb

Materials for Therapists and Clients: Google Maps, Google Earth, or Apple Maps (application or website browser).

Objective

In immigrant or mixed-status families, familial bonds can grow when parents share stories of their migration journey with their child(ren) and other members of their family (Dollahite, 2004; Frude & Killick, 2011). This chapter describes an experiential intervention with online maps to help families engage in conversations about their migration journeys, increase communication, validate one another's unique experience, and strengthen familial bonds.

Rationale for Use

Immigrant and mixed-legal-status families face unique challenges that impact familial relationships, including acculturation, language, and socioeconomic status (Brabeck & Xu, 2010; Capps et al., 2005; Rendón García, 2019). These factors can lead to familial rifts as children attempt to fit in with peers and parents attempt to hold on to cultural traditions. Many immigrant parents do not share their migration stories with their children unless prompted by external factors (Balderas et al., 2016). However, sharing these experiences can help family members gain understanding, increase empathy, and repair relationships.

Family life chronology is an experiential intervention that can help clients communicate about their family of origin's birthplace and ethnic background(s) to understand how these experiences impact their past and present (Banmen, 2002; Bermudez, 2008; Satir & Baldwin, 1984). In the assessment phase, therapists explore with clients the historical events and major life changes that have occurred and may be related to communication and other dynamics within the family (Shulman & Lamba, 2011; Yildirim, 2017). Through this experience, family members learn from one another about both unique and intersecting experiences

DOI: 10.4324/9781003289920-40

(Shulman & Lamba, 2011; Yildirim, 2017), allowing the opportunity for increased communication and validation of one another's experiences (Shulman & Lamba, 2011).

Mapping migration journeys is an alternative way to experientially assess a family's life chronology with families who have experienced migration. It allows those who have migrated from one or more location(s) to share their experience, both verbally and visually, while others actively listen (Yildirim, 2017). Through the process of listening and asking questions, this intervention helps to enhance understanding, empathy, and communication between family members.

The following explains how to conduct this intervention via telehealth with the use of online geographical maps and experiential therapeutic processing.

Setup

1. ***Discuss with clients their comfort and interest in sharing their migration story.*** There are many reasons that someone may not be comfortable sharing their migration story (e.g., cultural aspects, fear, trauma). Respect the client's desire to not share if this is their choice. If they are comfortable sharing, ensure that the information discussed will not be traumatic to the family, and collaborate with adults to share information in a way that is age appropriate for children.

2. ***Explain the intervention to the entire family.*** Explain that they will be using an online map to share their family members' migration journey. Tell children that they will have an opportunity to ask any questions that they might have and that you will help guide everyone in talking about their experience. Explain how this intervention will be helpful in practicing active listening and effective communication, increasing empathy between family members, and increasing familial bonding.

3. ***Determine who will guide the map.*** This intervention requires the use of Google Maps, Google Earth, or Apple Maps (application or website browser). Either the therapist or clients may take the lead in sharing their screen during this activity. Because clients will likely be more familiar with the location of their immigration journey, it may be best for clients to access the map through their own device being used for therapy. The following instructions assume that clients will guide the map. However, if clients are not as comfortable using this form of technology, you may access the map on your screen and find appropriate locations on the map with guidance from clients.

4. ***Obtain translation services if necessary.*** Because storytelling is an important part of this intervention, engage clients in the family's preferred language if possible. If you do not speak the clients' preferred language, a translator may be used with permission from the family. Otherwise, you may discuss with clients whether another member of the client system may be able to translate what is being said to allow the speaker to talk freely in whatever language they prefer.

Instructions

1. ***Instruct clients to find the location of the start of their journey on the map.*** You may have them enter a specific address if one is available to them. They may also use a landmark or something else specifically that they remember for their search. Before zooming in on this location, ask clients to begin with a view of the map in which their current location is still visible. This demonstrates the distance traveled throughout their journey. Then, instruct them to zoom in on their city of origin, possibly even their home location if this is available on the map.

2. ***Instruct clients to describe their experience living in this place.*** They may share what a typical day looked like when they lived here or describe things that they appreciated about this place.

3. ***Ask clients to show landmarks or specific places that they have special memories of in their hometown.*** If available, some maps may allow for a street view or let you see photographs of homes, parks, restaurants, or other locations. While sharing these locations, guide clients in sharing more about the significance of these locations. For example, you might ask, "Tell us about the significance of this place. What do you feel as you see this place on screen? What memories do you have of being there? Who else was there with you? What do you wish you could share with your children about this place?" Instruct clients to continue "traveling" through different locations within this place until they feel content in "beginning their migration journey." Some clients may spend an entire session just at this stage of the intervention. Others may be ready to move on earlier in the session. If clients have spent a substantial amount of time in discussing their hometown, consider waiting until the next session to continue with the remainder of the intervention so that clients don't have to stop midway through their "journey." In this case, simply process with clients what has been discussed up until this point and pick back up where you left off in a subsequent session.

4. ***Instruct clients to explain why and how they left.*** Ask why they decided to leave, how they decided where they would go, who would go with them, who would stay (if any), and how they prepared for their journey.

5. ***Ask clients to navigate the map in such a way that shows the specific geographical journey that they took as they traveled from there to their current location.*** Some clients may not know the details of their journey. If this is the case, assure them that this is okay and that they can simply share what they do know. Ask what modes of transportation they used to travel, who helped them along the way, if anything of significance happened during their journey, and what this experience was like for them.

6. ***Instruct clients to zoom out on the map to show the starting and end points of their journey again.*** Encourage them to share what their experience was like when they arrived at their final destination, what feelings they had, how they learned to adapt to their surroundings, and what they feel about it now.

Processing

Throughout the activity, help clients navigate any questions that children might have about their immigration journey. If children don't have specific questions while adults are sharing, the bulk of processing may occur after the activity has been completed.

Storytellers

The following prompts can be used to help storytellers reflect on their experience of sharing their journey with their family.

- How did it feel to share your story with your family?

- Can you paint me a picture of how your journey has impacted your relationship with [your parents/your children/others in your family]?

- What, if anything, do you wish that your [family/children/child] took away from your experience and your journey?

Listeners

The following prompts can be used to help listeners reflect on their experience of hearing someone else's migration journey story.

- How are you feeling right now?

- What emotions come up for you after learning more about your family's migration?

- How did you feel while your [mom/dad/grandmother/grandfather/family member] spoke about _____?

- What are some of the thoughts you have at this moment?

- What were you thinking when your [mom/dad/grandmother/grandfather/family member] spoke about _____?

- Are there any questions that might be running through your mind at this present moment?

- Can you paint me a picture of how your own experience growing up in a different country makes it difficult to relate to [this story/your mom/your dad/others in your family]?

- Are there other family members whose migration story you would like to know more about?

Everyone

The following prompts can be used to promote discussion and further reflection between everyone present in the session.

- Did you learn anything new about yourself or anyone else in your family while doing this activity? What did you learn?

- In what ways do you feel connected to your family right now in this moment? What does it feel like to be connected in this way? How might you imagine making this connection even stronger?

Vignette

Chelsea is a 14-year-old, cisgender Latina American who often argues with her mother, Rosa, a 39-year-old cisgender Latina and immigrant single mother from El Salvador. During the first session, Rosa explained to the therapist that Chelsea often disobeys rules at home and at school. Chelsea stated that her mother never understands that she hates school and wants to go out with her friends instead of helping with her younger sibling, Kathy, age 10.

Before engaging in the intervention with Chelsea and Rosa, the therapist engaged in a collateral session with Rosa to hear the migration story and determine whether it was age appropriate and if it contained traumatic events that she would not want to share with her daughter. After determining that the migration story was appropriate to share with Chelsea, the therapist spoke with Rosa about sharing her migration story using an online map and assessed her comfort using an application such as Google Earth.

During the next session, the therapist met with Chelsea and Rosa. Rosa already had the map pulled up on their computer before the session started, which made it easy to transition into the intervention after the therapist provided the instructions and rationale for the intervention.

At first, Chelsea seemed a little hesitant to participate but collaborated with her mom and helped her to share their screen with the therapist and zoom in and out of the map while her mom shared her experiences. Before discussing her migration story, Rosa shared with Chelsea what it was like growing up in El Salvador and even briefly discussed what it was like to grow up with Chelsea's grandparents. After providing some background on her upbringing, Rosa provided details of her migration journey using the map as a guide and point of focus. She shared the reason she decided to leave, the mode of transportation out of her town, and even explained how her experience was different from that of her siblings, as she was one of the last ones to immigrate. As her mom shared her story, Chelsea asked her mother follow-up questions without prompting from the therapist, and Rosa willingly answered every one of them.

Once Rosa felt that she had provided all the details that she could remember, she asked the therapist what to do next. The therapist then prompted the two to discuss how they felt in the moment, their thoughts, and their present understanding of each other's experiences. They discussed how their different upbringings and cultures currently impacted them. They further discussed how being open with one another in the present moment felt different than their usual communication.

The therapist found out that this was the first time that Rosa had provided detailed information about where she grew up or what her migration journey looked like. The therapist also learned that Chelsea had understood that her mother's upbringing was different but never really knew all the details, nor had they reflected on how her mom's story was different than her own. Chelsea was able to begin explaining to her mom why she behaved in certain ways – so that she could fit in with some of her friends who were given more freedom by their parents. Rosa mentioned to Chelsea that she understood that she wanted more freedom, which led to a discussion about Rosa's fear regarding her safety. In future sessions, the therapist further processed these fears and their relation to her own story. Through this discussion, Chelsea gained greater compassion for her mom and began to follow a few more rules at home. Likewise, Rosa gained greater compassion for Chelsea's own story and the ways in which it differed from her own.

Suggestions for Follow-Up

Experiential family therapy emphasizes that everyone in a family has a different experience (Banmen, 2002; Satir & Baldwin, 1984). Even if different family members traveled together on the same physical journey, each person has their own story and experience of that journey to share. Therefore, all members who have a migration story to share should have an opportunity to do so. Additional family members may share their stories following the same steps in subsequent sessions.

Contraindications

Ensure that the migration story is age appropriate for children before encouraging adults to share their stories with them. If the migration story is not age appropriate, discuss whether it can be modified without altering events that they find significant to their life experience. Refrain from using this intervention if the migration journey includes traumatic events that may be traumatizing/retraumatizing to any member of the family. Pause clients in telling their stories and take appropriate safety measures if any member of the family appears to be having significant difficulty in hearing the events of the story. The intervention should not be used if sharing details of the migration journey could raise risks to the family's safety due to their immigration status (e.g., if information could be shared outside of the session to put the family in danger of deportation or having their status be known to others).

References

Balderas, C. N., Delgado-Romero, E. A., & Singh, A. A. (2016). Sin papeles: Latino parent–child conversations about undocumented legal status. *Journal of Latina/o Psychology*, *4*(3), 158–172. https://doi.org/10.1037/lat0000060

Banmen, J. (2002). The Satir model: Yesterday and today. *Contemporary Family Therapy*, *24*(1), 7–22. https://doi.org/10.1023/A:1014365304082

Bermudez, D. (2008). Adapting Virginia Satir techniques to Hispanic families. *The Family Journal*, *16*(1), 51–57. https://doi.org/10.1177/1066480707309543

Brabeck, K., & Xu, Q. (2010). The impact of detention and deportation on Latino immigrant children and families: A quantitative exploration. *Hispanic Journal of Behavioral Sciences*, *32*(3), 341–361. https://doi.org/10.1177/0739986310374053

Capps, R., Fix, M., Murray, J., Ost, J., Passel, J. S., & Herwantoro, S. (2005, September 30). *The new demography of America's schools: Immigration and the No Child Left Behind Act*. Urban Institute. www.urban.org/sites/default/files/publication/51701/311230-The-New-Demography-of-America-s-Schools.PDF

Dollahite, D. C. (2004). Forging family bonds through storytelling. *Marriage & Families*, *13*(2), 1–7. https://scholarsarchive.byu.edu/cgi/viewcontent.cgi?article=1094&context=marriageandfamilies

Frude, N., & Killick, S. (2011). Family storytelling and the attachment relationship. *Psychodynamic Practice*, *17*(4), 441–455. https://doi.org/10.1080/14753634.2011.609025

Rendón García, S. A. (2019). "No vamos a tapar el sol con un dedo": Maternal communication concerning immigration status. *Journal of Latinx Psychology*, *7*(4), 284–303. https://doi.org/10.1037/lat0000131

Satir, V., & Baldwin, M. (1984). *Satir step by step: A guide to creating change in families*. Science and Behavior Books.

Shulman, J., & Lamba, G. (2011). Theories of family therapy. In A. Zagelbaum & J. Carlson (Eds.), *Working with immigrant families: A practical guide for counselors* (pp. 39–53). Taylor & Francis.

Yildirim, N. (2017). The updating in Satir's family therapy model. *European Journal of Multidisciplinary Studies*, *5*(1), 425–431. https://doi.org/10.26417/ejms.v5i1.p425-431

CHAPTER 35

MEDICAL FAMILY TELETHERAPY

EXPANDING CARE TO PROMOTE HEALTH EQUITY

Angela L. Lamson, Jennifer L. Hodgson, Betül Küçükardalı Cansever, and Irma Abrego Lappin

Materials for Therapists and Clients: None.

Objective

This chapter explains how medical family therapists (MedFTs) who practice teletherapy apply socioculturally attuned joining, assessment, diagnosis, and intervention. It also provides a method to extend socioculturally attuned medical family therapy treatment using the MED-STAT acronym (Giorlando & Schilling, 1997), a collection of solution-focused brief therapy interventions originally written for primary care physicians but well suited for MedFTs practicing via telehealth.

Rationale

Medical family therapy (MedFT) is a field grounded in systemic, biopsychosocial-spiritual, and relationally-oriented practice and research. MedFT addresses people's biological, psychological, social, and spiritual health (Engel, 1977, 1980; Wright et al., 1996) through a socioculturally attuned family therapy lens (McDowell et al., 2018). The application of MedFT most commonly occurs in primary, secondary, and tertiary care settings (Hodgson et al., 2014; McDaniel et al., 2014; Mendenhall et al., 2018). Regardless of context, those who identify as MedFTs fall somewhere within the medical family therapy healthcare continuum (Hodgson et al., 2014). In tandem with this continuum is an appreciation for the levels of integrated care ranging from separate practice locations with limited collaboration between providers to fully integrated models of care in which treatment plans are collaboratively written (e.g., Doherty et al., 1996; Heath et al., 2013). While these models were not created with teletherapy in mind, they do provide a framework for thinking through the numerous settings in which equitable teletherapy policies and practice strategies are necessary.

The success of integrated care in teletherapy is contingent upon the adoption of policies and practices that are ethically and socioculturally sound, patient- and family-centered, collaboratively designed, and

DOI: 10.4324/9781003289920-41

make services more accessible and effective for all parties involved in the care process (Hodgson et al., 2013). Teletherapy options in healthcare settings improve patient-centered services, provider-to-provider collaboration, and patients' continuity of care from the point of triage to treatment with a healthcare team. This gives people who might not otherwise get care for their physical, emotional, or relational health access to care. Therefore, it is essential for MedFTs to be prepared to extend teletherapy in a way that promotes and actively attends to health equity, especially in response to the growing need and demand for such services. The following provides a method to extend socioculturally attuned MedFT treatment using the MED-STAT acronym (Giorlando & Schilling, 1997), a collection of solution-focused brief therapy interventions originally written for primary care physicians but well suited for MedFTs practicing via telehealth.

Setup

Before implementing any teletherapy intervention in a healthcare context, particularly one grounded in socioculturally attuned care, therapists should be equipped with the skills and knowledge to practice as a MedFT (AAMFT, 2018). Therapists should consider the following:

- **Informed consent:** Prior to assessment in appointments within healthcare contexts, it is best practice for MedFTs to obtain three forms of consent from each patient.

  - Verify that the patient understands they are consenting to mental health treatment.

  - Clarify that the MedFT will share summative information with the healthcare provider through the electronic health record or verbally.

  - Ensure that the patient is comfortable discussing their mental health in front of anyone present in the patient's or MedFT's teletherapy location (e.g., other family members). It is essential to know who is present and will/may hear the patient(s) within each side of the teletherapy location (i.e., that of the patient(s) and that of the provider) prior to initiating treatment with each patient.

- **Confidentiality:** MedFTs, regardless of setting, must comply with HIPAA regulations, use appropriate precautions to protect patient data, and adhere to the highest ethical standards. It is important for MedFTs to remember that their code of ethics is distinct from that of other providers (e.g., nurse practitioners and laboratory technicians) when providing teletherapy via integrated care services or treatment in healthcare settings. Some staff in the healthcare industry (e.g., front-desk personnel and housekeepers) may not be subject to any professional code of ethics. As such, MedFTs may be required to take different steps or make different choices than their colleagues when interacting with patients.

- **Language accessibility:** MedFTs dedicated to providing socioculturally attuned care should recognize the importance of offering documentation and services in the patient's preferred language. Every medical practice maintains treatment consent documentation. However, patients might not always fully comprehend these materials due to language barriers or literacy needs. A MedFT with a sociocultural focus ensures that such documentation is available in multiple languages, catering to a patient's linguistic needs. In the absence of trained interpreters, reliable translation services (i.e., on-demand video remote interpretation) become crucial to ensure ethical and fair healthcare interactions, especially given the nuanced terminology often used in mental health and medical contexts.

- **Session duration:** Beyond logistical arrangements, MedFTs must be adept at managing the swift pace of integrated behavioral health teletherapy sessions. The joining, assessment, diagnosis, and intervention processes are often condensed into a concise 20-minute time frame. Extended sessions of 50 minutes are generally reserved for select cases.

Instructions

Within the MED-STAT acronym (Franklin et al., 2016; Giorlando & Schilling, 1997), each letter corresponds to a distinct intervention applicable throughout the various stages of the visit, encompassing joining, assessment, diagnosis, and intervention. The following briefly describes each component of the MED-STAT acronym:

- ***Miracle question:*** Help patients explore possibilities of life when their presenting concern is less present, overwhelming, or dominant in their life. For example, ask the patient what their morning would be like if they woke up and didn't notice their presenting concern at the start of their day.

- ***Exceptions:*** Ask patients to consider times when their symptom or concern wasn't happening or didn't happen much.

- ***Difference that makes a difference:*** Encourage patients to describe what was different when the symptom or concern was absent.

- ***Scaling:*** Quantify the patient's motivation for change and overall assessment of the problem's discomfort using scaling questions.

- ***Time-out:*** Allow patients to take a 30-second pause to reflect on what was discussed in the session to pivot toward accolades by the provider and tasks for the patient.

- ***Accolades:*** Extend genuine acknowledgment and praise for the patient's efforts. This promotes confidence and lays the stage for future triumphs.

- ***Task:*** Introduce a patient-tailored task that the patient agrees is achievable between appointments.

The following describes a teletherapy session with the process of joining, assessing, diagnosing, and intervening that uses the MED-STAT acronym (Franklin et al., 2016; Giorlando & Schilling, 1997) to extend socioculturally attuned MedFT treatment.

1. ***Joining.*** MedFTs introduce themselves to patients by articulating their role within the healthcare team and elucidating the array of services they can offer. This may encompass addressing behavioral health issues such as anxiety and depression and providing family support. As part of the initial interaction, verifying the patient's date of birth and their current address is essential. This precaution ensures that any unforeseen crises during the telehealth session can be promptly addressed. Following this introduction, it is advisable to provide a concise overview of integrated behavioral health care. Subsequently, MedFTs should obtain informed consent, adhering to the mentioned guidelines. Furthermore, employ open-ended questions tailored to the specific circumstances to facilitate a harmonious connection with the patient(s). These questions should be designed to elicit contextual information, enabling MedFTs to discern relevant concerns or strengths that might influence the necessity for particular screening tools or assessments. Example questions based on the MED-STAT acronym may include:

   - *Open-ended joining question:* Can you describe how you felt before logging in for your healthcare visit today?

- *Difference that makes a difference question:* Please share who or what is helpful to you on your better days.

- *Scaling question:* I see from your health records that the last time you had a healthcare visit, you were working on a goal to reduce your stress by practicing diaphragmatic breathing throughout the day. On a scale of 1 to 10, with 1 being "not very well" and 10 being "really well," how have those exercises been going for you?

2. **Assessing.** MedFTs typically have a series of indicated assessments that they use in healthcare contexts based on the populations that they serve (e.g., the Patient Health Questionnaire-9; Kroenke et al., 2001; or Generalized Anxiety Disorder-7; Spitzer et al., 2006). MedFTs should be equipped to send socioculturally adapted assessments via a patient portal during teletherapy, facilitating prompt sharing of scores with the patient's healthcare team to enhance the adoption of a biopsychosocial approach in all diagnoses. In addition, before making a diagnosis and implementing an intervention, assessing the patient's readiness and compliance level is essential. This assessment aids the MedFT in considering a holistic perspective that encompasses biopsychosocial-spiritual factors and allows for the tailored adaptation of the intervention, resulting in enhanced adherence (Prochaska, 1993). MedFTs can effectively gauge the patient's readiness through the utilization of scaling questions. Examples may include:

- *Miracle question:* If you woke up tomorrow morning and you noticed that the concerns that encouraged you to initiate therapy were no longer present, what would you notice about how you feel physically and emotionally?

- *Exceptions question:* When was the last time your family member realized you were not concerned with the challenges you have shared with me today?

- *Scaling question:* On a scale of 1 to 10, with 1 being the lowest energy you have experienced to navigate through your day and 10 being the best energy you have had to navigate through your day, how would you rate today?

3. **Diagnosing.** The DSM-5-TR (APA, 2022) is the leading diagnostic resource for mental health providers, but it is not the only way to view health. MedFTs are trained to deliver sociocultural assessments with patients while attending to biological, psychological, social, and spiritual health factors. At times, psychosocial issues present simultaneously with biological concerns (e.g., heart palpitations due to anxiety) and vice versa (e.g., depression that is really Parkinson's disease in its early stages). MedFTs must be highly skilled in the mental health diagnoses most commonly seen in their healthcare setting. Fortunately, with integrated behavioral health, MedFTs often find themselves in situations in which collaboration with other team members becomes pivotal, particularly when confronted with ambiguous diagnoses. Their distinctive approach to patient assessment affords them the opportunity to make meaningful contributions that can significantly enhance the diagnostic process and overall patient care. Teletherapy may not necessarily include more than one provider on the screen at one time, but electronic health record systems commonly offer instant options for email correspondence between providers to discuss possible treatment options. On the other hand, the frequency of symptoms holds equal importance alongside their presence when establishing a diagnosis. When patients have recently encountered a troubling complaint, it can preoccupy their thoughts, potentially hindering their awareness of symptom-free periods. Certain questions within the MED-STAT acronym can illuminate the precise nature of the patient's experiences and the specific circumstances in which they occur. This insight may prove invaluable for MedFTs in the diagnostic process, especially during time constraints. Example questions may include:

- *Exceptions question:* Are there ever times that you feel freed from symptoms associated with your diagnosis?

- *Difference that makes a difference question:* What sets apart the occasions when you experience your usual self/fewer symptoms from the times when you are more focused on your symptoms? What is the difference that makes the difference?

4. ***Intervening.*** There are numerous interventions that a MedFT can rely on in their work context. MedFTs should prioritize evidence-based treatment approaches that can be readily customized to suit various social contexts, such as age, race, ethnicity, and sexual identity, while also being suitable for delivery during concise teletherapy sessions. The MED-STAT acronym is grounded in solution-focused interventions that have been supported in healthcare contexts and easily disseminated through teletherapy (Franklin et al., 2016; Giorlando & Schilling, 1997). MED-STAT doesn't require a specific order or complete delivery during a single visit. Instead, it provides MedFTs with the flexibility to employ a range of interventions. These interventions are aimed at addressing a patient's, couple's, or family's biopsychosocial or spiritually related health issue through a solution-focused approach that is sensitive to sociocultural factors. Example interventions based on the MED-STAT acronym may include:

- *Accolades:* I'm genuinely impressed by your dedication to your baby's well-being, as evidenced by your willingness to make an effort to reduce smoking.

- *Task:* It appears that you're open to pushing your boundaries a bit further. Are you inclined to attempt [walking a single block daily/opting for stairs over the elevator/confining your smoking to outdoor areas/etc.]?

More specific examples of the MED-STAT acronym are used in the vignette that follows.

Vignette

Anna is a 43-year-old woman from Mexico. She has a 12th-grade education, is unemployed, and speaks limited English. Anna lives with her husband and three children (ages 5, 7, and 9) in a rural town. Anna is a stay-at-home mom and homeschools their children while her husband works out of town. Anna entered treatment due to feeling sad and stressed ever since she and her husband started having unresolved marital conflict. She reported recently experiencing headaches and an upset stomach. She shared that she is worried that something may be wrong with her health. Anna reported no interpersonal violence. She stated that they each have been upset about unmet intimacy needs. Anna reported that feeling unlovable and worthless is deeply rooted since her biological mother abandoned her at the age of 4. She shared that she was raised by her maternal grandparents, who live in Mexico and are more like parents to her. She had been unable to see them for years. Her husband's job brought them to the United States shortly after they were married. Anna stated, "I want to feel better and be a better wife for my husband."

Anna initiated care at her local primary care clinic. Her treatment plan included receiving teletherapy because she lives 70 minutes from the health center, and she could not leave her children unattended when coming to the center. Teletherapy also helped ensure she could receive treatment from one of the clinic's bilingual therapists in collaboration with her primary care provider, who was extending telehealth appointments to her as needed. The MedFT recommended that Anna invite her husband to the sessions to gain a greater systemic perspective for the therapist and additional treatment options for the patient(s).

At the start of each session, the therapist verified the patient's date of birth and address where the teletherapy session took place to match with the electronic health record. The address was also necessary in case emergency care was needed during the visit. The therapist used the camera to show the couple her office to verify that she was alone in a confidential space and then invited the couple to also share a visual of their space to verify there was no one in the space who had not consented to therapy.

The MedFT then engaged the couple by joining, assessing, and intervening through the MED-STAT acronym. Together, the couple and MedFT constructed a goal of identifying experiences that strengthened ways that they felt more connected as partners. The therapist asked the couple, "If you were to go to sleep this evening and something happened through the night that resolved the concerns you have been sharing with me, what might be the first thought that comes to your mind that lets you know that something is different? What would you notice about how you feel physically, emotionally, and spiritually? How could your husband tell that something must have happened through the night that resolved these concerns?" *(miracle question)*. The couple was also prompted to think of times when they felt most connected. "What was different in your physical, relational, and mental health during these times of connection?" *(exceptions)*. They then described in detail what was happening on those days *(difference that make a difference)*. The MedFT then *scaled* their motivation to "become more connected through positive and healthy communication, with 1 being 'low motivation to strengthen their relationship' and 10 being 'highly motivated to strengthen their relationship.'"

The provider then requested a *time-out* by saying, "We've talked about a lot today. Let's take a quiet pause for about 30 seconds to think about what stands out to the two of you and what you would like to work on from now until we meet again." If more than 30 seconds were available for a time-out, this time could also be used for the MedFT to briefly consult with others on the healthcare team.

Following the time-out, the MedFT extended *accolades*, such as, "It took a lot of courage to come to this session together with the commitment and motivation to strengthen your health and relationship." The MedFT encouraged the creation of a *task* to end the session. The MedFT and patients decided that the couple would notice times throughout the next week when they felt most connected with their partner *(exceptions)* and how they felt physically and emotionally during these times.

Over the first two weeks, Anna's stomachaches were reportedly even worse. She visited her primary care provider after the first session with the MedFT. No medication was offered for the pain, but her provider encouraged her to continue therapy with the MedFT. The therapist explained that when partners initiate therapy, physical symptoms often worsen before they get better. Typically, physical health and psychosocial symptoms improve as patients notice progress toward their goals. Anna's symptoms of depression and anxiety improved by session three (as evidenced by her PHQ-9 and GAD-7 scores), and her headaches and stomachaches decreased from five times a week to about once a week.

The MedFT stayed in communication with the patient's medical provider after each session to ensure that the patient's report of their physical symptoms did not warrant a telehealth visit with the medical provider. By session five, the couple was using a scaling question in their everyday conversations to gauge how they were feeling about their communication and connectedness.

Anna and her husband reported being extremely satisfied with teletherapy because of the noticeable improvements in their health and relationship. Anna mentioned that teletherapy saved her marriage because they lived over one hour away from the bilingual therapist's healthcare clinic, and her husband works out of town for several weeks each month. Having teletherapy as an option allowed them to participate in treatment, whether her husband was at home with Anna or on the road.

Processing

MedFTs who work via teletherapy may consider the following questions:

- How am I collaborating with other care team members, either virtually or in person? Have I obtained the necessary consent forms for interprovider disclosures?

- Is all my teletherapy documentation provided in the patient's dominant language? How do I ensure the accuracy and comprehensibility of translations?

- In what ways do my teletherapy procedures and policies, including patient referrals and retention practices, align with my commitment to being a socioculturally attuned MedFT?

- How do I assess the satisfaction of my teletherapy patients? Are my satisfaction inquiries culturally sensitive? For example, "How have we demonstrated our care for your physical, emotional, and relational well-being today?"

- Am I utilizing assessments and interventions suitable for my patient population in teletherapy? Are these tools available in the appropriate language and literacy level?

- Do I have knowledge of my health center's procedures and protocols in the event of a crisis during a telehealth visit?

Suggestions for Follow-Up

Integrated care in a teletherapy setting presents greater difficulties, yet it remains achievable. This necessitates establishing ethically sound policies and practices sensitive to sociocultural factors, prioritizing patients and families, and aiming to enhance accessibility and service efficiency for everyone involved (Hodgson et al., 2013). MedFTs working via telehealth should regularly self-assess the following:

- *Follow-up protocols.* Evaluate and adapt follow-up protocols, recognizing the distinctions in teletherapy compared to private practice or in-person healthcare settings.

- *Collaboration.* Address potential challenges in collaboration among healthcare team members in a virtual environment and seek ways to improve cohesion.

- *Timeliness.* Be aware of potential time delays during virtual visits and find strategies to minimize them.

- *Patient–provider interaction.* Understand that healthcare visits, especially in teletherapy, are driven by patient needs and provider availability, necessitating a flexible approach.

- *Communication.* Recognize the limitations of not sharing the same physical space with other providers, and develop strategies for effective communication, such as scheduling joint appointments or utilizing electronic health records.

- *Integration of care.* Emphasize the importance of integrated care in a teletherapy context, ensuring ethical policies and practices that prioritize patients and families while promoting accessibility and efficiency.

- *Advocacy.* Advocate for teletherapy options within healthcare settings to enhance patient-centered care, facilitate provider collaboration, and improve continuity of care for patients, particularly those who may otherwise lack access to adequate healthcare services.

Contraindications

A critical aspect of telehealth with MedFTs is to clarify that teletherapy is not suitable for addressing mental health or physical healthcare emergencies. In situations in which patients are at risk of suicide, homicide, or child or elder maltreatment or are experiencing a health crisis, they should promptly seek assistance from their local emergency services or relevant emergency number to ensure an appropriate and timely response to their concerns.

References

American Association for Marriage and Family Therapy. (2018). *Competencies for family therapists working in healthcare settings*. www.aamft.org/healthcare

American Psychiatric Association. (2022). *Diagnostic and statistical manual of mental disorders* (5th ed., text Rev.). https://doi.org/10.1176/appi.books.9780890425787

Doherty, W., McDaniel, S., & Baird, M. (1996). Five levels of primary care/behavioral healthcare collaboration. *Behavioral Healthcare Tomorrow, 5*(5), 25–27.

Engel, G. L. (1977). The need for a new medical model: A challenge for biomedicine. *Science, 196*, 129–136.

Engel, G. L. (1980). The clinical application of the biopsychosocial model. *The American Journal of Psychiatry, 137*, 535–534.

Franklin, C., Zhang, A., Froerer, A., & Johnson, S. (2016). Solution focused brief therapy: A systematic review and meta-summary of process research. *Journal of Marital and Family Therapy, 43*(1), 16–30. https://doi.org/10.1111/jmft.12193

Giorlando, M. E., & Schilling, R. J. (1997). On becoming a solution-focused physician: The MED-STAT acronym. *Families, Systems, & Health, 15*(4), 361–373. https://doi.org/10.1037/h0090137

Heath, B., Wise, R. P., & Reynolds, K. (2013). *A standard framework for levels of integrated healthcare*. SAMHSA-HRSA Center for Integrated Health Solutions.

Hodgson, J., Lamson, A., Mendenhall, T., & Crane, D. R. (2014). *Medical family therapy: Advanced applications*. Springer.

Hodgson, J., Mendenhall, T., & Lamson, A. (2013). Patient and provider relationships: Consent, confidentiality, and managing mistakes in integrated primary care settings. *Families, Systems, & Health, 31*(1), 28–40. https://doi.org/10.1037/a0031771

Kroenke, K., Spitzer, R. L., & Williams, J. B. (2001). The PHQ-9: Validity of a brief depression severity measure. *Journal of General Internal Medicine, 16*(9), 606–613. https://doi.org/10.1046/j.1525-1497.2001.016009606.x

McDaniel, S. H., Doherty, W. J., & Hepworth, J. (2014). *Medical family therapy and integrated care*. American Psychological Association.

McDowell, T., Knudson-Martin, C., & Bermudez, J. M. (2018). *Socioculturally attuned family therapy: Guidelines for equitable theory and practice*. Routledge/Taylor & Francis Group.

Mendenhall, T., Lamson, A., Hodgson, J., & Baird, M. A. (2018). *Clinical methods in medical family therapy*. Springer.

Prochaska, J. O. (1993). Working in harmony with how people quit smoking naturally. *Rhode Island Medicine, 76*(10), 493–495.

Spitzer, R. L., Kroenke, K., Williams, J. B., & Löwe, B. (2006). A brief measure for assessing generalized anxiety disorder: The GAD-7. *Archives of Internal Medicine, 166*(10), 1092–1097. https://doi.org/10.1001/archinte.166.10.1092

Wright, L. M., Watson, W. L., & Bell, J. M. (1996). *Beliefs: The heart of healing in family health and illness*. Basic Books.

Part 7
Training and Supervision

CHAPTER 36

SUPPORTING THERAPISTS THROUGH DELIBERATE PRACTICE IN SYSTEMIC TELETHERAPY

Debra L. Miller, Gianna M. Casaburo, and Melissa M. Yzaguirre

Materials for Supervisors and Supervisees: None.

Objective

This chapter introduces research and best practices that guide clinical supervisors in supporting the development of skills for systemic teletherapy practice. Steps for implementing deliberate practice (DP), a systemic teletherapy skill development strategy, are reviewed.

Rationale for Use

Providing treatment via teletherapy creates unique challenges that must be addressed in clinical supervision. Therapists can benefit from opportunities for skill-building and intervention development specific to teletherapy practice. Generally, systemic therapists who practice interventions or rehearse new skills before implementing them fare better in adopting family-focused, evidence-based practices (Miller, 2021). DP can be used to achieve this goal.

Practicing a skill to develop mastery is a reliable way to improve one's performance on that skill (Ericsson, 2006). When used for honing therapeutic skills, DP allows clinicians to practice rehearsing their response to a particular stimulus or statement likely to be heard in a treatment setting. Two things guide the clinician's response to the stimulus: (1) a specific set of criteria that describes the therapeutic skill and (2) an opportunity for rehearsal or practice coupled with feedback from a supervisor or coach. This specific attention to skill criteria and rehearsal of a response to one statement or stimulus differs from role-plays that often involve more extended dialogues or additional context of the therapeutic interaction. This process is best described by examples later in this chapter.

DP is a helpful tool in therapist skill development that can lead to improved client outcomes (Chow et al., 2015). Built on the premise that excellent performance is achieved through practicing a skill in reliable ways, DP is an evidence-based method of improving performance that can be applied to many activities, including therapeutic practice. Subsequently, the American Psychological Association has produced a series of DP books and videos that target different models of therapeutic practice, including systemic family therapy (Blow et al., 2022), motivational interviewing (Manuel et al., 2022), and emotionally focused therapy

DOI: 10.4324/9781003289920-43

(Goldman et al., 2021). While each target skill is akin to different models of practice, the premise of improving therapist skills through practice and feedback loops remains the goal (Ericsson & Pool, 2016).

Supporting therapists in active, engaging opportunities for coaching helps improve systemic therapy skills (Casaburo et al., 2023) and can be facilitated face-to-face or virtually. Emerging research notes specific benefits to telesupervision practices, such as clinical growth for practitioners and increased access to supervisors for support (Soheilian et al., 2023). Together, these strategies support interactive learning processes, which can lead to greater implementation of new skills (Beidas & Kendall, 2010).

Setup

DP and active coaching strategies can be applied in both in-person and online supervision settings. However, conducting these supervision strategies in a virtual format automatically simulates experiences relevant to the practice of teletherapy. Fortunately, proactive consideration and discussion about these adjustments can promote communication among supervisors and their supervisees.

Before implementing the following supervision strategies, supervisors must remain aware of the diverse identities that may be present in virtual supervision and create inclusive environments. In many instances, considering the nuances related to language, worldview, and context can promote safety and understanding in the supervisory and treatment process (Bernal & Sáez-Santiago, 2006; Gutierrez, 2018; Maier et al., 2022; Reese & Vera, 2007). For example, supervisors can open conversation and solicit feedback about cultural norms to create awareness and set the stage for respectful interactions. Nuances in communication (e.g., facial expressions, hand movements, or other body language) may need to be asked about directly because the context of seeing a supervisee in their environment is limited in the virtual supervision space. Additionally, supervisors can take proactive measures to promote an inclusive environment. For instance, supervisors may enable the closed caption feature or the ability to "react" (e.g., click and display a heart, smiley face, or other emoji to communicate a response to something someone else has said) on virtual platforms.

Instructions

Whether applied to teletherapy specifically or more generally to specific therapeutic skills, DP starts by taking a specific skill or concept and breaking it down into a few (usually no more than three) descriptive steps or criteria that can be practiced to support that skill's development. Skill criteria are generally short, uncomplicated, and descriptive statements that guide supervisees into actionable steps that support mastery of the skill. Then, a series of stimuli or prompts that mimic a real client scenario are created to necessitate that skill being used. Prompts are brief and created in varying levels of difficulty (i.e., beginner, intermediate, advanced) so that supervisees have an opportunity to practice at the level most suited for them. Next, in pairs (or small groups) with a supervisor or mentor facilitating, one person reads the prompt in the tone and manner instructed, and the other responds to the prompt, rehearsing the skill criteria. Once completed, the supervisor or mentor debriefs with the supervisee and the person providing the prompt. This process is repeated so that the supervisee can continue to improve their delivery of the skill criteria to the client stimulus or prompts each time.

DP is facilitated in such a way that supervisees can rehearse the skill criteria and debrief with a supervisor or trusted mentor following the practice. This becomes a feedback loop or cycle in which the practice is observed, expert feedback is given from a supervisor or mentor, small learning goals or tweaks pertinent to the mastery of the skill criteria are discussed, behavioral rehearsal happens again, and performance is again assessed (Goldman et al., 2021). This continuous loop provides an ongoing opportunity for supervisees to gain mastery through small learning goals and practice. In these ways, DP uniquely creates a learning space in which skill criteria and behavioral rehearsal challenges supervisees to practice the skill and continue to build mastery (Rousmaniere, 2019). DP books and online resources guide specific therapeutic skills such as systemic family therapy, emotionally focused therapy, and motivational interviewing. Prompts such as those designed in these books can be facilitated through supervisor/supervisee virtual interactions to replicate the context in which teletherapy interventions would be delivered. Supervisors can also be creative in coming up with prompts that fit the needs of their supervisees, given the spirit of a DP approach to therapist development.

DP for teletherapy can be conducted utilizing the following steps (Rousmaniere, 2016). A set of skill criteria and client prompts are included for reference.

1. ***Review a series of skill criteria pertinent to the therapeutic skill being supported.*** For example, if the therapeutic skill is "assessing a client's virtual safety," the identified skill criteria might be:

   - Criteria 1: "Pause and observe your client's virtual environment at the start of the session."

   - Criteria 2: "Provide a reflection or observation that captures the client's affect, behavior, or words."

   - Criteria 3: "Use an open-ended question to inquire about the client's environment."

2. ***Expose the therapist to a stimulus.*** DP works by exposing therapists to a scenario common in therapeutic practice – one likely to evoke a response of what could happen in a real-life situation (Ericsson, 2006; McGaghie et al., 2014). DP prompts could include specific teletherapy topics, such as assessing a client's environment. In this example, a stimulus might be as follows:

   - "A client, sounding distracted, quietly says, 'I almost didn't jump on our call today. I wasn't sure if I should keep the appointment.'"

3. ***Practice the skill.*** DP is an experiential process that allows practice of common systemic therapy skills (Blow et al., 2022). Once a supervisee has had someone give the stimulus or prompt acting as the client, they should respond using the skill criteria. An example response might look like this:

   - [silence/pause] (criteria 1) "As you talk about coming to session today, I notice your voice is low and you seem distracted." (criteria 2) "What are some things that are happening in your home environment right now?" (criteria 3)

4. ***Provide corrective feedback.*** Once the supervisee responds, the supervisor or mentor provides expert feedback. Expert feedback relates specifically to the skill criteria. An example of corrective feedback might look like this:

   - "Nice work pausing and looking at your client's environment before offering a reflection. This allows some space to take in what you are seeing on screen and addresses criteria 1. For criteria 2, you noticed the client's low voice tone and that your client seemed distracted. However, when you delivered that observation, you sounded uncertain. Remember, reflections or observations are important to help clients understand how you see them and their situation. You also asked an open-ended question that was connected to the distraction that you observed, which addresses criteria 3. I'd like you to try this again, this time with a focus on criteria 2 and giving a clear observation of how you see the client's environment."

5. ***Assess the response.*** Supervisors should help supervisees assess their reaction to corrective feedback. This provides an important and necessary pause and reflection to understand the supervisee's experience and what they might need for their next iteration of rehearsal. This also assures supervisors can support a supervisee to practice the skill in a way that is challenging to them but not too overwhelming. Assessing the response might look like this:

   - "What was it like for you to try that skill again with more certainty about your observation of the client's environment?"

Feedback from the supervisee would guide the next steps and assure that the practice was challenging but not too hard. There are a number of possible reactions from the supervisee that would require the supervisor to respond in different ways. If the supervisee reflected feeling confident, and that was the supervisor's observation, they might support and reinforce the skill acquisition as follows:

- "I could hear your confidence when you shared with the client your observation of their environment. Great work!"

If the supervisee indicated they were still feeling uncertain, or there were other indicators that the skill was too hard, the supervisor would take a step back to further assess how to develop that skill. This might mean engaging the supervisee in repetition of the skill criteria or breaking down the skill into smaller, more manageable learning goals.

6. ***Repeat steps as needed.*** Finally, the supervisor should ask the supervisee to repeat steps 2 and 3, (i.e., exposing the supervisee to a practice stimulus or prompt and engaging them in practicing the skill). This is important because the repetition and practice of the skill paired with corrective feedback enhances skill mastery. This cycle of DP emphasizes career-long repetition of skill development (Goldman et al., 2021). In each new repetition, the supervisor should continue to observe, assess performance, and provide corrective feedback.

Let's say from the previous example that the supervisor observed hesitancy of the supervisee to offer an observation of the client's environment, or the supervisee reflected that they still felt a bit uncertain about offering that environmental observation to the client, as indicated in skill criteria 2. The supervisor could offer additional corrective feedback on the skill criteria, engage the supervisee in how they could correct their response, and then prompt the supervisee to try another rehearsal. For example, the supervisor might say the following:

- "You described the client's environment in a way that was easy to understand and met skill criteria 2. However, I hear you say it still feels a little hard to deliver. Slowing down to offer this reflection to a client is a new skill specific to teletherapy practice, and repetition can help us when we are learning new skills. Let's repeat this same prompt again to see if your confidence improves this next time."

Suggestions for Follow-Up

When using this activity in group supervision, rotate positions held by each member of the group in the practice exercise (e.g., role of client, role of therapist) to allow each person the opportunity to practice skills and to provide feedback.

If supervision occurs in person, utilizing a video platform to practice teletherapy-specific skills during DP can provide an opportunity to model and reinforce the kinds of teletherapy skills you want supervisees to promote. For example, in Chapter 5, Springer, Taylor, and Bischoff encourage the frequent use of clients' names as a way to increase attention in virtual sessions and clearly communicate to one person when working with a family system. Offering the opportunity for supervisees to practice this skill via a teletherapy platform in supervision can help to reinforce the importance of this skill and support supervisees in using it in an organic setting.

DP exercises are available through Sentio University (sentio.edu). These materials are open source and offer video prompts for DP practice specific to teletherapy. You can also create your own DP exercises. This can happen quite naturally within a supervision group and with a little planning. First, you would need to identify a specific therapeutic skill – one that can be broken down into no more than three specific skill criteria. You can model this from the example prompt provided. Next, think of a few client statements that would elicit the need for that skill. You can use examples that you have come across in your own practice or listen to your supervisee's feedback on what has come up for them. Last, use the skill criteria and prompt in the DP cycle identified earlier in this chapter.

Contraindications

DP is a well-established method of therapist skill training (Rousmaniere, 2016). When utilizing DP for systemic teletherapy supervision, supervisors should be mindful of technological limitations that can disrupt or hinder the effectiveness of the exercise (e.g., poor internet connections) or virtual distractions that could inadvertently limit the ability to follow the steps of DP to their fullest. For example, all parties practicing the DP cycle should have their cameras on and assure good sound quality while practicing skills so that skill mastery can be assessed and corrective feedback given in thoughtful and considerate ways.

DP is contraindicated if not done in a way that supports a supervisee's proximal zone of development (Zaretskii, 2009). A desirable space for learning is one that is just outside the supervisee's current capacity (Wass & Golding, 2014). Supervisees will not benefit from skills that are too easy, and skills that are too hard could potentially be harmful to the supervisees' experience and learning (Blow et al., 2022). It is important to note that if the supervisee were to appear or report feeling overwhelmed by the skill rehearsal or appear to not be grasping the skill, the supervisor should shift to focusing on smaller, more obtainable learning goals. Practice should be challenging but not overwhelming (Blow et al., 2022). Supervisor observation and supervisees' feedback during practice and debriefing are important indicators to assessing the fit of the exercise. DP diary forms are available through the American Psychological Association (apa.org) and can also be used to facilitate feedback on practice exercises.

Further, if the DP prompt involves culturally sensitive scenarios, there's a risk of unintentionally reinforcing stereotypes or offending participants from specific cultural backgrounds. Sensitivity to cultural differences is crucial. Any new DP stimulus should be designed with this in mind.

References

Beidas, R. S., & Kendall, P. C. (2010). Training therapists in evidence-based practice: A critical review of studies from a systems-contextual perspective. *Clinical Psychology: Science and Practice, 17*(1), 1–30. https://doi.org/10.1111/j.1468-2850.2009.01187.x

Bernal, G., & Sáez-Santiago, E. (2006). Culturally centered psychosocial interventions. *Journal of Community Psychology, 34*(2), 121–132. https://doi.org/10.1002/jcop.20096

Blow, A., Seedall, R., Miller, D. L., Vaz, A., & Rousmaniere, T. G. (2022). *Deliberate practice in systemic family therapy.* American Psychological Association.

Casaburo, G. M., Asiimwe, R., Yzaguirre, M. M., Fang, M., & Holtrop, K. (2023). Identifying beneficial training elements: Clinician perceptions of learning the evidence-based GenerationPMTO intervention. *Journal of Child and Family Studies, 32*(8) 2331–2346. https://doi.org/10.1007/s10826-023-02600-5

Chow, D. L., Miller, S. D., Seidel, J. A., Kane, R. T., Thornton, J. A., & Andrews, W. P. (2015). The role of deliberate practice in the development of highly effective psychotherapists. *Psychotherapy, 52*(3), 337–345. https://doi.org/10.1037/pst0000015

Ericsson, A., & Pool, R. (2016). *Peak: Secrets from the new science of expertise.* Random House.

Ericsson, K. A. (2006). The influence of experience and deliberate practice on the development of superior expert performance. In K. A. Ericsson, N. Charness, P. J. Feltovich, & R. R. Hoffman (Eds.), *The Cambridge handbook of expertise and expert performance* (pp. 683–703). Cambridge University Press.

Goldman, R. N., Vaz, A., & Rousmaniere, T. (2021). *Deliberate practice in emotion-focused therapy.* American Psychological Association.

Gutierrez, D. (2018). The role of intersectionality in marriage and family therapy multicultural supervision. *The American Journal of Family Therapy, 46*(1), 14–26. https://doi.org/10.1080/01926187.2018.1437573

Maier, C. A., Prouty, A. M., & Söylemez, Y. (2022). Zooming into feminist family therapy telesupervision: Experiences of supervisors during the COVID-19 pandemic. *Journal of Feminist Family Therapy, 35*(1), 1–24. https://doi.org/10.1080/08952833.2022.2141986

Manuel, J. K., Ernst, D. B., Vaz, A., & Rousmaniere, T. (2022). *Deliberate practice in motivational interviewing.* American Psychological Association.

McGaghie, W. C., Issenberg, S. B., Barsuk, J. H., & Wayne, D. B. (2014). A critical review of simulation-based mastery learning with translational outcomes. *Medical Education, 48*(4), 375–385. https://doi.org/10.1111/medu.12391

Miller, D. L. (2021). *Core therapist skills supporting implementation of evidence-based practices with serious emotionally disturbed children in community mental health settings: A modified mixed methods Delphi study* (Publication No. 28866649) [Doctoral dissertation, Michigan State University]. Michigan State University ProQuest Dissertations Publishing.

Reese, L. R. E., & Vera, E. M. (2007). Culturally relevant prevention: The scientific and practical considerations of community-based programs. *The Counseling Psychologist, 35*(6), 763–778. https://doi.org/10.1177/0011000007304588

Rousmaniere, T. (2016). *Deliberate practice for psychotherapists: A guide to improving clinical effectiveness.* Taylor & Francis.

Rousmaniere, T. (2019). *Mastering the inner skills of psychotherapy: A deliberate practice manual.* Gold Lantern Books.

Soheilian, S. S., O'Shaughnessy, T., Lehmann, J. S., & Rivero, M. (2023). Examining the impact of COVID-19 on supervisees' experiences of clinical supervision. *Training and Education in Professional Psychology, 17*(2), 167–175. https://doi.org/10.1037/tep0000418

Wass, R., & Golding, C. (2014). Sharpening a tool for teaching: The zone of proximal development. *Teaching in Higher Education, 19*(6), 671–684. https://doi.org/10.1080/13562517.2014.901958

Zaretskii, V. K. (2009). The zone of proximal development: What Vygotsky did not have time to write. *Journal of Russian & East European Psychology, 47*(6), 70–93. https://doi.org/10.753/RP01061-0405470604

CHAPTER 37

ROUND-ROBIN CASE CONCEPTUALIZATION FOR THEORETICALLY GROUNDED VIRTUAL SUPERVISION

Kelly Duggan Shearer

Materials for Supervisors and Supervisees: HIPAA-consistent videoconferencing platform that allows participants to toggle between gallery view of all participants and "pinned" speaker views. Platforms that allow participants to be temporarily removed from the screen when their video feed is off are also useful (e.g., "hide non-video participants" on Zoom).

Objective

Round-robin case conceptualization assists therapists in thinking systemically about cases and creating theoretically grounded treatment plans by privileging multiple perspectives in group supervision. The following provides instructions for implementing this approach in virtual supervision settings.

Rationale for Use

Round-robin case conceptualization is an adaptation of Andersen's (1987) reflecting teams. Traditionally, reflecting teams involve a group of therapists and/or supervisees watching a live therapy session and stopping it midway through the session to discuss their thoughts in front of the therapist and clients (Andersen, 1987).

Although intended for use in the treatment relationship, reflecting teams have also been used in supervision when clients are absent (Reichelt & Skjerve, 2013). In round-robin case conceptualization, case report and/or video are used rather than watching a live therapy session so that clinicians can feel free to make mistakes without negatively impacting clients. Videoconferencing platforms allow those who are "on camera" to navigate the fast-paced, independent thinking of the treatment room without the pressure of the client being present. Slower, more thoughtful evaluation of those "off camera" mimics the one-way-mirror experience of traditional reflecting teams without the challenge of securing physical space.

Round-robin case conceptualization builds a bridge between positivist and postmodern values (Lowe et al., 2008) by integrating the guidance of a seasoned supervisor with the wisdom of supervisees. Supervisors act as guides, keeping track of time and offering feedback to enhance supervisees' conceptualization of client systems. The supervisee (i.e., therapist) who is working with the client system shares relevant case information and/or shows a video of their work. Afterward, other supervisees in the group discuss priorities

DOI: 10.4324/9781003289920-44

for treatment, theoretical case conceptualization, and treatment planning ideas, while the therapist observes their conversation. A signature element of round-robin case conceptualization that differs from traditional reflecting teams is the intentional use of theoretical models to guide conceptualization. Having supervisees share theoretically grounded ideas for treatment as they unfold allows the treating therapist to see the thought process behind treatment recommendations, promoting a more nuanced and critical evaluation of theoretical constructs. Supervisees are exposed to their peers' flow of ideas, normalizing their own struggle to work with client systems. This increases supervisees' willingness to engage in the reflective and imperfect practice of case conceptualization with their own clients (Shurts et al., 2006).

Setup

The following steps should be done a week prior to round-robin case conceptualization. This allows supervisees to prepare a brief presentation and to review chosen theories as per their defined roles, ensuring a robust discussion.

1. ***Introduce the concept of round-robin case conceptualization.*** Framing the activity as a collaborative effort to support the treating therapist and the client system is important. For example, the supervisor might say, "Next week, we will think together about what is happening for [supervisee]'s client from two different theoretical perspectives. The intent is that [supervisee] has multiple ways to conceptualize this case, and the group develops a deeper understanding of these theories. The purpose of the activity is to think critically together, so there is no right or wrong way to do this. To prepare, we will establish our discussion 'ground rules.'"

2. ***Have the group collaboratively decide upon discussion "ground rules."*** Trust and cohesion between supervision group members should be considered before engaging in this activity. Rules should explicitly address power differences and actions to take when disagreements occur.

   The following prompts may be used to assist supervisees in determining what ground rules are critical in their own work:

   - What are some concerns that you have about participating in this exercise?

   - How do you best receive feedback?

   - What actions might the group need to take in order for you to feel like your ideas are important?

   - What are you willing to do to make other people feel like their ideas are important?

   There are some important ground rules that should be brought up by the supervisor if supervisees do not come up with them on their own. Examples of these might include:

   - Information about the clients and supervisees' personal responses to the activity should be kept confidential.

   - Formulate responses tentatively rather than as objective truths to avoid judging the family and treating clinician (Reichelt & Skjerve, 2013).

   - Responses should promote understanding rather than defending one's position.

   - Expression of nondominant narratives should be supported. Supervisees who hold privileged identities should be encouraged to monitor the ways they might unintentionally dominate the conversation.

- When differences of perspective occur, use experience-honoring language. For example, "Thank you for that perspective. My experience of this is different . . ."

- Feedback should be behaviorally focused. For example, "I appreciated that you valued the family's intention when you said . . ."

3. ***Identify one supervisee to prepare a brief case write-up to share with the supervision group.*** A video of the therapist in session with the client(s) may be requested, though it is not necessary.

   Instruct the supervisee to report the following:

   - How long they have been seeing the client(s) in therapy

   - The social location of each member of the client system

   - The presenting problem(s)

   - Any relevant diagnoses

   - Outcomes of any relevant assessments

   - Ethical or safety concerns

   - Current goals of therapy

4. ***Divide group members into three teams.*** These teams should include a "treatment team," "reflection team A," and "reflection team B." Each reflection team will be assigned a different task to orient their discussion of the case. Supervisees may select their own team based on their interest. Alternatively, supervisors may assign supervisees to teams based on supervisees' strengths or areas in need of growth. To create a noncompetitive atmosphere, explicitly frame each team as a collaborative unit (Fine, 2003).

   Each team has the following tasks:

   - ***Treatment team:*** Articulate a systemic conceptualization of the presenting problem that includes interpersonal, developmental, and sociocultural factors. Also provide a critique of reflections provided by reflection teams A and B.

   - ***Reflection team A:*** Conceptualize the presenting problem identified by the treatment team. Create a treatment plan using a theoretical perspective that differs from that of reflection team B.

   - ***Reflection team B:*** Conceptualize the presenting problem identified by the treatment team. Create a treatment plan using a theoretical perspective that differs from that of reflection team A.

   - ***Treating therapist:*** Share relevant case information and/or show a video of their clinical work. The treating therapist is not assigned to a team.

5. ***Identify two theories from which the case will be conceptualized.*** The supervisor may select the theories or may engage supervisees in a collaborative discussion to determine which theory each reflection team will use to conceptualize the case. Some considerations for theory choice include:

   - Relevance of particular theories to the case

   - Treating therapist's current theoretical grounding or conceptualization of the case

   - Supervisees' need to develop competence in working with particular theories

6. ***Send a written list of discussion prompts to each supervisee.*** The discussion prompts may be sent via email or in the chat box to reference as they discuss the case. Example prompts are provided in the instructions that follow.

Instructions

The following instructions for round-robin case conceptualization are for a three-hour supervision group. Suggested times for each stage of the activity are provided based on this overall time frame. Length of time can be modified as needed.

1. ***Review previously determined ground rules.*** Check in with supervisees to see if any adjustments should be made, and send the updated ground rules in the chat box. All participants should have their videos on. Approximately 5 minutes should be allotted for this task.

2. ***Explain instructions related to video and microphone use.*** Use speaker view with videos "pinned" for those who are actively speaking. This allows the team that is talking to feel as if they are in a room together. As each team is called upon to discuss the case, they restart or "pin" their video, while nonparticipants hide or "unpin" themselves. All participants should have their videos on while instructions are explained. Approximately 5 minutes should be allotted for this task.

3. ***Ask if supervisees need clarification on discussion prompts and send the first set of prompts in the group chat.*** New prompts should be sent prior to the step in which it is utilized. All participants should have their videos on. Approximately 5 minutes should be allotted for this task.

4. ***Ask the treating therapist to present their case summary and/or video.*** Request that they focus on how they feel "stuck" with their client(s) (Andersen, 1987). All participants should have their videos on. Approximately 10 to 15 minutes should be allotted for this task.

5. ***Ask the treatment team to discuss their initial impressions of the presenting problem from a systemic perspective.*** The treatment team should avoid suggestions for intervention. The treating therapist listens but does not join in the conversation. The treatment team should discuss their responses to the following discussion prompts:

   - What interpersonal or family interactions are most urgent to address?

   - How does development or culture influence the expression of the presenting problem?

   - What interpersonal, familial, or macrosystemic factors influence the expression of the presenting problem?

   - What is the client system doing that promotes stability? What strengths, resources, and coping strategies does the client system exhibit?

   - State two or three possible areas to be addressed in treatment.

   The treatment team and treating therapist should keep their videos on while everyone else turns theirs off. Approximately 20 to 25 minutes should be allotted for this task.

6. ***Ask the treating therapist to decide which of the treatment team's suggestions reflecting teams A and B should focus on.*** All members of the supervision group, including the supervisor, should have videos on. Approximately 5 minutes should be allotted to this task.

7. ***Ask reflection team A to discuss the presenting problem.*** The team should use the chosen theory (i.e., theory A) to frame their conversation. The reflection team should discuss their responses to the following discussion prompts:

   - What core concepts of theory A describe why people have problems? Do any of these concepts explain what is happening in the client system?

   - Using these theoretical concepts, what could help alleviate the problem for the client system? Think specifically about recursive, interpersonal processes that, if altered, might contribute to resolution of the presenting concern.

   - Write a treatment goal that focuses on a change in the client system that might alleviate the presenting issue. This goal should be grounded in theory A.

   - Suggest one or two interventions that the therapist could implement to help the client system make this change. Interventions should be grounded in theory A.

   Reflection team A should have their videos on while everyone else has theirs off. Approximately 25 minutes should be allotted to this task.

8. ***Ask reflection team B to discuss the presenting problem.*** The team should use the chosen theory (i.e., theory B) to frame their conversation. The reflection team should discuss their responses to the following discussion prompts:

   - What core concepts of theory B describe why people have problems? Do any of these concepts explain what is happening in the client system?

   - Using these theoretical concepts, what could help alleviate the problem for the client system? Think specifically about recursive, interpersonal processes that, if altered, might contribute to resolution of the presenting concern.

   - Write a treatment goal that focuses on a change in the client system that might alleviate the presenting issue. This goal should be grounded in theory B.

   - Suggest one or two interventions that the therapist could implement to help the client system make this change. Interventions should be grounded in theory B.

   Reflection team B should have their videos on while everyone else has theirs off. Approximately 25 minutes should be allotted to this task.

9. ***Ask the treatment team and treating therapist to discuss the strengths and limitations of each reflection team's case conceptualizations.*** The treatment team and treating therapist should discuss their responses to the following questions:

   - How do theories A and B help us to see the presenting problem differently?

   - What are common elements that theories A and B use to conceptualize the problem?

   - Does theory A or B help to conceptualize the case better?

   - How does theory A or B seem more fitting for this client system?

   - What concerns might you have about using either theory A or B with this client system?

   - What are additional suggestions you might have for treatment?

   - Do you have any questions you want to ask reflection team A or B? If so, each team should respond with their answer(s).

Supervisors should provide strong support as ideas are critiqued to preserve group cohesion.

Every member of the supervision group should have their videos turned on. Approximately 25 minutes should be allotted to this task.

10. ***Ask all participants to reflect on their experience.*** Supervisees should discuss their responses to the following questions:

- What seems clearer to you about the case after doing this exercise?

- What is something that you learned that could be applied to other cases? How might you implement suggestions from today's activity?

- What theoretical concepts presented today would you like to learn more about?

- What did you learn about yourself as a therapist?

It is also essential to discuss relational dynamics following round-robin case conceptualization. Fine (2003) suggests explicitly inviting supervisees who hold marginalized identities to share previously unspoken comments so that an equitable supervision environment is maintained. Encourage supervisees to reflect on the following questions either verbally or in the virtual supervision platform's chat feature.

- In what ways did you feel most like a part of the team?

- At what times did you feel least like a part of the team?

- What feelings or thoughts arose when your suggestion was accepted?

- What feelings or thoughts arose when your response was not acknowledged?

- Think about how you interacted with the other group members during this activity. What does this suggest about how you participate in the supervision system? What might your interactions teach you about your role in the therapy system?

Every member of the supervision group should have their videos turned on. Approximately 15 minutes should be allotted to this task.

Initially, participating in reflection teams may feel intimidating to supervisees, especially those who identify with marginalized groups (Fine, 2003). Supervisors should attune to the developmental needs of supervisees and provide higher levels of support for more novice clinicians. Encourage a positive focus on what the client and treating clinician are doing well (Costa, 1994). This helps to develop compassionate perspectives that reduce judgment.

Throughout this process, supervisors may remain visible or hide their video. Consider the developmental needs of supervisees in making this decision. Also consider how supervisees will feel supported. Supervisors may have a conversation with supervisees about the decision to remain visible or to hide their video and consider feedback from supervisees in making this choice. Some supervisees may be more anxious seeing their supervisor on screen. Others may feel less anxious and more supported if their supervisor is visible. Regardless, supervisors should keep track of time and help the group transition from one task to the next. To help track timing and video instructions for this activity, see Table 37.1. Supervisors should also provide guidance verbally or via chat when the conversation is not productive or is inaccurate.

Table 37.1 Timing and video instructions for round-robin case conceptualization.

Step	Time Allotted for the Step	Video Pinned/On	Video Hidden/Off
Setup (1 week prior)	TBD by Supervisor	Supervisor Supervisees	None
1	5 minutes	Supervisor Supervisees	None
2	5 minutes	Supervisor Supervisees	None
3	5 minutes	Supervisor Supervisees	None
4	10–15 minutes	Supervisor Treating Therapist Treatment Team Reflection Team A Reflection Team B	None
5	20–25 minutes	Supervisor (optional) Treatment Team Treating Therapist	Reflection Team A Reflection Team B
6	5 minutes	Supervisor (optional) Treating Therapist	Treatment Team Reflection Team A Reflection Team B
7	25 minutes	Supervisor (optional) Reflection Team A	Treating Therapist Treatment Team Reflection Team B
8	25 minutes	Supervisor (optional) Reflection Team B	Treating Therapist Treatment Team Reflection Team A
9	25 minutes	Supervisor Treating Therapist Treatment Team Reflection Team A Reflection Team B	None
10	15 minutes	Supervisor Treating Therapist Treatment Team Reflection Team A Reflection Team B	None
Processing	15 minutes	Supervisor Supervisees	None

Vignette

The week before this activity, Doreen (the supervisor), facilitated a discussion between the supervisees to establish ground rules to promote participation. At that time, the group also decided to use narrative and structural theories to conceptualize the case.

Sam, a 38-year-old student clinician who identified as a Black, cisgender male, had been working in his university's clinic for 8 months. He stated that he felt particularly frustrated and discouraged because his work with a client, Guillermo, had stalled. Guillermo, a 17-year-old, Latino, cisgender male, reported heightened conflict with his family related to his desire to attend college in another state rather than living at home and working to contribute to the family's financial needs. Guillermo insisted that the long-term benefit of a college education was worth the risk, but his parents, who immigrated from Guatemala in their 20s, said that they needed the additional income immediately. Sam felt stuck because although he supported his client, he aligned more with Guillermo's parents.

Doreen reminded the group of the previously agreed-upon ground rules for round-robin case conceptualization and typed them in the chat box. She invited Sam to share his case summary and video with the supervision group. Doreen asked Sam and two other supervisees (i.e., the treatment team) to identify the primary clinical focus for the reflection teams, which they identified as helping Guillermo and his family speak about Guillermo's desire to attend college in another state without heated conflict or shutdown. During this portion, all other supervisees hid their video, leaving Doreen, Sam, and the treatment team on screen.

Then, reflection team A discussed the case using narrative theory. During this time, reflection team A turned on their videos as everyone else stopped and hid their videos. The three members of reflection team A deconstructed how systemic oppression and the family's immigration history created a dominant story that was limiting. Reflection team A noted that the parents' experiences with discrimination made them fearful that their son would also experience discrimination. Initially, reflection team A described this as a cognitive distortion. Doreen turned on her video and guided them toward a description more consistent with narrative theory by asking, "How is a cognitive distortion similar to a dominant discourse? Are there ways that we can use narrative terms to describe this so that we honor that similarity?" In response, reflection team A identified the "cognitive distortion" as having veracity in light of racism and named it as a social force contributing to the dominant discourse. They named the discourse "dangerous discrimination," externalizing the problem. The team mapped the influence of the problem, stating that the parents attempted to protect Guillermo by forbidding him from moving away. The team also noticed "sparkling moments" throughout Guillermo's high school career when Guillermo's parents were able to support him through loving conversations. Reflection team A suggested that these previously unnoticed successes could be utilized to build a rich narrative of support that transcended geographic distance. Reflection team A concluded and turned off their videos.

The four members of reflection team B turned on their videos and discussed the case from the perspective of structural theory. They acknowledged how the family's collectivistic values promoted a mutual commitment between children and parents. When Guillermo was younger, the boundary between Guillermo and the parental subsystem was protective yet clear. However, as Guillermo grew up, the boundary that once was clear became rigid (i.e., an adaptive relic), prohibiting Guillermo's mature ideas from being expressed. Reflection team B noted the similarities between narrative theory's "sparkling moments" and structural theory's focus on underutilized family strengths. Reflection team B suggested that reframing Guillermo's education as an extension of the parents' values could change the family's worldview and lead to a renegotiation of parent–child boundaries.

Throughout the activity, Doreen offered guiding questions, both verbally and in the chat box, that helped reflection teams A and B explore how social location factors were dealt with in each of the theories.

She asked, "I wonder if there are ways that Guillermo's ethnicity might be impacting each member of the family system? Are there strengths that can be capitalized upon to promote second-order change? How might Guillermo's experience as a first-generation student be influencing the presenting problem? How might Guillermo's parents' experience as immigrants be informing the presenting problem?"

At the conclusion of the discussion, Sam, Doreen, and all other supervisees turned on their videos, offered questions, and explored further "curiosities" about the reflection teams' conceptualizations. Doreen guided Sam to identify how the reflection teams' suggestions informed his conceptualization of the client. Sam stated that he now viewed the family's conflict as a desire to remain emotionally connected – a strength that can be utilized regardless of Guillermo's physical location. Doreen concluded the activity and asked the supervision group to talk about how the activity impacted them personally and professionally, noting places of relational connection and disconnection with other group members and concepts they could apply to their own clinical work.

Suggestions for Follow-Up

Adult learners benefit from repeated discussions focused on application of theoretical material to "real-life" situations (Vella, 2008). Encouraging all supervisees to discuss how their clinical work was informed by the exercise deepens their ability to apply conceptual material.

Contraindications

Supervisors should consider the needs of each supervisee and client system before implementing round-robin case conceptualization. The discussion prompts listed in this chapter may not be fitting for all supervision groups. Supervisors may adjust prompts or other details of this activity as they see fit to meet the needs of each supervision group. Cases requiring crisis management may not be appropriate for this approach if a more direct supervision method is necessary.

References

Andersen, T. (1987). The reflecting team: Dialogue and meta-dialogue in clinical work. *Family Process, 26*(4), 415–428. https://doi.org/10.1111/j.1545-5300.1987.00415.x

Costa, L. (1994). Reducing anxiety in live supervision. *Counselor Education & Supervision, 34*(1), 30–40. https://doi.org/10.1002/j.1556-6978.1994.tb00308.x

Fine, M. (2003). Reflections on the intersection of power and competition in reflecting teams as applied to academic settings. *Journal of Marital and Family Therapy, 29*(3), 339–351. https://doi.org/10.1111/j.1752-0606.2003.tb01211.x

Lowe, R., Hunt, C., & Simmons, P. (2008). Towards multi-positioned live supervision in family therapy: Combining treatment and observation teams with first-and second-order perspectives. *Contemporary Family Therapy, 30*(1), 3–14. https://doi.org/10.1007/s10591-007-9052-0

Reichelt, S., & Skjerve, J. (2013). The reflecting team model used for clinical group supervision without clients present. *Journal of Marital and Family Therapy, 39*(2), 244–255. https://doi.org/10.1111/j.1752-0606.2012.00298.x

Shurts, W. M., Cashwell, C. S., Spurgeon, S. L., Degges-White, S., Barrio, C. A., & Kardatzke, K. N. (2006). Preparing counselors-in-training to work with couples: Using role-plays and reflecting teams. *The Family Journal, 14*(2), 151–157. https://doi.org/10.1177/1066480705285731

Vella, J. (2008). *On teaching and learning: Putting the principles and practices of dialogue education into action.* Jossey-Bass.

CHAPTER 38

VIRTUAL REFLECTING TEAMS

A MILAN APPROACH TO TELETHERAPY INTERVENTION

Rebecca A. Cobb, Stephanie Brownell, Samantha J. Camera, and Camille Chapin

Materials for Therapists: Recording device.

Materials for Clients: None.

Objective

Reflecting teams are a common therapeutic approach utilized within the context of group supervision. After witnessing a therapy session, a team of therapists discusses their observations either in front of the clients or with the lead therapist, who delivers a message from the team back to the clients. Developed by the Milan systemic school (Selvini et al., 1979) and further developed to be more collaborative by Andersen (1987), reflecting teams help clients to gain insight (Coulehan et al., 1998; de Oliveira, 2003), break repetitive patterns, and explore new ones (Jenkins, 1996). This chapter will present an approach to using asynchronous reflecting teams in teletherapy.

Rationale for Use

Traditionally, reflecting teams are conducted in real-time settings. After discussion about the method and receipt of client consent, therapists work with clients as they would in a normal therapy session. Meanwhile, a therapeutic treatment team watches from behind a one-way mirror. The therapist leaves the room mid-session and engages in a reflective discussion with the team while the clients take a break. The therapist then decides which part of the conversation would be most useful for the clients to hear (Selvini et al., 1979) and reenters the therapy room with the team (Andersen, 1987). The team then discusses in front of the clients the previously agreed-upon points of conversation. During this time, clients listen but do not engage in the conversation. The team leaves the room, and the therapist processes with the clients what they heard and discusses key takeaways. The process can then repeat in subsequent sessions.

Virtual reflecting teams may be conducted either synchronously or asynchronously. Synchronous reflecting teams observe the therapy session virtually as it is taking place, much like traditional in-person

DOI: 10.4324/9781003289920-45

reflecting teams, and may reflect on client stories and interactions while clients observe virtually in real time (see Chapter 39 on plurilinguistic virtual reflecting teams with Latino/a families). Asynchronous teams discuss the case after the session has taken place, and the therapist brings messages from the team to clients in subsequent sessions. For asynchronous teams, the therapist may either provide the team with audio or video recordings of session(s), or they may simply provide a verbal description of the clients and their session(s) to the team. When audio or video is used, the therapist may either show the entire session, or they may choose parts of the session to show the team that they think are particularly relevant or challenging.

Tenets of the Milan Approach

Regardless of the approach, reflecting teams are conducted utilizing core tenets of the Milan approach, including neutrality, hypothesizing, and circularity (Selvini et al., 1979).

- *Neutrality.* Neutrality refers to the nonpathologizing and impartial stance of the therapist regarding all elements of the system (Selvini et al., 1979). It is neutrality that guides the therapist as a balanced witness (Simon, 1992) to the dynamic causal chain of influence at play in systemic patterns of interaction. The therapist must conduct themselves in such a way that preference or judgment isn't communicated to any individual that could suggest favoring one client over another. The commitment to impartiality is nonpathologizing and consistent with the theoretical orientation of the Milan group's assumption of the social construction of reality.

- *Hypothesizing.* The team formulates an a priori hypothesis of what is going on within the entire relational system based solely on the initial presenting information. They then participate in "a continual interactive process of speculation and making assumptions about the family situation" (Adams, 2015, p. 184). For the reflecting team, the hypothesizing process is "living" (Sampson et al., 2021) and is subject to change as the system evolves. The veracity of the hypothesis is irrelevant because even a supposition proven to be false will deliver valuable information in support of or in refutation of the hypothesis. The function of the hypothesis is to challenge the system's homeostasis or pattern of functioning (Adams, 2015).

- *Circularity.* Circularity brings forth change through stimulating the relational system in reaction to the continually refined hypothesis (Selvini et al., 1979). The positive feedback loop stimulates the system's potential to change. If needed, the team can further refine the hypothesis, which can be tested again and repeated in quest of the difference sought (Selvini et al., 1979).

Benefits of Reflecting Teams

The following describes a few of the many benefits of traditional reflecting teams:

- *Multiple perspectives.* Reflecting teams work from the assumption that reality is socially constructed (Lange, 2010). Through their conversations with one another, reflecting team members offer clients a multiplicity of views and ideas regarding change as different experiences and strategies for change are considered (Lange, 2010).

- *Unique conversations.* Clients may engage in unique conversations with one another and their therapist as a result of things they have heard from the team (Lange, 2010).

- *Generation of new ideas, meaning, and solutions.* Through hearing new perspectives and engaging in unique conversations, both clients and the therapist may come up with new ideas, generate new meanings, and come up with possible solutions to presenting problems (Barbetta & Telfener, 2020).

- **Getting unstuck.** Reflecting teams can be particularly helpful when therapists and clients feel stuck and there is a halt in therapeutic progress. Insights gained from the team can provide unique insight to the therapist, which may offer suggestions for future directions of therapy well beyond the implementation of the reflecting team (Prest et al., 1990).

- **Compatibility with other approaches.** Though rooted in the Milan approach, reflecting teams are compatible with many theoretical orientations.

Virtual reflecting teams offer a few of their own unique benefits:

- **More diverse perspectives.** Research indicates that reflecting teams are more effective when teams represent a diverse group of professional and social locations (Harris & Crossley, 2021). Typically, reflecting teams are conducted in academic settings or within the confines of one practice. Virtual reflecting teams allow for a more diverse group of therapists to participate in the team by allowing therapists and clients to join from any location without requiring additional time for travel. This allows for greater diversity in terms of location (e.g., rural, suburban, urban) and practice setting (e.g., therapists from different practices may participate within the context of virtual supervision without disrupting the remainder of their caseload for the day). Of particular benefit to clients, therapists may be selective in the generation of a reflecting team that they think would be helpful for the clients with whom they are working.

- **Multiple methods.** Virtual reflecting teams may be conducted either synchronously or asynchronously. Clients who are hesitant to participate in synchronous reflecting teams may be more comfortable participating in an asynchronous format.

Unique benefits specific to asynchronous virtual reflecting teams also include the following:

- **Saving time.** Reflecting teams are typically expected to commit to observing the entire therapy session and are often expected to participate each time that the clients meet with the therapist. For in-person sessions, this typically requires a minimum of an hour weekly, not including travel time. When reflecting teams participate asynchronously, therapists may choose to share just parts of the session that they think are particularly relevant. This allows the team to reflect on things that they have seen without having to participate in the entire session.

- **Additional processing time.** When reflecting teams participate asynchronously, teams are also afforded more time to discuss the case. Likewise, therapists have more time to process this discussion prior to returning to their work with their clients.

Setup

The following outlines steps for setting up a virtual reflecting team prior to session.

1. **Decide if a reflecting team might be appropriate.** Before introducing the idea of a reflecting team to clients, first decide if a virtual reflecting team might be appropriate and beneficial to them. For example, past traumatic experiences or breaches of trust might make some clients hesitant about the idea of a reflecting team. In some instances, even suggesting the possibility of one might not be appropriate. Carefully consider each client's unique needs before introducing the activity.

2. ***Introduce the activity to clients.*** Discuss with clients that you have a unique opportunity for them to participate in a reflecting team. Explain the activity step by step and outline the expectations of confidentiality (i.e., the therapist may discuss confidential information from therapy with the team, but the team may not share information with anyone else).

3. ***Decide on an approach.*** Discuss with clients the various approaches to a virtual reflecting team that are possible (i.e., real time participation, video recording, audio recording).

4. ***Gather a team.*** In most cases, the team is formed within the context of a group supervision setting. When this is the case, the team is gathered as the first step in this process, prior to identifying clients that may want to participate in the intervention. However, virtual reflecting teams may also occur outside of the context of supervision with an appropriate release of information. When creating a team, gather a diverse group of therapists who speak from a place of collaboration, validation, support, and hope (Harris & Crossley, 2021).

5. ***Receive written consent.*** If the reflecting team is not part of a supervision meeting, clients must sign a release of information prior to sharing any information, audio, or videos with the team. Written consent for audio/video recording must also be received prior to recording anything in session.

Instructions

The following specifies instructions for conducting an asynchronous virtual reflecting team:

1. ***Record the session.*** Record the entire therapy session(s) using a HIPAA-consistent telehealth platform.

2. ***Select a portion of the session to show the team.*** Though the team may choose to view the entire therapy session, selecting a portion/portions of the session to show the team or editing out parts that are irrelevant saves time for all members and allows more time for hypothesizing and discussion. The portion shown to the team will frame hypotheses and invite diverse perspectives from the team.

3. ***Provide context to the team.*** Once the team meets, the therapist should provide context regarding the case to the team, much like a therapist would do in a typical supervision meeting. For example, the therapist should provide general information regarding the clients' social locations, presenting problem(s), and goals for therapy.

4. ***Play video or audio.*** After providing client context, the therapist should play the selected video or audio clips to the team. The therapist may choose to pause the video and discuss at multiple points or wait until the end of the video or audio to discuss.

5. ***Discuss with the team.*** Utilizing key components of the Milan approach, the team then discusses and conceptualizes the case through the use of neutrality, circularity, and hypothesizing. The therapist and team may choose to record this discussion and show it to the client(s) in the next session.

6. ***Select and send a message from the team.*** If the discussion with the team is not recorded and brought back to the clients, the team may instead choose to send a message or messages back to the client(s). This message may be written and given to the therapist to read, or it may be recorded and played for the client(s) to see or hear in session. Research indicates that effective reflections include those of positive regard, validation, and hope (Harris & Crossley, 2021).

7. ***Give the message to the client(s).*** In the next session, the therapist may then play the video or audio of the team's discussion or message or verbally share a written message from the team. Even if the team has already recorded a video or audio recording to share with the clients, the therapist

should check with the clients first to see if they prefer to see or hear the recording of the team's message or if they prefer to have the therapist relay the message. Some clients may not want to see or hear the team directly, even if they want to know what they have to say.

8. ***Discuss with the client(s).*** A critical component of a successful reflecting team is the discussion that takes place between the therapist and client(s) about their experience and insights provided by the team.

Processing

The following is a list of processing questions that the therapist might ask:

- What is it like for you to know that the team has heard your story?
- What was it like for you to hear the team say _____?
- What insights did you gain about one another through this experience?
- Did the team say anything that surprised you?
- Did the team say anything that had already occurred to you?
- Is there anything you think the team missed?
- Do you have any questions about the team's message?
- Do you have any messages that you would like to send back to the team?
- Would you like to try this again?

Vignette

Leslie is a 30-year-old cisgender, bisexual, white, single, Jewish woman with a history of sexual and religious trauma. Leslie took on the role of caregiver for others in her career and experienced a dominant narrative in her personal life of people not believing or validating her trauma experience. Leslie discussed this narrative in individual therapy with her therapist, who was participating in group supervision at the time. Upon discussion of Leslie's case in group supervision, a reflecting team was formed with the belief that by hearing the voices of a group of people who believed her story and grew to care for her, Leslie's dominant story might begin to shift. Team members represented a diverse group of a clinical supervisor and five family therapy student interns who practiced from differing theoretical orientations. Upon identification of the possibility of this intervention, the therapist asked the client if she would be interested in hearing from the therapist's supervision "team." Leslie agreed to try this new approach. Because Leslie's therapist was a student intern, consent for video recording and informed consent regarding case discussion within the context of supervision was already signed with other intake paperwork.

The next time that the therapist saw Leslie, she recorded their session and brought several video clips of the session back to the team to watch during supervision. Supervision occurred virtually over a HIPAA-consistent platform, and the team chose to type their reflections into the chat function as they watched the videos. After the completion of the selected video clips, everyone in the team read one another's comments. They then participated in further discussion and decided what messages would be most helpful for the client to hear. The team's selected messages included validating comments, words of affirmation, and hope for her future. Some of these messages included, "I hear in her voice the desire to be understood and believed," "The people that she loves most should believe her," "How incredible that she has made a career of supporting others in their truths," and "I believe her." The team also decided to ask Leslie a question: "In your work supporting others, what advice might you give to someone who was dismissed and discounted by those they loved?" The team's hope was to offer Leslie validation and support while also corroborating her understanding of herself as the expert in her own life. The therapist took the team's messages back to Leslie and read them aloud during their next session. As the messages were read, Leslie's posture visibly relaxed, and she exhaled deeply. The therapist discussed with Leslie what it was like for her to hear the team's messages and asked if she wanted to continue the conversation with the team, and she agreed.

During the next supervision meeting, the therapist played the recording of her sharing the team's message with Leslie and her response to it. Based on this video clip, the team provided a new message to Leslie using the same approach initially described. Leslie, who appeared down in initial sessions, enthusiastically asked if the team had any new messages for her at the start of the next session. Ultimately, the team provided their reflections a total of three times.

Having a group of people validate Leslie's past traumas and dismissal of those traumas by others began to create a new story of growth and healing. This was further supported by reflections and hypotheses regarding Leslie's current occupation and expert role, both as a caregiver and in her own life. As Leslie experienced herself in new ways, she reported that her experience of the world was also changing. She reported feeling more energetic, excited about her future, and unburdened by her family's expectations and limiting beliefs.

Suggestions for Follow-Up

Between sessions, clients may develop new insights based on what they heard from the team the previous week. In subsequent sessions, therapists are encouraged to follow up with clients on their experience of the reflecting team from the previous session and check in to see if they would like to continue the participation of the team. Therapists may continue discussion with the team and relay messages between the team and clients as the experience proves to be useful and clients continue to express interest in continuing the intervention.

Contraindications

Client experiences with reflecting teams can vary. A systematic review indicated that reflecting teams can feel unusual and strange for clients. Many clients reported that they felt more self-aware during the process but that they gained more comfort with time (Harris & Crossley, 2021). Although usually a positive experience, reflecting teams may not always be a positive intervention (Brownlee et al., 2009; Tseliou et al., 2020), especially if too much information is shared or if the reflections don't feel relevant to the client(s) (Lax, 1995). As with any potential intervention, it is important to be aware of how an existing systemic power imbalance may be compounded by the social location of both the team and the client, as well as language used and general context of the sessions. Relatedly, some participants may not experience reflecting teams as collaborative. Asynchronous reflecting teams in particular may limit the felt experience of a collaborative stance without the physical presence of the team during the therapy session.

References

Adams, J. (2015). Milan systemic therapy. In J. L. Wetchler & L. L. Hecker (Eds.), *An introduction to marriage and family therapy* (2nd ed., pp. 182–205). Routledge.

Andersen, T. (1987). The reflecting team: Dialogue and meta-dialogue in clinical work. *Family Process, 26*(4), 415–428. https://doi.org/10.1111/j.1545-5300.1987.00415.x

Barbetta, P., & Telfener, U. (2020). The Milan approach, history, and evolution. *Family Process*, *60*(1), 4–16. https://doi.org/10.1111/famp.12612

Brownlee, K., Vis, J., & McKenna, A. (2009). Review of the reflecting team process: Strengths, challenges, and clinical implications. *The Family Journal*, *17*(2), 139–145. https://doi.org/10.1177/1066480709332713

Coulehan, R., Friedlander, M. L., & Heatherington, L. (1998). Transforming narratives: A change event in constructivist family therapy. *Family Process*, *37*(1), 17–33. https://doi.org/10.1111/j.1545-5300.1998.00017.x

De Oliveira, A. S. (2003). An "Appropriated unusual" reflecting team. *Journal of Family Psychotherapy*, *14*(2), 85–88. https://doi.org/10.1300/j085v14n02_07

Harris, R., & Crossley, J. (2021). A systematic review and meta-synthesis exploring client experience of reflecting teams in clinical practice. *Journal of Family Therapy*, *43*(4), 687–710. https://doi.org/10.1111/1467-6427.12346

Jenkins, D. (1996). A reflecting team approach to family therapy: A Delphi study. *Journal of Marital and Family Therapy*, *22*(2), 219–238. https://doi.org/10.1111/j.1752-0606.1996.tb00200.x

Lange, R. (2010). The family as its own reflecting team: A family therapy method. *Journal of Family Therapy*, *32*(4), 398–408. https://doi.org/10.1111/j.1467-6427.2010.00512.x

Lax, W. D. (1995). Offering reflections: Some theoretical and practical considerations. In S. Friedman (Ed.), *The reflecting team in action: Collaborative practice in family therapy* (pp. 145–166). Guilford Press.

Prest, L. A., Darden, E. C., & Keller, J. F. (1990). "The fly on the wall" reflecting team supervision. *Journal of Marital and Family Therapy*, *16*(3), 265–273. https://doi.org/10.1111/j.1752-0606.1990.tb00847.x

Sampson, J. M., Hughes, R. L., Wallace, L. B., & Finley, M. A. (2021). Integration of teaming therapy and mixed-reality simulation as remote learning modality for couple and family therapy graduate training programs. *Journal of Marital and Family Therapy*, *47*(2), 392–407. https://doi.org/10.1111/jmft.12494

Selvini, M. P., Cecchin, G., Prata, G., & Coscolo, L. (1979). *Paradox and counterparadox*. Jason Aronson.

Simon, R. (1992). *One on one conversations with the shapers of family therapy*. Guilford Press.

Tseliou, E., Burck, C., Forbat, L., Strong, T., & O'Reilly, M. (2020). How is systemic and constructionist therapy change process narrated in retrospective accounts of therapy? A systematic meta-synthesis review. *Family Process*, *60*(1), 64–83. https://doi.org/10.1111/famp.12562

CHAPTER 39

PLURILINGUISTIC VIRTUAL REFLECTING TEAMS WITH LATINO/A FAMILIES

Carlos A. Ramos, Julian F. Crespo, and Ezequiel Peña

Materials for Therapists: HIPAA-consistent videoconferencing platform that has virtual waiting room capabilities.

Materials for Clients: None.

Objective

In reflecting teams, an observing team of therapists joins the therapy session around the halfway point and shares their curiosities and reflections while clients silently listen. This chapter provides instructions on ways in which to adapt traditional reflecting teams specifically for use with Latino/a clients via virtual platforms.

Rationale for Use

Reflecting teams are used around the world, in many languages, and across many cultures (Pender & Stinchfield, 2012). Virtual reflecting teams have anecdotally shown to be particularly effective in working with Spanish-speaking and bilingual clients. Immigrant or transnational families frequently use digital means for staying connected across long distances, including internationally (Falicov, 2014). The use of virtual reflecting teams allows geographically distant family members to join family conversations. In a traditional in-person reflecting team, family members who live farther away would not be able to participate. One of the main core values for Latino/a families is *familism*, meaning family connection, support, and unity. Zafra (2016) underscores the importance of therapists working with Latino/a families through an interpersonal lens because most "decisions are made as a family" (p. 14), and there is an expectation for families to be emotionally and geographically united. Because of the visually proximal and familial nature of virtual reflecting teams, this platform can be of great use in creatively using digital means with Latino/a and Spanish-speaking families who demonstrate an affinity for narrative, metaphor, and story sharing (Ondish et al., 2019).

Chismorreo, chusmear, and *chismear* are forms of social and dialogical practice in Latino/a culture, in which participants tell, create, and reconstruct information that is passed on (Tanaka, 2007). The practice of

DOI: 10.4324/9781003289920-46

chismorreo usually happens in small groups in which participants know and trust each other. The accuracy or the truthfulness of the stories is irrelevant. In the process of sharing them, they become real and part of learning about life lessons.

In addition to its social function, the practice of *chismorrear* has therapeutic value. It opens the dialogical space for participants to connect with each other and embrace the interactional complexities of human thought and emotion (Tanaka, 2007). This practice allows participants to understand themselves within the context of a community (Fasano et al., 2009).

Given the relational realities and complexities of Spanish-speaking clients, traditional reflecting teams can be taken one step further to make them even more dialogical. Rather than suggesting to clients that they simply listen and keep their thoughts, questions, and ideas private, they can be invited to join the reflecting team conversations through a therapeutic *chismorreo* or story-sharing (Ramos et al., 2021). This polyphonic chorus, a form of dialogical practice, reflects Anderson's (1997) notion of a shared inquiry or conversational partnership, which she describes as "an in-there-together, two-way, give-and-take exchange" (p. 112).

The following ways of therapeutically engaging are closely connected with Anderson's (1997) collaborative stance. She defines therapy as a "dialogical conversation [or] generative process in which new meanings – different ways of understanding, making sense of, or punctuating one's lived experiences – emerge and are mutually constructed" (p. 109). Each conversation is unique with experiential, contextual, cultural, and linguistic differences and is "formed on a moment-by-moment basis" (Anderson, 1997, p. 111). The sharing and resharing of stories and experiences facilitates the telling of new stories, which then influences how clients change in relation to these new narratives (Anderson, 2012). The same hermeneutic process holds true for bilingual families when virtual reflecting teams are employed as a means of eliciting the sharing of new stories, a generative process that allows new meanings and different ways of understanding and engaging to emerge (Anderson, 2012). This is particularly effective with highly interactional and relational members of diverse Latino/a communities.

Setup

To set up a plurilinguistic virtual reflecting team, take the following steps:

1. ***Set up the virtual platform.*** Team participation includes live observation of sessions by the team via a HIPAA-consistent virtual platform. The platform should have a meeting license that does not have time restraints and does not limit the number of participants.

2. ***Form the team.*** Plurilinguistic virtual reflecting teams consist of three to six team members who are therapist(s) or observing team members in the therapy process. A team may be made up of a group of therapy supervisees and a supervising therapist. Supervisors, however, should be mindful of the number of reflecting team members and voices included. The intention is to inspire a therapeutic *chismorreo* without overwhelming clients with shared stories and experiences. All team members must be conversationally fluent in Spanish and English, meaning they are comfortable understanding and communicating in both languages. This fluid approach allows clients and therapists to exist in "two worlds of thought simultaneously" (Polanco, 2021, p. 61). The theme of conversation should also be considered as it relates to the composition of the reflecting team. For example, a virtual reflecting team consisting of a group of mothers exchanging stories about the challenges of motherhood may help normalize a client's experience of feeling ashamed and guilty for having a child who is experiencing behavioral challenges.

3. ***Obtain consent for team observation.*** Consent for team observation should be initially described on consent forms. Consent for team observation differs from consent for team reflection in that this

written consent allows the team to observe therapy sessions and provides an initial introduction to the team process. Clients should sign these forms prior to attending sessions. The therapist(s) should review the team process at the beginning of the first session to ensure that clients understand and feel comfortable with the reflecting team format. Therapists should revisit this again when they plan on reflecting in the presence of the clients for the first time.

4. ***Schedule a team discussion approximately halfway through the session.*** This conversation should not be visible or audible to clients. During this time, clients should wait in the virtual waiting room. The team shares thoughts, questions, and curiosities behind the virtual screen.

5. ***Decide when to reflect.*** Discuss the possibility of a story-sharing reflecting team during the consultation break while clients wait in a virtual waiting room. The decision to pursue a story-sharing reflecting team should be inspired by the theme of conversation, overall therapeutic process, and conversation among the team members during the consultation break. The decision to include a reflecting team should consider the topic of conversation, clients' processes and experiences, timing, and team input and observations. They can also be improvisational or in-the-moment discussions that are driven by and reflect current, live sessions. The team should also consider therapeutic intentions in relation to therapeutic change. How would a shift in the therapy context that embraces a back-and-forth story-sharing interaction facilitate a meaningful experience or a change in relationship to new narratives (Anderson, 2012)?

6. ***Discuss with clients.*** The supervisor invites the clients back from the virtual waiting room. Prior to the team reflecting in front of the clients, clients must verbally consent to and be aware of the reflecting team process. This is different than the initial informed consent in that the primary therapist(s) verbally discusses the desire for the observing team to have a conversation in their presence. Therapists share that the team would like to facilitate a team conversation that reflects their curiosities and thoughts about the session. Therapists also share that the clients are welcome to join the reflection if there is something that they would like to contribute to the conversation. They have the option of both listening and contributing if there is an experience, question, or theme they find meaningful. The observing team members keep their cameras off until they have consent from clients to join.

Instructions

1. ***Initiate a plurilinguistic engagement.*** Once the client(s) consent to a story-sharing experience, therapists invite the observing team members to turn on their cameras. The therapist(s) and/or supervisor revisit the process for the reflecting team interactions. Mention that the team wishes to share their thoughts and stories. Encourage clients to sit back and observe as if they are watching their favorite TV show or "telenovela." If they, however, at any point hear something that they would like to respond to, they are welcome to share. The team then improvises based on the client's response and continues to build on this conversation. Thus, rather than concluding the conversation and then asking the clients to reflect on the team's reflections after they have finished (Andersen, 1991), this approach provides clients the opportunity to actively engage in the process. Both team members and clients are valued as conversational participants (Goolishian, 1990).

2. ***Begin team reflections and story-sharing.*** Story-sharing from team members normally involves a sense of trust among the group and a sharing of personal experiences that may relate to clients' experiences (Anderson, 1997). The accuracy or the truthfulness of the stories is irrelevant. In the process of sharing them, they become real and part of learning about life lessons. The stories shared should be "relative to the audience and . . . fit the attitude and questions the audience brings to the

conversation" (Becvar et al., 1997, p. 119). Share diverse experiences in the form of stories with the intention to facilitate new client narratives via a wide range of personal narratives. The intention is also to challenge some contextual restraints (Bateson, 2000) that may limit the narratives shared by both clients and team members during therapy.

3. ***Move with the narratives.*** For this approach, the reflecting team is encouraged to "move *with* the narrative" (Anderson, 1997, p. 139) as it unfolds during the plurilinguistic engagement. That is, embrace the exchanges during the reflecting team discussion as meaningful experiences. Generate questions to add or expand on the conversation and/or ideas that were discussed. Continue to embrace this moment-by-moment approach and move with the presented stories, ideas, and topics. Avoid challenging or assuming that the present narrative is irrelevant or nonsense (Anderson, 1997). What may seem like nonsense may be meaningful to clients. Thus, questions should be influenced by in-the-moment curiosity intended to generate meaningful experiences.

Processing

Following the conclusion of the session, the reflecting team should discuss their experience and perceptions of the client experience. Supervisors may consider asking the following questions:

- What stood out about the conversation?

- What do you think inspired the client(s) to join the conversation?

- How do you think client participation influenced the reflecting team conversation?

- How did client participation with the reflecting team influence the therapeutic process?

- How do you think our plurilinguistic engagement inspired a therapeutic moment of movement?

- What were we able to talk about in this context that may have not been possible in a traditional reflecting team?

- What was it like for the team to exchange personal, therapeutic narratives and stories in a group format?

Vignette

A Latino/a couple, Adrian (33) and Izzy (28), presented in therapy wanting to improve their communication. The couple had been together for over 10 years but described their relationship as "unstable," meaning they were constantly arguing and "never on the same page." The couple and therapist communicated in session through a combination of both Spanish and English.

As part of a training clinic, the couple consented to therapy being observed within the context of live supervision. About halfway through the second session, the supervision group wondered if a reflecting team might be of benefit to the couple. The therapist discussed this option with the couple, and they consented to team participation in subsequent sessions. The team consisted of six therapy interns from the supervision group and their supervisor, who were all fluent in both Spanish and English.

In the next session, the therapist asked the couple for their permission for the team to join them and to reflect. The couple agreed. The team turned their cameras on and then proceeded with a reflecting conversation.

The supervisor initiated the conversation by setting the context for a therapeutic *chismorreo*. He described the reflecting team as something like watching a captivating telenovela or television show. The difference being that if they heard something meaningful, they were welcome to chime in and share their thoughts.

The team initiated the reflecting process with the notion of commitment, highlighting different examples of how the couple continued to commit to their relationship given all their challenges. The idea of commitment evolved into a discussion about trust after one of the team members wondered about the couple's meaning of trust and if trust and commitment were related. Adrian and Izzy both immediately chimed in and responded to this curiosity. Adrian shared that he did not "fully trust" Izzy because of previous infidelity, causing him to consistently "check" her phone logs and text messages. He did not share this relationship experience with friends or family because of fear of judgment. Infidelity would indicate "weakness" as a Latino male. This was the first time he was able to openly talk with others about this experience. Similarly, Izzy mentioned that Adrian also was "not faithful," which led to her worrying and constantly asking for his "whereabouts." There was a shift in the couple's demeanor after sharing these vulnerable experiences; they seemed to be more receptive and sensitive toward each other.

The reflecting team followed the couple's narrative of infidelity and trust. They did this from a strengths-based perspective and included comments and stories to intentionally reflect the couple's strengths and resources. They asked the couple if they were both committed to working on trust and if so, in what ways they would do so. Adrian and Izzy both confirmed that they were committed and provided a variety of ways they could achieve this goal. At the end of the session, the couple expressed their appreciation for everyone's participation and noted that this was a "very helpful" and "unique" conversation. They explained that normally, when they ask their friends for advice, they are repeatedly told to "move on from each other. You're wasting your time." This time, however, the couple's experience was different; they felt heard, understood, and hopeful for their relationship.

During the fourth and last session the following week, Izzy described a variety of intra- and interpersonal changes right from the start. She mentioned that Adrian had changed his Facebook status to "engaged," which was a "huge deal" for her, and that they were talking about marriage for the first time. They were not questioning each other's "whereabouts," but rather, they were sending each other pictures of "old memories" throughout the day when they were apart. Izzy also mentioned that her "kids" noticed something was different about her. They noticed that she was "giddy," meaning she was "blushing and smiling more often." Halfway through the session, the therapist asked, "How has this conversation been helpful so far?" Izzy responded that she "liked that the therapists wanted to hear about the changes and found these changes important."

Suggestions for Follow-Up

Shortly after the plurilinguistic reflecting team has concluded or during the following session, therapists should inquire about the clients' experiences with the conversation. Therapists may ask:

- What was your experience like listening to the team's stories?
- What was helpful about the different ideas shared?
- What inspired you to join the conversation?
- How was this experience different from previous therapy conversations?

Based on the clients' feedback, the team can then decide how to move forward with future team participation and collaboration.

Contraindications

There are certain situations and/or clients for which this approach is not a good fit and should not be implemented. For instance, some clients may not be comfortable with others viewing their therapy sessions. If they do consent to this, they may prefer that observers remain silent and out of sight rather than discuss their observations in front of them. Clients experiencing high-conflict situations or other safety concerns may also not be appropriate.

References

Andersen, T. (1991). *The reflecting team: Dialogues and dialogues about the dialogues.* Norton.

Anderson, H. (1997). *Conversation, language, and possibilities: A postmodern approach to therapy.* Basic Books. https://doi.org/10.1177/070674379704200715

Anderson, H. (2012). Collaborative relationships and dialogic conversations: Ideas for a relationally responsive practice. *Family Process, 51*(1), 8–24. https://doi.org/10.1111/j.1545-5300.2012.01385.x

Bateson, G. (2000). *Steps to an ecology of mind.* The University of Chicago Press.

Becvar, R. J., Canfield, B. S., & Becvar, D. S. (1997). *Group work: Cybernetic, constructivist, and social constructionist perspectives.* Love Publishing.

Falicov, C. J. (2014). *Latino families in therapy* (2nd ed.). The Guilford Press.

Fasano, P., Ruiu, A., Giménez, J. M., Ramírez, A., Aymá, A., & Savulsky, N. (2009). El sentido del chisme en una comunidad de pobres urbanos. *Ciencia, Docencia y Tecnología, 20*(39), 49–85.

Goolishian, H. A. (1990). Family therapy: An evolving story. *Contemporary Family Therapy, 12*(3), 173–180. https://doi.org/10.1007/bf00891242

Ondish, P., Cohen, D., Lucas, K. W., & Vandello, J. (2019). The resonance of metaphor: Evidence for Latino preferences for metaphor and analogy. *Personality and Social Psychology Bulletin, 45*(11), 1531–1548. https://doi.org/10.1177/0146167219833390

Pender, R. L., & Stinchfield, T. (2012). A reflective look at reflecting teams. *The Family Journal, 20*(2), 117–122. https://doi.org/10.1177/1066480712438526

Polanco, M. (2021). Rethinking narrative therapy: An examination of bilingualism and magical realism. *Journal of Systemic Therapies, 40*(1), 61–74. https://doi.org/10.1521/jsyt.2021.40.1.59

Ramos, C. A., Castro, J., & Velez, J. A. G. (2021). Therapeutic Latinx story-sharing or chismorreo. In M. Polanco, N. Zamani, & C. D. H. Kim (Eds.), *Bilingualism, culture, and social justice in family therapy* (pp. 47–54). AFTA Springer Briefs in Family Therapy.

Tanaka, C. (2007). El chisme como fenómeno social: Un campo-tema desde la perspectiva construccionista. *Fermentum. Revista Venezolana de Sociología y Antropología, 17*(50), 646–672.

Zafra, J. (2016). The use of structural family therapy with a Latino family: A case study. *Journal of Systemic Therapies, 35*(4), 11–21. https://doi.org/10.1521/jsyt.2016.35.4.11

CHAPTER 40

"REAL" PRACTICE WITH CLIENTS

USING SIMULATION IN VIRTUAL GROUP SUPERVISION

Dana J. Stone and Deborah J. Buttitta

Materials for Supervisors and Supervisees:

- Access to simulation platform

- Vignettes/scenarios

- Computer or tablet with access to a web camera

- Wi-Fi internet (hard-wired internet connections produce the best results)

- Telehealth platform

Objective

Simulation mirrors real-life clinical scenarios to offer an experiential tool for supporting therapist development in online group supervision. The recommended process engages the entire supervision group, with supervisees rotating into set roles as the clinician, consultants, and, within role-play format, as clients. The supervisor functions as the facilitator of the process. The main objective of simulation is to offer supervised opportunities for deliberate practice of clinical skills. The simulation processes described in this chapter are adapted from an in-person format to fit online supervision. Two formats are outlined. The first uses mixed-reality technology. The second uses traditional role-play as a "mock" simulation utilizing case vignettes or real client scenarios.

Rationale for Use

Simulation has historically been used as an effective tool in the training of medical care providers by enabling the practice of real-life emergency situations without jeopardizing the health of actual patients (Lighthall & Barr, 2007; McMahon et al., 2005; Schwindt & McNelis, 2015). More recently, the mental health field has used simulation, including mixed-reality simulation, in the training and supervision of therapists (Sampson et al., 2021; Satter et al., 2012; Washburn et al., 2018). Simulation utilized through a mixed-reality platform involves the integration of artificial intelligence (i.e., an avatar) along with trained

DOI: 10.4324/9781003289920-47

live actors who control the avatars and speak for them from a different location. The use of live actors is what differentiates mixed-reality simulation from traditional simulation platforms. For example, a live traditional simulation includes real people acting in person to simulate a scenario, while a virtual simulation involves real people working in a fully simulated or digital environment (Lighthall & Barr, 2007). The mixed-reality platform, which involves a simulated environment and avatar with an actor, offers spontaneity, flexibility, and more human elements in the process, which fosters stronger engagement from clinicians in training.

Mixed-reality simulation may offer simulation experiences that replicate work with individuals, couples, parent–child, or small groups of clients. Scenarios or vignettes are often prepared by subject matter experts for the specific purpose of the simulation exercise. For example, a solution-focused therapist might write a clinical vignette and provide information about the types of questions a solution-focused therapist would ask and the types of answers a client in the vignette situation might provide. The avatar actors are prepared for the scenario in advance of the simulation through consultation with the subject matter expert (when available) and by doing their own research on the topic if needed. Actors are provided a vignette with detailed information to help them understand the character and nuances of the scenario so they know how to respond to the therapist with whom they are interacting. Avatar actors are trained to understand the stated objectives of each scenario and interact with therapists in an effort to meet those objectives. For example, the scenario used in this chapter is focused on conducting a thorough assessment of suspected child abuse within a complex family situation. During the simulation, if the therapist fails to ask appropriate assessment questions or misses suspected child abuse, the avatar is instructed to increase the level of distress or offer more focused cues. Alternatively, if the therapist is too aggressive in their assessment and fails to consider the therapeutic relationship or important cultural or systemic factors, the avatar is directed to stop being forthcoming and reflect a guarded presentation.

Mixed-reality simulation can be used to develop and strengthen basic microskills (e.g., active listening, circular questioning, rapport building), increase the accuracy of diagnostic questioning, and improve competency in the assessment and management of crises (Satter et al., 2012; Washburn et al., 2018) in a safe and supportive environment. This ultimately increases the potential for therapist self-efficacy and confidence building (Ajaz et al., 2016; Krach & Hanline, 2017). In more complex simulated sessions, supervisees can practice not only navigating a difficult clinical scenario but also managing anxiety by allowing the supervisor to attend to both professional and personal aspects of therapist development.

When simulation is used for therapist development in supervision, it is informed by three interrelated frameworks:

1. The competency-based supervision model, which attends to the knowledge, skills, and values of specific competencies (Falender & Shafranske, 2007, 2014)

2. Self of the therapist, which focuses on awareness of personal responses to clinical challenges and managing reactivity (Aponte & Kissil, 2016)

3. Deliberate practice, which focuses on practicing skills to improve performance and clinical outcomes (Chow et al., 2015; see Chapter 36)

All three frameworks are considered simultaneously to provide a lens for the supervisor to guide and support therapist development. Because the competency-based supervision model is utilized across multiple theoretical orientations, it allows supervisees and supervisors a broad range of theoretical applications (Falender & Shafranske, 2007, 2014). In terms of self of the therapist, this process provides opportunities for increased awareness regarding how a supervisee's automatic responses may influence both their therapeutic presence and clinical choices while also inviting moments of pause and reflection in a supportive context (Aponte & Kissil, 2014). Mixed-reality simulation engages supervisees in deliberate and targeted practice of core competencies considered foundational and essential in clinical practice. Miller and colleagues (2020) highlight the value of intentional or deliberate practicing to attain varying levels of mastery, which is helpful as supervisees move from academic learning to application of theory with clients.

The group context offers opportunity for growth as supervisees learn from doing, observing, and engaging in critical thinking as consultants to their peers. Group supervision encourages collaborative learning, and the simulation process requires a level of vulnerability, as supervisees take turns as the clinician. As the group engages in the process, supervisees learn from mistakes and celebrate successes, individually and collectively. Most importantly, this process can create a community of support early on in professional development, which is a protective factor related to perseverance and longevity in many helping professions (Skovholt & Trotter-Mathison, 2016).

Online supervision with simulation and role-plays may allow access to simulation technologies for supervisors who may not otherwise have access. Additionally, simulation during online supervision allows supervisors to address the application of skills directly for use in the context of teletherapy. Providing supervision online using simulations and role-plays could meet the required "training or coursework regarding delivery of mental health services to clients via telehealth" required by many mental health state licensing boards (Sampson et al., 2021; Sodergren, 2023).

Setup

The choice to use simulation is often based on availability of resources. Both traditional and mixed-reality simulation systems are typically housed in professional organizations (e.g., the American Association for Marriage and Family Therapy) and universities. Clinics and universities without their own simulation software need to contact such organizations to gain access to simulation technology, typically through a paid subscription. Once access is established, supervisors may receive brief training to learn how to fully utilize the simulation experience. If access to simulation is unavailable (e.g., lack of available funding), role-play may be used as an alternative option.

For this training experience to be effective in both simulation and role-play, safety must be created in group supervision. Supervisees must also be oriented to the simulation or role-play process and prepared for specific scenarios in advance.

Creating Safety in Group Supervision

It is critical that the supervisor cultivate a supervision relationship conducive for learning and growth. Several factors help to build confidence in supervisees who will participate in the simulation or role-play exercises:

- Establish a safe and supportive learning environment.

- Foster group cohesion.

- Encourage persistence and risk-taking.

- Know when to "direct" and when to gently guide.

- Note strengths of each supervisee as they develop skills and demonstrate them in the group space.

- Ongoingly monitor safety in the supervision environment through a collaborative process with all supervisees (Rigazio-DiGilio, 2016).

Orienting Supervisees to Simulation Process

Early in the supervision relationship, supervisors should prepare supervisees for the simulation or role-play experience by educating the group regarding the benefits of their participation in simulation and tie related discussions to skill development. Depending on the developmental level of each therapist, supervisees may be hesitant or concerned about participating as the lead therapist. Supervisors may model skills as the lead therapist in role-plays with supervisees as the clients and identify which skills to focus on during the upcoming simulation or role-play exercises. Supervisors can review the skills in more specific detail by describing nonverbal skills, reviewing reflecting skills, providing examples of appropriate questions that could be used for the clinical situation, or reminding supervisees of relevant policies and procedures (e.g., legal and ethical guidelines).

Planning for Specific Scenarios

Supervisors should prepare supervisees prior to the simulation or role-play by explaining simulation, what it is, and how to use it. Supervisors may use vignettes relevant to the training stage of the supervisees. Scenarios may focus on various topics in clinical training such as learning how to manage crises like child abuse reporting or a suicide assessment. Crisis management is an excellent choice for the use of simulation because supervisees can work on ethical decision-making, implementing legal mandates effectively, and managing anxiety during critical incidents. Alternatively, they could focus on the supervisee's use of interventions from a specific model of therapy such as a genogram from Bowen's intergenerational therapy or the miracle question from solution-focused therapy. Supervisors should share the vignette that will be utilized in each simulation experience in advance so supervisees know what skills they will be implementing and how to prepare for the session. Supervisors should also explain that supervisees who are not in the role of the therapist should support the therapist in consultation related to the skills outlined in the review session.

When a simulation environment is not accessible and role-play will be utilized, supervisors also need to prepare one or more supervisees to be in the role of the client(s). Supervisors should have a set of standardized vignettes with enough information for supervisees to embody the role of the client(s). Supervisors should meet with supervisees individually to prepare them for the role-play. In supervision spaces in which more than one role-play will happen over the course of the supervision experience, supervisors should ask supervisees to rotate out of the client position so they may also play the role of the therapist. The choice to use simulation versus role-play may be based on access, but more often, simulation is used as supervisees begin to practice newly acquired skills. Advanced supervisees might benefit more from using their actual cases, which are used within the context of role-play.

Instructions

The following provides detailed instructions for implementing simulation and role-plays in the context of virtual group supervision.

Simulation

Simulation utilizes a program that offers mixed-reality technology with actors behind avatar clients. Supervisees take turns as the therapist. If the entire simulation exercise is scheduled for two hours, the first 20 minutes should be set aside for review and prep for the session. The next 75 to 90 minutes should be for engagement in the simulation. The final 25 to 30 minutes should be for individual reflection and group processing. The following explains these steps in detail.

1. When supervisees and supervisors enter the online supervision environment, there will be an "extra" participant box in the group; this will be for the avatar client(s). Before the avatar(s) appear(s) on screen, supervisors prepare supervisees by explaining the simulation exercises and providing an outline or review of each of the following:

   • Simulation exercise plan

   • Clinical scenario

   • Session learning objectives

   • Role of the therapist

   • Role of the observers as collaborators and consultants

   • Additional logistics (e.g., therapist is able to stop and start the simulation as needed for support from the supervisor and supervisee team)

2. Assure that supervisees understand basic clinical skills necessary for implementation with the scenario. This may include:

   • Empathy and active listening skills

   • Establishing and/or maintaining therapeutic alliance

   • Basic clinical assessment skills

   • Crisis assessment skills

   • Review and disclosure of legal and ethical mandates to clients

   • Managing personal reactivity to client reports of trauma or possible crisis

3. Work with supervisees to determine the order of when each person will play the role of the therapist.

4. When the first supervisee is ready in the therapist role, they say "start simulation" to begin the mock therapy session. The client avatar comes onto the screen, and the therapist begins the session by following the plan laid out by the group before they started. At any point, the therapist may say "pause session" to ask for support or help from the group. Supervisors may also pause the session if they think the supervisee is going off track or is struggling. After consultation, the therapist rejoins the session by saying "start session" again.

5. Supervisees take turns by rotating into the role of therapist approximately every 7 to 10 minutes, depending on the number of supervisees in the supervision group. Each supervisee continues the conversation where the last therapist left off. The supervisor or another supervisee manages time. When the 7- to 10-minute period is over, the session is paused, and the next therapist takes over.

Role-Play

When access to mixed-reality simulation is unavailable, supervisees can role-play clients from a vignette or a real case dilemma. Unlike traditional role-play, this "mock" simulation includes a group of supervisees taking turns being the therapist and having the opportunity to pause for help. The remaining supervisees and the supervisor act as consultants and provide guidance and support to the therapist. Supervisees take turns as the therapist.

The steps for role-play are similar to the steps required for simulation, with designated supervisees as clients. Supervisors prepare supervisees who will engage in the role-play as the clients in advance of the role-play simulation. This can typically be done by creating a breakout room in the online supervision platform so conversations between supervisors and supervisees in client roles are not overheard by other supervisees.

During pauses by the therapist, "clients" should be placed into a "breakout" or separate room while the therapist, supervisees, and supervisors consult. The separation of the clients from the group discussion allows for more authentic responses from the client actors and mimics simulation. Supervisors are responsible for moving clients to breakout rooms and bringing them back when the session starts again.

Example Vignette

The following is an example of a scenario with specific learning objectives that might be provided to a supervision group for application in either simulation or role-play. This scenario was created to help beginning clinicians practice culturally relevant assessment and crisis-management skills and would be used in a supervision group that is composed of trainees.

This is your third individual session with Ana, who is age 11 and in fifth grade. While building rapport and getting to know Ana, you have learned that she is the oldest child of two siblings and currently lives with her younger sister, age 8, mother, father, and maternal uncle. Ana has shared with you that she identifies as Persian, that her parents emigrated from Iran with her when she was 3 years old, and that she, her sister, and her mother are bilingual and her father and uncle speak monolingual Farsi. Ana was referred to therapy because she has been an active and high-achieving student but recently has become less participatory during classroom learning, stays inside during recess to rest her head on her desk, and has not been engaging with her peers socially as she used to. Both parents and teachers have expressed concern.

Ana's mother's youngest brother, Arash, age 19, just moved in with the family after his recent immigration to the U.S. Ana's adjustment to this new person in their household has been difficult. Arash is not currently attending school and is having trouble finding employment. During a previous intake with the parents, they reported that Arash is home most of the day, struggling with depressed mood and isolation. Ana's parents indicate that Arash is taking care of their daughters after school and on most weekends, since they are both working extra shifts to compensate for the extra person to provide for in the household.

During the first few sessions with Ana, she was quiet and more reserved, but she has since started to share more openly. She reports that her little sister is her best friend and that she "protects" her at home. Having her uncle Arash around has been difficult. In this session, Ana shares that she and Arash do not get along, especially when her parents are not home. Ana shared in the last session that Arash yells at her and her sister and is constantly telling her what to do. Today, Ana told the therapist that Arash grabs her by the arm sometimes when she is trying to walk away from him.

Sample Learning Objectives

The following are sample instructions supervisors might give to the supervisees in preparation for the simulation or role-play. The instructions make clear the objectives of the simulation and what the therapist should be doing during the session.

Therapists will:

- Maintain the therapeutic alliance
- Demonstrate empathy

- Demonstrate active listening

- Conduct an assessment of suspected child abuse

- If child abuse appears to be present:

  - Assess level of immediate safety

  - Assess frequency, severity, and pattern of abuse

  - Assess for other risks (e.g., other minors in home, substance use)

- Use questions and communication skills appropriately to gather enough information to file a report

- Demonstrate appropriate disclosure of legal and ethical mandates with consideration of the client's age

- Manage their own reactivity during discovery of suspected abuse

Processing

Processing allows supervisees to reflect on their experience both individually and as a group. Supervisees should have some time to reflect on their own work. If they were not the therapist, supervisees should reflect on their experience of observing and providing feedback for those who were in the role of the therapist. Group members and supervisors should also provide feedback for all people who acted in the role of therapist. Throughout the process, the supervisor should lead group processing and remind supervisees that feedback should be strength based and growth oriented. The following are sample questions for processing simulation or role-play exercises at the individual and group levels.

Individual processing questions may be focused on self-assessment of competency, deliberate practice, implementation of theory, or self of the therapist. Group processing questions may also be asked.

Self-Assessment of Competency

- In what ways were you successful in keeping the client(s) engaged?

- What did you do well specific to the skills we set out to practice today?

- What is one skill you would like to work on or improve?

Deliberate Practice

- Can you identify an area of your clinical skills that you would like to improve?

- What came easy to you? What was difficult?

- What will you take from this practice session into a future session with a client?

- In what ways were you able to implement your chosen theoretical orientation or intervention?

Implementation of Theory

- In what ways did the clinician effectively use [the selected theory-specific intervention]?

- How did the intervention help or hinder the achievement of the session goal?

- In what other ways, besides the use of [the theory-specific intervention], did the theoretical orientation show up in the process?

Self of the Therapist

- What was going on for you personally as you were in the therapist's seat?

- What were you feeling?

- Did you notice any reactivity or default responses that you may need to attend to personally?

Group Processing Questions

- What did you notice your colleagues doing well as the therapist? As consultants?

- What are some of the ways the group did well to support each therapist?

- What are some of the ways the group might improve as consultants to the therapist in future sessions?

Suggestions for Follow-Up

Simulation can be used throughout training and supervision to build upon skills and to expand feedback-informed practice for supervisees. In a simulation, the therapist supervisee can get feedback in real time, as the session is unfolding. Supervisors can also integrate the learning gained from simulation into action steps for future sessions with clients. For example, after participation with the aforementioned scenario, the supervisor could outline specific steps in child abuse assessment and reporting for the supervisee's future interactions with clients. In addition, the same group could use similar scenarios across time and development to deepen learning and possible outcomes.

Contraindications

In educational settings, if supervisees are required to purchase vouchers to participate in simulation, it may be cost prohibitive. In addition, in other training environments, the organization may not have funds available to purchase simulation packages for their clinicians in training. Role-plays may be conducted when simulation is not an affordable option.

Using simulation with deaf supervisees in training can be prohibitive when the deaf supervisee is in the role of therapist because the avatar cannot use sign language. Use of interpreters does not provide the deaf supervisee with equal access to the simulation experience. In cases where a deaf supervisee is working with an interpreter, role-play scenarios might be better suited.

References

Ajaz, A., David, R., & Bhat, M. (2016). The PsychSimCentre: Teaching out-of-hours psychiatry to non-psychiatrists. *Clinical Teacher, 13*(1), 13–17. https://doi.org/10.1111/tct.12382

Aponte, H. J., & Kissil, K. (2014). "If I can grapple with this I can truly be of use in the therapy room": Using the therapist's own emotional struggles to facilitate effective therapy. *Journal of Marital and Family Therapy, 40*(2), 152–164. https://doi.org/10.1111/jmft.12011

Aponte, H. J., & Kissil, K. (2016). *The person of the therapist training model: Mastering the use of the self.* Routledge.

Chow, D. L., Miller, S. D., Seidel, J. A., Kane, R. T., & Thorton, J. A. (2015). The role of deliberate practice in the development of highly effective psychotherapists. *Psychotherapy, 52*(3), 337–345. https://doi.org/10.1037/pst0000015

Falender, C. A., & Shafranske, E. P. (2007). Competence in competency-based supervision practice: Construct and application. *Professional Psychology: Research and Practice, 38*(3), 232–240. https://doi.org/10.1037/0735-7028.38.3.232

Falender, C. A., & Shafranske, E. P. (2014). Clinical supervision: The state of the art. *Journal of Clinical Psychology, 70*(11), 1030–1041. https://doi.org/10.1002/jclp.22124

Krach, S. K., & Hanline, M. F. (2017). Teaching consultation skills using interdepartmental collaboration and supervision with a mixed-reality simulator. *Journal of Educational and Psychological Consultation, 28*(2), 190–218. https://doi.org/10.1080/10474412.2017.1301818

Lighthall, G. K., & Barr, J. (2007). The use of clinical simulation systems to train critical care physicians. *Journal of Intensive Care Medicine, 22*(5), 257–269. https://doi.org/10.1177/0885066607304273

McMahon, G. T., Monaghan, C., Falchuk, K., Gordon, J. A., & Alexander, E. K. (2005). A simulator-based curriculum to promote comparative and reflective analysis in an internal medicine clerkship. *Academic Medicine, 80*(1), 84–89. https://doi.org/10.1097/00001888-200501000-00021

Miller, S., Chow, D., Wampold, B. E., Hubble, M. A., Del Re, A. C., Bargmann, M., & Bargmann, S. (2020). To be or not to be (an expert?): Revisiting the role of deliberate practice in improving performance. *High Abilities Studies, 31*(1), 5–15. https://doi.org/10.1080/13598139.2018.151910

Rigazio-DiGilio, S. A. (2016). MFT supervision: An overview. In K. Jordan (Ed.), *Couple, marriage, and family therapy supervision* (pp. 25–49). Springer. https://doi.org/10.1891/9780826126795

Sampson, J. M., Hughes, R. L., Wallace, L. B., & Finley, M. A. (2021). Integration of teaming therapy and mixed-reality simulation as remote learning modality for couple and family therapy graduate training programs. *Journal of Marital Family Therapy, 47*(2), 392–407. https://doi.org/10.1111/jmft.12494

Satter, R. M., Cohen, T., Ortiz, P., Kahol, K., Mackenzie, J., Olson, C., Johnson, M., & Patel, V. L. (2012). Avatar-based simulation in the evaluation of diagnosis and management of mental health disorders in primary care. *Journal of Biomedical Informatics, 45*(6), 1137–1150. https://doi.org/10.1016/j.jbi.2012.07.009

Schwindt, R., & McNelis, A. (2015). Integrating simulation into reflection-centered graduate psychiatric/mental health nursing curriculum. *Nursing Education Perspectives, 36*(5), 328–328. https://doi.org/10.5480/15-1614

Skovholt, T. M., & Trotter-Mathison, M. (2016). *The resilient practitioner: Burnout and compassion fatigue prevention and self-care strategies for the helping professions* (5th ed.). Routledge. https://doi.org/10.4324/9781315737447

Sodergren, S. (2023). *Statutes and regulations relating to the practices of professional, clinical counseling, marriage and family therapy, educational psychology, clinical social work.* Board of Behavioral Sciences. www.bbs.ca.gov/pdf/publications/lawsregs.pdf

Washburn, M., Parrish, D. E., & Bordnick, P. S. (2018). Virtual patient simulations for brief assessment of mental health disorders in integrated care settings. *Social Work in Mental Health, 18*(2), 121–148. https://doi.org/10.1080/15332985.2017.1336743

INDEX

5-4-3-2-1 grounding technique 115–120; *see also* grounding

abstract thoughts 61
abuse 19, 81, 89, 183, 263, 264; *see also* child abuse; cyberbullying; domestic violence; intimate partner violence; neglect; trauma; violence
accessibility: alternate services 3, 8; consultation 46; in-home therapy 131; in-person services 8; private spaces 15, 20; supervision 46, 230; therapy 11, 44, 46, 56, 138, 220, 225
accolades 221, 223–224
accomplishment 44–46, 123, 139
acculturation 214
active listening 214, 258, 261, 263
ADHD *see* attention-deficit/hyperactivity disorder
adjustment disorder 7
adoption 53, 83
advocacy 225
affirmation 22, 39, 63, 249
affirming 22, 30–31, 70
alliance *see* therapeutic alliance
altar-making *see* virtual altar making
Andersen, T. 235, 238, 244, 253
Anderson, H. 252–254
anger: management 7; client 67–68, 76–77, 118, 134, 152, 170–171; therapist 44
animals: therapist 23, 30, 40; client 23, 151, 155, 208–209; cognitive stimulation therapy 141; puppets 70, 76; sand tray 67; stuffed animals 195, 197; *see also* dogs; pets
animosity 156, 158
antiracism 30; *see also* discrimination; racism
anxiety: death 75–76; diagnosing 222; efficacy of solution-focused therapy 121; efficacy of teletherapy treatment 7; evaluation 83; externalization of 93, 95–96; Generalized Anxiety Disorder-7 222; hoarding disorder 132–135; incarceration 118–119; intimate relationships 162, 171–172, 176, 178; medical family therapy 221–222, 224; sand tray 69; scholastic testing 80; school 88, 205–206; sensory reduction and deprivation 118; separation anxiety 23, 205–206; supervisee 240, 258, 260; teletherapy 23; therapist 44; timed tests 80–81; transition 53

app 18, 20, 36; for compilation of images 209; for maps 213–214, 216; for meditation 161; for phone service 56; sand tray 62–68, 208; spyware 181
application *see* app
art 29–30, 208, 212
artificial intelligence 257
asynchronous 184, 244–249
attachment: attachment-based injuries 27; bonds 165–166, 171; injuries 172; insecurity 172; needs 165–166, 169–171; secure attachment 165
attending skills 45
attention-deficit/hyperactivity disorder (ADHD) 162
attunement 22, 35–36, 161, 240
auditory cues 22, 25–27, 199
autism 30, 62
avatar 257–258, 260–261, 264

baby 52–53, 57, 75, 77, 157–158, 191–193, 223
background 23, 37, 70, 116; *see also* virtual background
bilingual 223–224, 251–252, 262
biopsychosocial-spiritual 219, 222–223
body language 22, 25, 103, 119, 152, 160, 230; *see also* nonverbal communication
books 23, 29–31, 54, 197, 229, 231
boundaries 53, 204, 223; behavior in session 27; chess 79–84; clear 16, 56–57, 79–80, 84, 151, 158, 242; contraindication of therapy 158; diffuse 80, 150–151; grief 210; intimate relationship therapy 149–153, 161; legal and ethical 6; parent-child 242; physical environment 16, 103, 197–198; rigid 150–152, 242; telehealth family sculpt 196–198; therapist self-care 41–42, 44–45, 50, 56–57
Bowen, M. 190, 260; *see also* transgenerational theories
breakout rooms 12, 262
breathing exercises 39, 49, 116, 135, 161, 222
bullying *see* cyberbullying
burnout 41, 43–46, 50
Burnout Clinical Subtype Questionnaire 44
business management 52, 54–56

car 15–16, 88, 192–193, 205, 211
cartoons 30, 107
case conceptualization 235–243
cat 40, 124, 142, 192, 206
Catholicism 95, 104, 111, 203; *see also* religion

centering 36
chat function 152; choosing a platform 11; confidentiality 16, 18, 20, 80, 85; educating clients 13; sharing links 71, 81, 109; supervision 238, 240, 242, 249
chess 79–85, 192–193
child abuse 16, 61, 258, 260, 263–264; *see also* abuse
chismorreo 251–252, 255
Christianity 125, 203; *see also* religion
circularity 245, 247
circular questions 123, 258
clay 195, 197
clip art 93, 189, 191
closed captioning 12, 27, 230
closure 36, 39–40
CMN *see* consensual nonmonogamy
coaching 150, 230
coalitions 198
code of ethics *see* ethics
cognitive distortion 242
cognitive stimulation therapy (CST) 137–144; *see also* virtual cognitive stimulation therapy (vCST)
collage 107, 209, 211
"commute home" *see* end-of-day letting-go rituals
compassion 41, 46, 48–49, 161–162, 164, 176, 217, 240; self-compassion 39, 50, 161
compassion fatigue 41
competency-based supervision 258
concentration 138
confidentiality 18, 56, 124, 157, 220; client devices 19, 181–183; client physical environment 14, 16, 19–20, 156; confidentiality agreement 139; ethics codes 20, 220; reflecting teams 247; safety 7; screen sharing 71; supervision 236; teletherapy platform 11, 18; therapist's physical environment 14, 19, 223; websites and applications 18, 40; *see also* HIPAA
consensual nonmonogamy (CMN) 165; *see also* ethical nonmonogamy
consultation 41–42, 44, 46, 48, 54, 172, 224, 253, 260–262; *see also* supervision
continuing education 6–7, 42, 48, 172
continuity of care 6, 8, 220, 225
contraindications 3, 7; assessing appropriateness of teletherapy for IPV 184; background images 31; chess 85; deliberate practice 233; digital play genograms 194; digital sand therapy 69; distractions as metaphors 158; guided grounding 119–120; intimate relationship deescalation 164; mapping the cycle 172; medical family teletherapy 225; migration journeys 217–218; mindfulness-based sex therapy 178; plurilinguistic virtual reflecting teams 256; round-robin case conceptualization 243; simulation 264; solution-focused scavenger hunt 89; stacking the deck 207; structural interventions for intimate relationship therapy 154; suicide intervention 128; telehealth family sculpt 201; teletherapy poetry 97; transformational teletherapy chairs 105; vCST 144; virtual altar-making 212; virtual home visits for hoarding disorder 135; virtual puppet play 78; virtual reflecting teams 249; virtual vision boards 113–114
coping 81, 209; coping mechanisms 97, 117–119, 123; coping skills 238; coping strategies 133, 135

core competencies 259
corrective feedback 231–233
COVID 75, 77, 88; *see also* pandemic
crisis 121–122, 125, 128, 255, 262; *see also* emergency; trauma
crisis management 243, 260, 262
CST *see* cognitive stimulation therapy
cultural attunement 22, 27, 92, 189, 203, 207, 212, 214
culturally relevant assessment 210, 238, 258, 262
cultural norms 22, 209, 230, 251–252
cultural sensitivity 225, 233
cultural traditions 213
culture 83, 217
cyberbullying 181; *see also* technology-facilitated intimate partner violence
cyberstalking 7, 16, 19, 181–183; *see also* technology-facilitated intimate partner violence

danger 135, 183, 218, 242
Day of the Dead *see Día de los Muertos*
DBT *see* dialectical behavioral therapy
death 75, 92, 203, 208–211
deconstruction 61, 91, 242; *see also* narrative therapy
deescalation 153, 158, 160–164, 197
degenerative disorders 62
deliberate practice (DP) 229–233, 257–258, 263
delusions 118
dementia 137–138
depersonalization 44–45
deportation 218
depression 7, 118, 121, 125, 132, 134, 165, 211, 224
Día de los Muertos 211–212
diagnosis 7, 132, 162, 219–222, 237
diagnostic assessment 131–132, 135, 222, 258
dialectical behavioral therapy (DBT) 44
difference that makes a difference 221–224
digital play genograms 189–194; *see also* genograms
disability 135
discrimination 242–243; *see also* antiracism; racism
dissociation 7, 16, 105, 115–116, 118–119
distractions as metaphors 155–158
diversity 30, 70, 230, 246–248, 252
divorce 66, 203–204
documentation 11, 62, 166, 171, 198, 222, 224
dogs 14, 35, 37, 40, 153, 155–156; *see also* animals; pets
domestic violence (DV) 16, 121; *see also* intimate partner violence
domestic violence shelter 16, 183
dominant story 91, 107, 236, 242, 248
double bind 157
DP *see* deliberate practice
drawing 97, 141, 168–169
DV *see* domestic violence
dysregulation 7, 103, 134, 161; *see also* flooding

eating disorder 7
EFT *see* emotionally focused therapy
ego strength 105
electronic surveillance 180; *see also* technology-facilitated intimate partner violence

EMDR *see* eye movement desensitization and reprocessing
emergency 4, 16, 55, 122, 125, 151, 223, 225, 257; *see also* crisis
emergency contacts 54, 124–125
emotionally focused therapy (EFT) 165–172
emotional regulation 133–135, 149, 158, 160
empty-chair technique *see* transformational teletherapy chairs
enactments 150–151
end-of-day letting-go rituals 38–40
equity 30, 219–220, 240
ethical nonmonogamy 162; *see also* consensual nonmonogamy
ethics 3–9, 18–20, 42, 44, 48, 219–220, 225; in supervision 6, 237, 260–261, 263
exceptions 124, 221–224; *see also* solution-focused therapy
executive functioning 118, 138
experiential therapy 115–120, 153, 195–201, 213–218
externalization 91–97, 101–105, 110, 190, 208, 210, 242; *see also* narrative therapy
eye contact 21–22; *see also* nonverbal communication
eye movement desensitization and reprocessing (EMDR) 63

facial expressions 15, 21–22, 25, 27, 82, 170, 230; *see also* nonverbal communication
familism 251
family life chronology 213
fear 64, 74, 169, 171, 176, 206, 214, 217, 242
flooding 103, 105, 160–163; *see also* dysregulation

gender-affirmative care 31
gender diversity 30
gender expression 204
gender identity 31, 203–204
Generalized Anxiety Disorder-7 222
genograms 260; *see also* digital play genograms
geographical maps 213–218; *see also* Google Earth; Google Maps
Gestalt therapy 101; *see also* transformational teletherapy chairs
Google Earth 213–214, 216; *see also* geographical maps
Google Maps 213–214; *see also* geographical maps
gratitude 22, 39, 45, 162–163, 215, 219, 255
grief 49, 77, 104, 119, 208–212
grounding 49, 97, 103, 134–135, 154; *see also* guided grounding
group norms 138–139
group therapy 54, 61, 70–74, 92, 115, 137–144, 208–210
guided grounding 115–120; *see also* grounding; mindfulness
guilt 103–105, 200, 252

hallucinations 118
harm reduction 133, 135
health equity 219–220
hierarchy 79–80, 84, 149–150, 152, 196, 198, 210; *see also* structural therapy
hinge partner 171; *see also* consensual nonmonogamy; ethical nonmonogamy

HIPAA 220; teletherapy platform 11, 18; websites and applications 18, 78, 80, 85; *see also* confidentiality
hoarding 130–135
Hoarding Assessment Tool 132
Hoarding Rating Scale 132
holistic 137, 198, 222
homework: structured pause 163; sensate focus 174–178
hypothesizing 150, 194, 245, 247, 249

immigration 213–318, 242–243, 251, 262; *see also* migration
impulse control 79–83
incarceration 118–119
inclusion 29–31, 138, 142, 207, 230
infertility 53, 104; *see also* in-vitro fertilization
infidelity 225
informed consent 6, 19, 171, 220–221, 249, 253
integrated care 219–220, 225
intergenerational patterns 189
intergenerational therapy 260; *see also* Bowen, M.
intergenerational trauma 62; *see also* trauma
internal family systems (IFS) 174, 176–178
internalization 110, 177
internalized biases 172
international teletherapy 5
interpreter 220, 264
intimate partner violence (IPV) 16, 19, 180–184; *see also* abuse; domestic violence; intimate terrorism; situational couples violence; violent resistance; technology-facilitated; trauma
intimate relationships: distractions as metaphors 155–158; intimate partner violence 180–184; mapping the cycle 165–172; mindfulness-based sex therapy 174–178; sand therapy 61; sculpting 195; structural interventions 149–154; structured pause 160–164
intimate terrorism 180–181, 184; *see also* domestic violence; intimate partner violence
in-vitro fertilization 104
IPV *see* intimate partner violence
isolation 41, 44, 209, 262

jail *see* incarceration
joining 80, 219–221, 224; *see also* rapport; therapeutic alliance; therapeutic relationship
journaling 39
justice 206–207

law 3–9, 166, 171, 260–261, 263
LGBTQ+ 30–31, 127
licensure 4–6, 53, 259
lighting 15, 25, 177
limbic system 115, 118
literacy 69, 108, 220, 225
loneliness 119, 169, 171, 177, 193

managing distractions 35–37
mapping 84, 165–172, 214, 243
map *see* geographical maps; mapping
maternity leave *see* parental leave
MedFT *see* medical family therapy

medical family therapy (MedFT) 219–225
medical family therapy healthcare continuum 219
meditation 14, 39, 49, 116, 161, 163; *see also* grounding;
    mindfulness
MED-STAT 219–224
memory loss 137–144
mental stimulation 138
metaphors 82, 92, 155–158, 189–195, 197–200, 210
microphones 13, 27, 153, 238
migration 212; *see also* immigration; migration journeys
migration journeys 213–218
Milan 244–247
military combat trauma 62; *see also* trauma
mindfulness 42, 49, 174–178; *see also* grounding;
    meditation
mindfulness-based sex therapy 174–178
miracle question 86–87, 89, 122–123, 128, 221–222,
    224, 260; *see also* solution-focused therapy
mixed-reality simulation 257–264
motivational interviewing 229, 231
multitasking 22, 26, 36, 44–45, 156
music 27, 39, 139–143, 163, 211
mute 12–13, 15, 25, 56, 149, 152–153

narrative therapy 91–97, 107–113, 190, 210
natural disaster 5, 212
negative cognitions 62–64, 68
neglect 61, 89; *see also* abuse
neurodiversity 30
neurolinguistic programming (NPL) 63
neurological changes 62
neurotypical 75
neutrality 245, 247
night terrors 211
noise machine 15, 19–20, 35, 180–181
nonbinary 125, 127, 204
nonmonogamy *see* consensual nonmonogamy; ethical
    nonmonogamy
nonpathologizing 245
nonverbal communication 21–29, 63, 103, 105, 144,
    170, 189; *see also* body language; eye contact; facial
    expressions; tone of voice; visual cues
NPL *see* neurolinguistic programming

Oaklander, V. 70–77
obsessive symptoms 75
ODD *see* oppositional defiant disorder
offerings *see* ofrendas
ofrendas 212
older adults 137–144
one-way mirror 235, 244
oppositional defiant disorder (ODD) 83
outsider witnessing 111; *see also* narrative therapy

pandemic 75, 77, 88, 208; *see also* COVID
paradoxical intervention 157; *see also* strategic therapy
parental leave 52–57
Patient Health Questionnaire-9 222
personal maintenance 39–40
personal needs 35–36, 45, 56
pets 23, 156, 157, 161; *see also* animals; dogs

photographs *see* pictures
physical movement 36, 138
pictures: background images 30; cognitive stimulation
    therapy 140–142; digital play genograms 190;
    intimate partner violence 181; migration journeys
    215; telehealth family sculpt 195–196, 198–199, 201;
    teletherapy chairs 102–103; therapeutic relationships
    23; virtual altar making 208–209, 211–212; vision
    boards 107–114
playfulness 29, 70, 189, 190, 192, 194, 202, 72,74
play genograms *see* digital play genograms
plurilinguistic virtual reflecting teams 251–256; *see also*
    reflecting teams
poetry 208–209; *see also* poetry therapy; teletherapy
    poetry
poetry therapy 92
police 124–125, 205–207
polyamory *see* consensual nonmonogamy; ethical
    nonmonogamy
portability 5
positive cognitions 63–64
postmodern 86, 235
postpartum depression 121
posttraumatic stress 7
power imbalance 249
PowerPoint 91, 93, 102, 107–108, 165–166, 189, 191,
    202–204, 207–209
prayer 49, 208–209; *see also* religion
preferred outcomes 91, 107; *see also* narrative therapy
preferred story 91, 110, 113, 190; *see also* narrative
    therapy
pregnancy 51–57
prison *see* incarceration
problem-saturated stories 91, 97, 107, 110; *see also*
    narrative therapy
problem solving 23, 79–84, 118, 134, 156
professionalism 45
pronouns 30–31
proximal zone of development 233
psychoeducation 183
PTSD 165
puppets 70–78

racism 30, 242; *see also* antiracism; discrimination
rapport 30, 80–81, 258, 262; *see also* joining; therapeutic
    alliance; therapeutic relationship
reality orientation 137, 140
reflecting teams *see* plurilinguistic virtual reflecting
    teams; round-robin case conceptualization; virtual
    reflecting teams
reframing 63, 119, 150, 152, 156–157, 165, 171, 212, 242
release of information 53–54, 247
religion 48–49, 189, 203, 212, 248; *see also* Catholicism;
    Christianity; prayer; spirituality
reminiscence therapy 137
resilience 14, 38, 50, 208
resistance 74, 127, 134, 189
restructuring 79, 149–150, 198, 200; *see also* structural
    therapy
rituals 23, 38–40, 48
role-play 229, 257, 259–264

round-robin case conceptualization 235–243; *see also* reflecting teams

safety 61, 68, 115; contraindications 7, 31, 89, 154, 164, 178, 217–218, 256; deliberate practice 230–231, 237; hoarding disorder 131–135; intimate partner violence 180–184; safety planning 124–125; suicide intervention 122–126; supervision 259, 263; therapeutic environments 11, 15–16
sand therapy 61–69
sand tray *see* sand therapy
scaling questions 123–124, 128, 221–222, 224; *see also* solution-focused therapy
scavenger hunt 86–89
sculpting *see* telehealth family sculpt
secondary traumatic stress 41
self-awareness 36, 61
self-care 36, 46; assessment 41–43; tips and tricks 47–50; *see also* end-of-day letting-go rituals
self-compassion 39, 50, 161
self-concept 63, 66
self-disclosure 52–53, 57
self-harm 7
self-of-the-therapist 36, 258, 263–264; *see also* self-care
self-regulation 161
self-sooth 135, 160, 161–164
self-talk 63–64, 110; sensate focus 174–178
sensory experience 35, 62, 115, 117–119
sex therapy 174–175
sexual identity 223
sexuality 170, 177, 203
sexual orientation 31
sexual pain 177
sexual trauma 248; *see also* trauma
sexual violence 180; *see also* trauma; violence
shadow box 208, 210–211
shame 118, 134
simulation 257–264
situational couples violence 180; *see also* domestic violence; intimate partner violence
sleep: miracle question 88, 224; personal needs 36; poor sleep 134; self-care 42, 47, 55
slowing down 21–23, 232
social construction 245
social location 237, 242, 246–247, 249
social skills 81
socioculturally attuned 219–221, 225, 237
socioeconomic status 213
solution-focused therapy: genograms 190; medical family therapy 219–225; scavenger hunt 86–89; suicide intervention 121–128; supervision 258, 260
Spanish 209, 251–252, 254
sparkling moments 242; *see also* narrative therapy
spirituality 209, 212; connection 197; self care 41–42, 47–49; spiritual health 219, 222–224; *see also* religion
spyware 181; *see also* stalking
stacking the deck 202–207
stalking 180–181; *see also* domestic violence; intimate partner violence
stereotypes 223
stimulus 229–233

Stranger Things 65
strategic therapy 155–158, 202–203
stress 41, 44, 50, 68, 88–89, 134, 222; *see also* posttraumatic stress; secondary traumatic stress
stressors 38, 41, 54, 117–118
structural therapy 79–84, 149–154, 198, 210, 242
Structured Interview for Hoarding Disorder 132
structured pause 160–164
stuffed animal 195, 197, 200
substance use 7, 119, 121, 263
subsystems 150–152, 195, 197, 200, 242
suicide 16, 55, 121–128, 260
supervision 6, 12, 56, 69, 172; deliberate practice 229–233; plurilinguistic virtual reflecting teams 251–256; round-robin case conceptualization 235–243; self care 42, 44, 46, 48; using simulation in virtual group supervision 257–264; virtual reflecting teams 244–249
supplemental materials 101–102, 107–108, 165–166, 189, 195–196, 202–203
symbolic projection 70, 74

technology-facilitated intimate partner violence (t-IPV) 180–184
telehealth family sculpt 195–201
telenovela 253, 255; *see also* television
teletherapy poetry 91–97
television (TV) 30, 125, 155, 253, 255; *see also* telenovela
temporary licensure 5
temporary practice 4–6, 8
text messaging 11, 56, 161, 163, 181, 184, 255
therapeutic alliance 7, 21–24, 27, 29, 132, 211, 261–262; *see also* joining; rapport; therapeutic relationship
therapeutic environment 11–16
therapeutic relationship 21–25, 29, 35–36, 53, 152, 258; *see also* joining; rapport; therapeutic alliance
therapy interfering behavior 44–46
thickening the plot 110, 190, 210; *see also* narrative therapy
time-out 221, 224
t-IPV *see* technology-facilitated intimate partner violence
tone of voice 22, 25–27, 45, 82, 105, 231; *see also* nonverbal communication
training: sand tray 69; simulation 257–260, 264; skill 233; teletherapy 3, 6–9, 182; vCST 139, 144
transformational teletherapy chairs 101–105
transgenerational theories 190; *see also* Bowen, M.
translation services 214, 220
trauma 14, 83, 97, 108, 115–116, 214, 261; complex 62; religious 248; responses 207; *see also* abuse; crisis; intergenerational trauma; military combat trauma; neglect; posttraumatic stress; PTSD; sexual trauma; suicide; traumatic; vicarious trauma; violence
traumatic 13, 16, 63, 214, 216–217, 246
treatment teams 237–243, 244; *see also* reflecting teams
triangulation 157, 160
TV *see* television

unbalancing 150
Underworld Technique 62, 65–68

Ungame 202–207
Uniform Inspection Checklist 132–134
unique outcomes 110, 210; *see also* narrative therapy
upside-down 65; *see also Stranger Things*

validation therapy 137, 140
vehicles 45, 133
verbal transparency 22, 25–27
violence 7, 16, 154, 170; interpersonal violence 178, 223; *see also* abuse; domestic violence; intimate partner violence; sexual violence; trauma
violent resistance 180–181; *see also* domestic violence; intimate partner violence
virtual altar making 208–212
virtual background 29–31, 48, 62, 132, 203; *see also* background
virtual cognitive stimulation therapy (vCST) 137–144
virtual environment 3, 11–16, 23, 225, 231
virtual home visits for hoarding disorder 130–135
virtual reflecting teams 244–249
Virtual Sandtray®© App 62–63, 65–68
virtual vision boards 107–114

vision 26, 144, 197
vision board 107–114
vision boards *see* virtual vision boards
visual contact 16, 21, 116, 167
visual cues 29–31, 53; *see also* nonverbal communication
Volunteer Burnout Questionnaire 44

waiting room 23, 35, 251, 253
websites: chess 79–81, 85; confidentiality 18; digital sand therapy 63; migration journeys 213–214; virtual puppet play 70–71; virtual vision boards 108, 113–114
wellness 41, 44, 47–48, 50, 223, 225
wellness check 16
whiteboard 12, 91, 93–96, 167–169
window of tolerance 115, 119, 160
withdrawal 104, 118–119, 163
workstation 42, 47

yoga 39, 47, 49

Zoom 95–96, 138, 235

For Product Safety Concerns and Information please contact our
EU representative GPSR@taylorandfrancis.com Taylor & Francis
Verlag GmbH, Kaufingerstraße 24, 80331 München, Germany